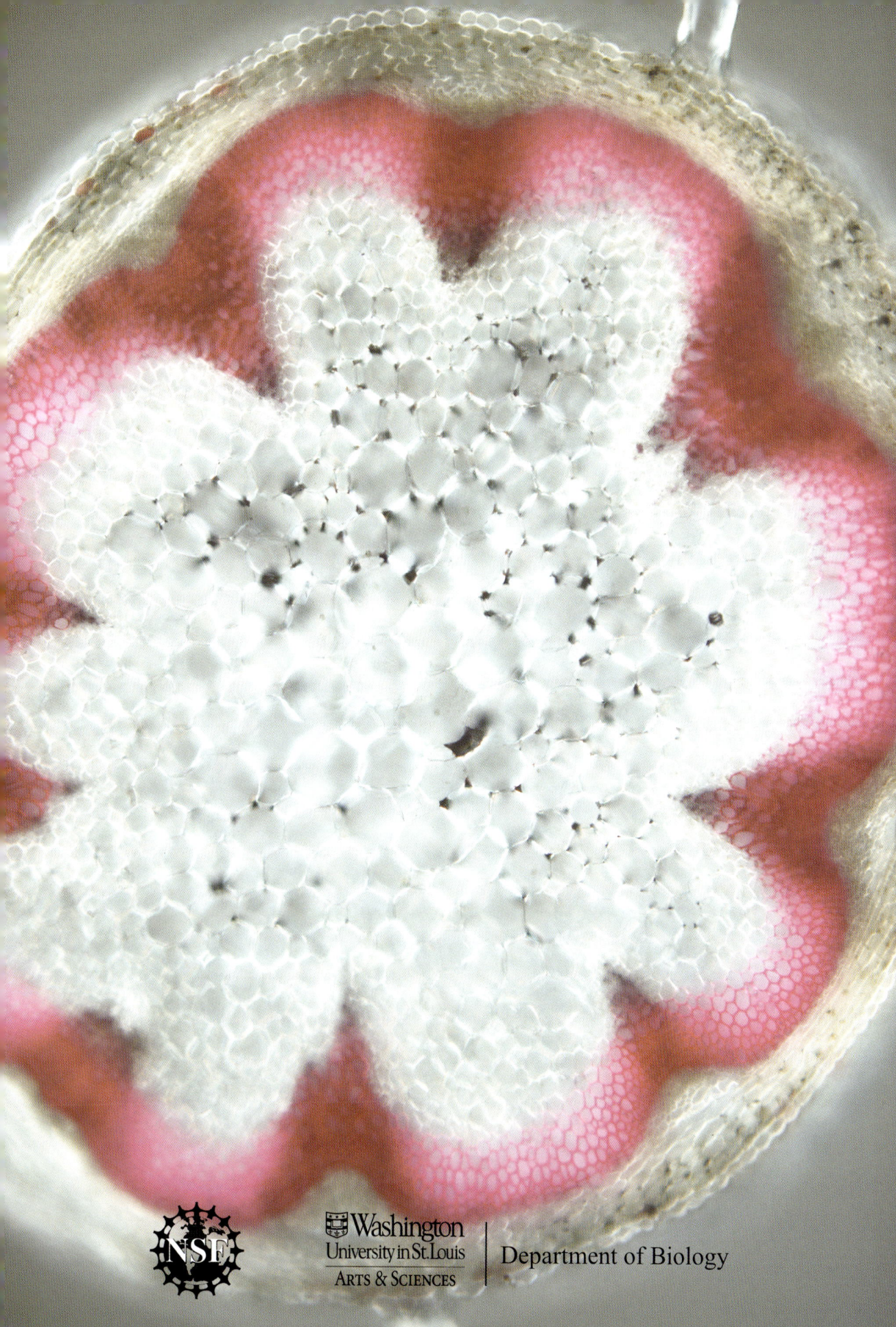

CELLULAR TRANSFORMATIONS
BETWEEN ARCHITECTURE AND BIOLOGY

초판 발행	2021.09.08	First Edition Published	2021.09.08
지은이	Ram Dixit, Sung Ho Kim	Authors	Ram Dixit, Sung Ho Kim
펴낸이	KyongWon Suh	Publisher	KyongWon Suh
레이아웃 디자인	Ryan Do	Layout and Design	Ryan Do
에디터	Younsil Jeon	Editing	Younsil Jeon
펴낸 곳	DAMDI Publishing Co.	Publishing Office	DAMDI Publishing Co.
	2F, 88, Samgaksan-ro, Gangbuk-gu,	Address	2F, 88, Samgaksan-ro, Gangbuk-gu,
	Seoul 01083, Republic of Korea		Seoul 01083, Republic of Korea
Tel	+82-2-900-0652	Tel	+82-2-900-0652
Fax	+82-2-900-0657	Fax	+82-2-900-0657
E-mail	damdi_book@naver.com	E-mail	damdi_book@naver.com
Homepage	www.damdi.co.kr	Homepage	www.damdi.co.kr

All rights are reserved. No part of this publication may be reproduced, transmitted or stored in a retrieval system, photocopied in any form or by any means, without permission in writing from Ram Dixit and Sung Ho Kim. Copyright © Ram Dixit, Sung Ho Kim 2021.

All images developed by undergraduate and graduate students of Washington University in St. Louis with Ram Dixit and Sung Ho Kim.

정가 25,000원

Printed in Korea
ISBN 978-89-6801-103-0 [94540]
ISBN 978-89-6801-015-6 (Set) [94540]

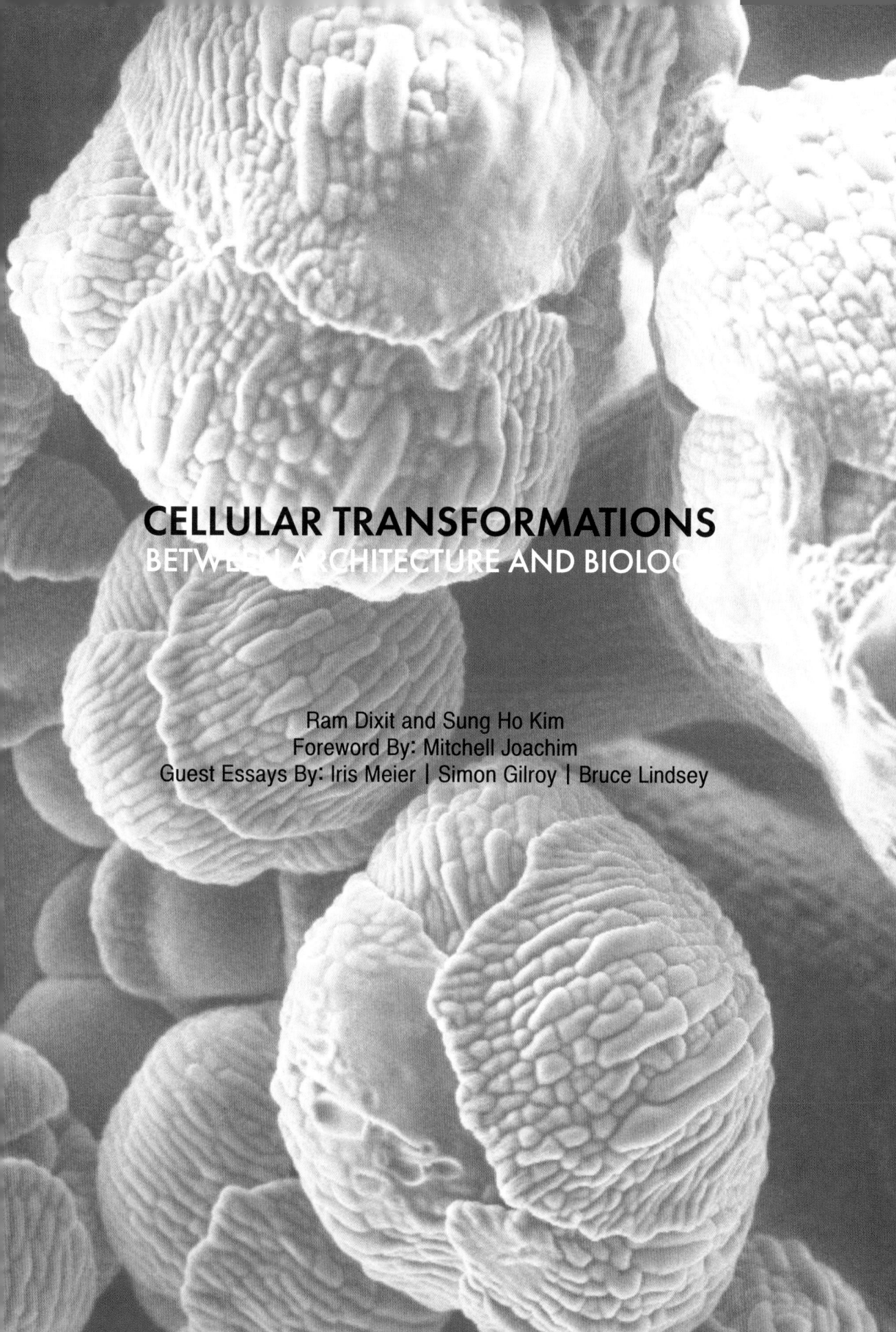

CELLULAR TRANSFORMATIONS
BETWEEN ARCHITECTURE AND BIOLOGY

Ram Dixit and Sung Ho Kim
Foreword By: Mitchell Joachim
Guest Essays By: Iris Meier | Simon Gilroy | Bruce Lindsey

TABLE OF CONTENTS

01 | 001 **ACKNOWLEDGMENTS**
     002 Ram Dixit and Sung Ho Kim

02 | 003 **CELLULAR TRANSFORMATIONS**
     006 Introduction | Ram Dixit and Sung Ho Kim

03 | 007 **BUILT FOR BIOTA**
     010 Foreword | Mitchell Joachim

04 | 011 **PLANT CELL MORPHOGENESIS**
     018 Biology Research | Ram Dixit

05 | 019 **ARCHITECTURE OF SKIN**
     054 Architecture Research | Sung Ho Kim and Andrew Yoo

06 | 055 **MAPPING SOFT BODIES**
     064 Beginnings: 2011

07 | 065 **MOBILE CELL LAB**
     078 Catalyst: 2013

08 | 079 **SCAFFOLDING RESEARCH**
     102 Emerging: 2013

09 | 103 **MICRO-ENVIRONMENTS**
     122 Scaffoldings: 2013

10 | 123 **ADVANCED CELL ANALYSIS 01**
     140 Transformation: 2014

11 | 141 **CHERNOBYL RESEARCH**
     154 Remediation: 2014

| 12 | 155 | ADVANCED CELL ANALYSIS 02 |
| | 170 | Transformation: 2015 |

| 13 | 171 | MISSION TO MARS RESEARCH |
| | 182 | Inhabitation: 2015 |

| 14 | 183 | ADVANCED CELL ANALYSIS 03 |
| | 188 | Transformation: 2018 |

| 15 | 189 | 3D PRINTED CELLS |
| | 206 | Replication: 2017-2020 |

| 16 | 207 | ADVANCED CELL ANALYSIS 04 |
| | 214 | Transformation: 2020 |

| 17 | 215 | SAFEGUARDS AGAINST COVID-19 RESEARCH |
| | 228 | Pandemic: 2020 |

| 18 | 229 | DESIGNING AND STRUCTURING THE INTERDISCIPLINARY |
| | 232 | Iris Meier |

| 19 | 233 | BUILDING NEW PERSPECTIVES |
| | 236 | Simon Gilroy |

| 20 | 237 | A BIOLOGICAL COMPUTATIONAL MODEL OF DESIGN |
| | 246 | Bruce Lindsey |

| 21 | 247 | BIOGRAPHY |
| | 250 | Contributors |

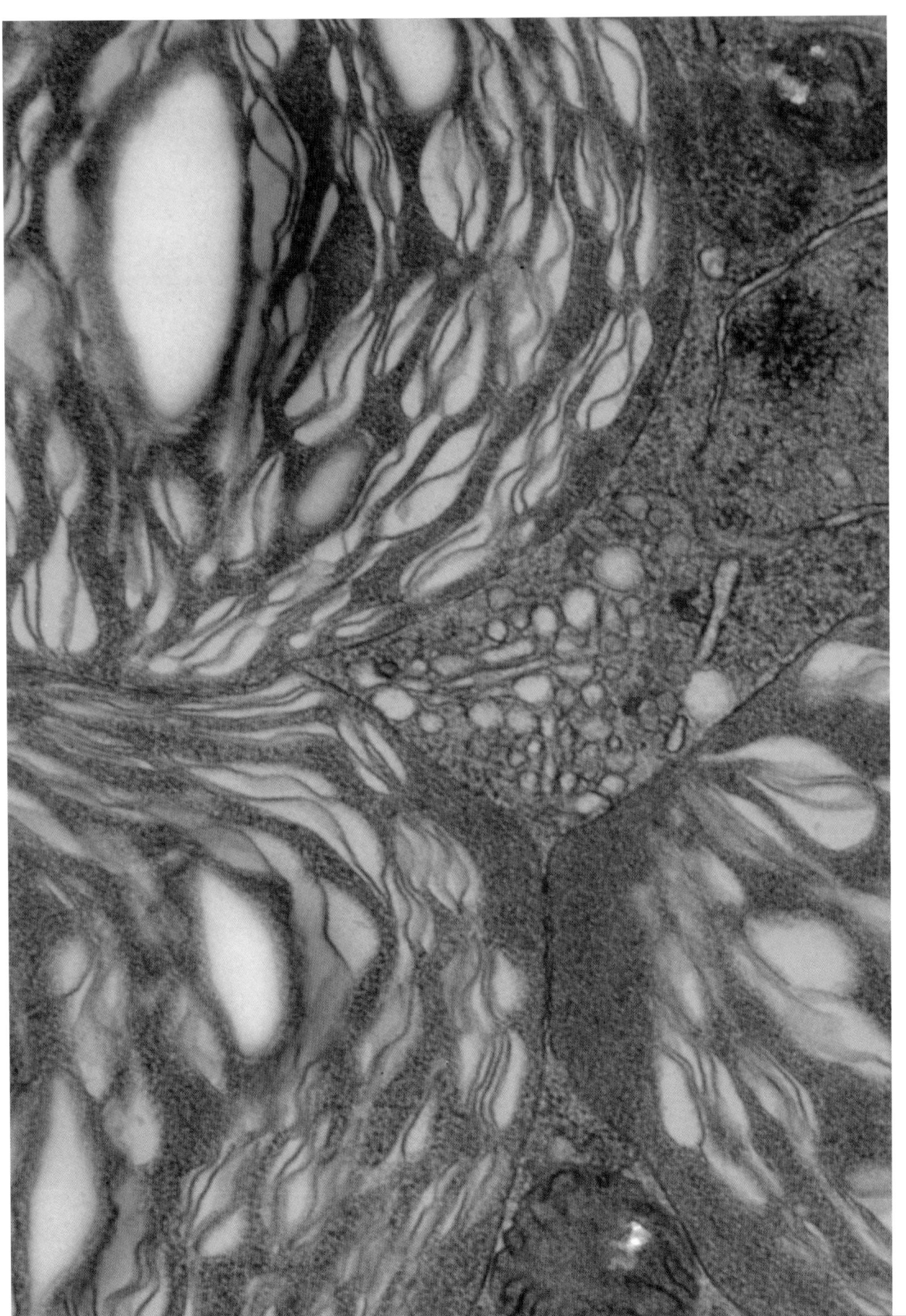

ACKNOWLEDGMENTS

Cellular Transformations emerged from our passion and commitment to exploring alternative learning processes within the context of a research university. This journey has demanded a lot of sacrifice over the past 10 years to maintain high standards of teaching, research, and practice. Much of our time commitment to this course was borrowed from our personal and family lives, and therefore we would like to thank the Dixit and Woofter-Kim families for their support and understanding of our late-night classes and frequent meetings.

We extend a heartfelt thanks to our biology and architecture students who took a leap of faith with this course. They endured working well outside their respective comfort zones and prevailed, excelled in teamwork, and exceeded our expectations for creative thinking and learning.

Along the way, we have benefited from many collaborators who gladly extended their intellectual and technical expertise to enhance this course. We thank Dr. Dan Chitwood and Dr. Chris Topp at the Donald Danforth Plant Science Center for giving talks on plant developmental biology; Kevin Reilly, director of the plant growth facility at the Donald Danforth Plant Science Center, for his excellent tours of the plant growth, characterization and automated phenotyping facilities; members of the Sakiyama-Elbert lab in Biomedical Engineering at Washington University in St. Louis for leading the ever-popular tour of their animal cell engineering and imaging facilities; and Dr. Pierre-François Perroud in Dr. Ralph Quatrano's lab for generously teaching students how to culture moss under axenic conditions.

We would like to recognize the following students of Spring 2020: Ethan Chiang, Zhengran Xu, Zhuoxian Deng, Xinfei Tao and Patrick Murray for working beyond our expectations and delivering high-quality research projects in the middle of a pandemic. Also, great thanks to Ryan Do for his keen eyes for the layout design of the book and text editing. Thank you to Damdi for working with us through these complex illustrations and graphics. To KyongWan Suh of Damdi for his patience and time that allowed us to assemble a strong manuscript.

We thank Mitchell Joachim, Iris Meier, Simon Gilroy, and Bruce Lindsey for their support and critical evaluation of our research. Thanks to Gay Lorberbaum for connecting us 11 years ago, Heather Woofter, previously as Chair of the Graduate School of Architecture and currently as Director of the College of Architecture, for the flexibility to improve our partnership over the years. To Dr. Kathy Miller, previous Chair of the Biology Department, and Dr. Joseph Jez, current Chair of the Biology Department, for supporting our teaching and recognizing its value.

We would like to thank the National Science Foundation for their generous support and funding to develop the production of this book. Thank you to the Biology Department at Washington University in St. Louis for financially supporting the 3D printed models as a learning tool for students to explore the physical properties of cellular structures.

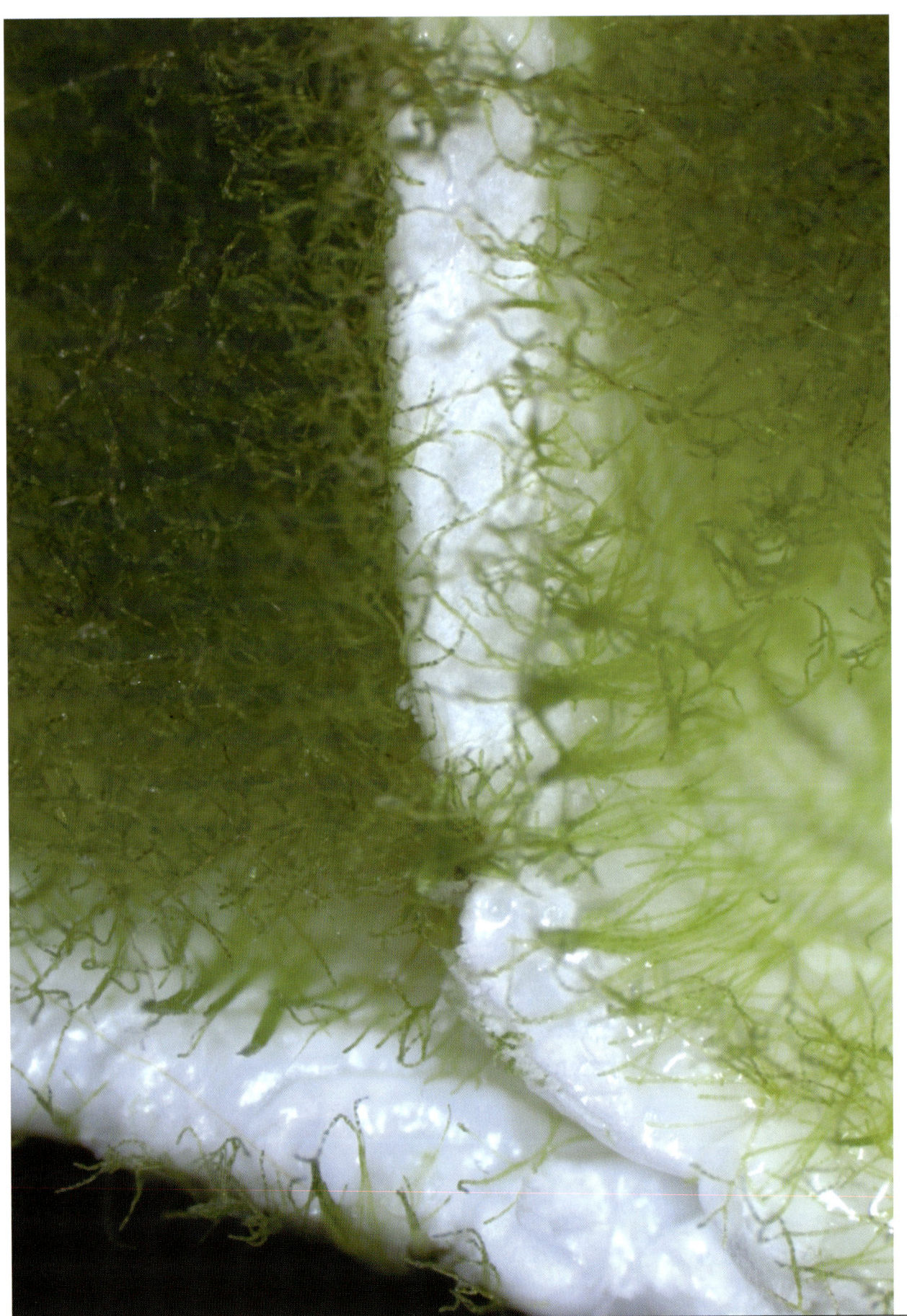

INTRODUCTION
CELLULAR TRANSFORMATIONS

Ordered structures are ubiquitous in nature, among both living and non-living materials. Complex architectures in nature often do not require a template or blueprint for their construction. Rather, their assembly occurs through interactions between building blocks that are defined by their inherent physical and chemical properties and the constraints posed by the external environment. Life is the epitome of nature's efforts against the thermodynamic tendency towards disorder. All living organisms use energy to construct elaborate structures to adapt, survive and reproduce. Order in life occurs hierarchically, with higher-level order emerging from the pattern of arrangement of lower-level elements.

Cells use macromolecules to build complex machines and architectures to organize their interior and orchestrate various activities needed for their growth and survival. While the DNA genome encodes the recipe for individual proteins, it does not specify how multiple proteins and other molecules come together to form complex structures. Another defining feature of biological structures is that they are dynamic. The time scales of dynamics can vary from nanoseconds to weeks, depending on the biological structure and its components.

In addition, external factors such as temperature or pathogens can cause these timescales to transform dramatically. These transformations are a kind of metamorphosis that leads to an altered state that enables organisms to adapt to prevailing conditions.

Architecture inspired by biology is not a new concept; the ancient Greeks and Romans incorporated plant leaf motifs into architectural ornamentations and structures. The Art Nouveau decorative design arts and Frank Lloyd Wright's architecture that blurs the boundary between building and organic formation is a conceptual and metaphoric understanding of biology. Typically, architecture has imitated the imagery of biology and nature without awareness of the underlying mechanisms of formation and functionality. Collaboration between architecture and biology could be further strengthened by a deeper knowledge of the inner workings of biological structures. The emerging possibilities from new biotechnologies that are advancing at an incredible pace inspire new methods of thinking in design. Integrating the knowledge of biological transformation with design could have profound consequences for shaping the built environment.

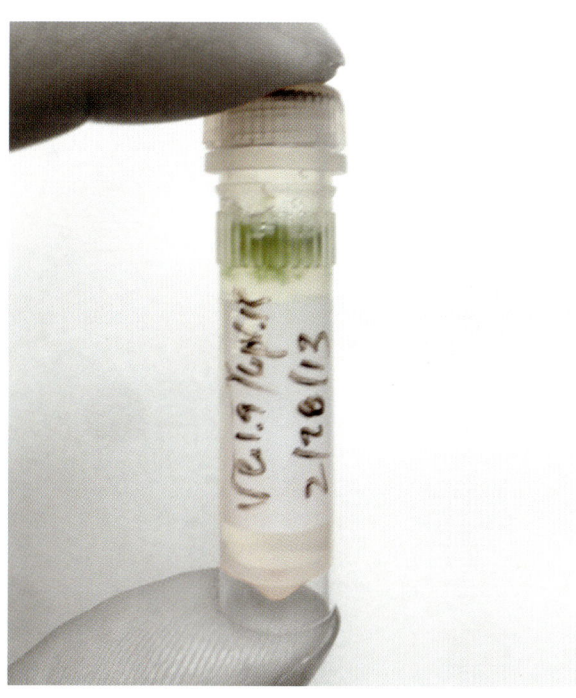
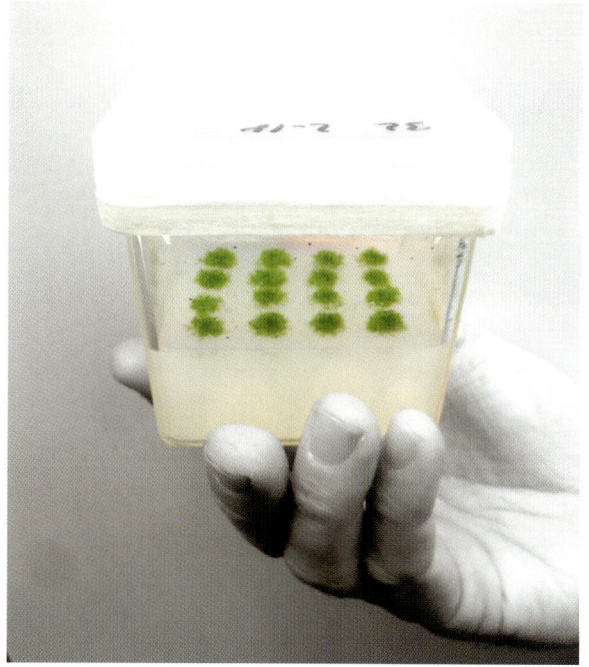

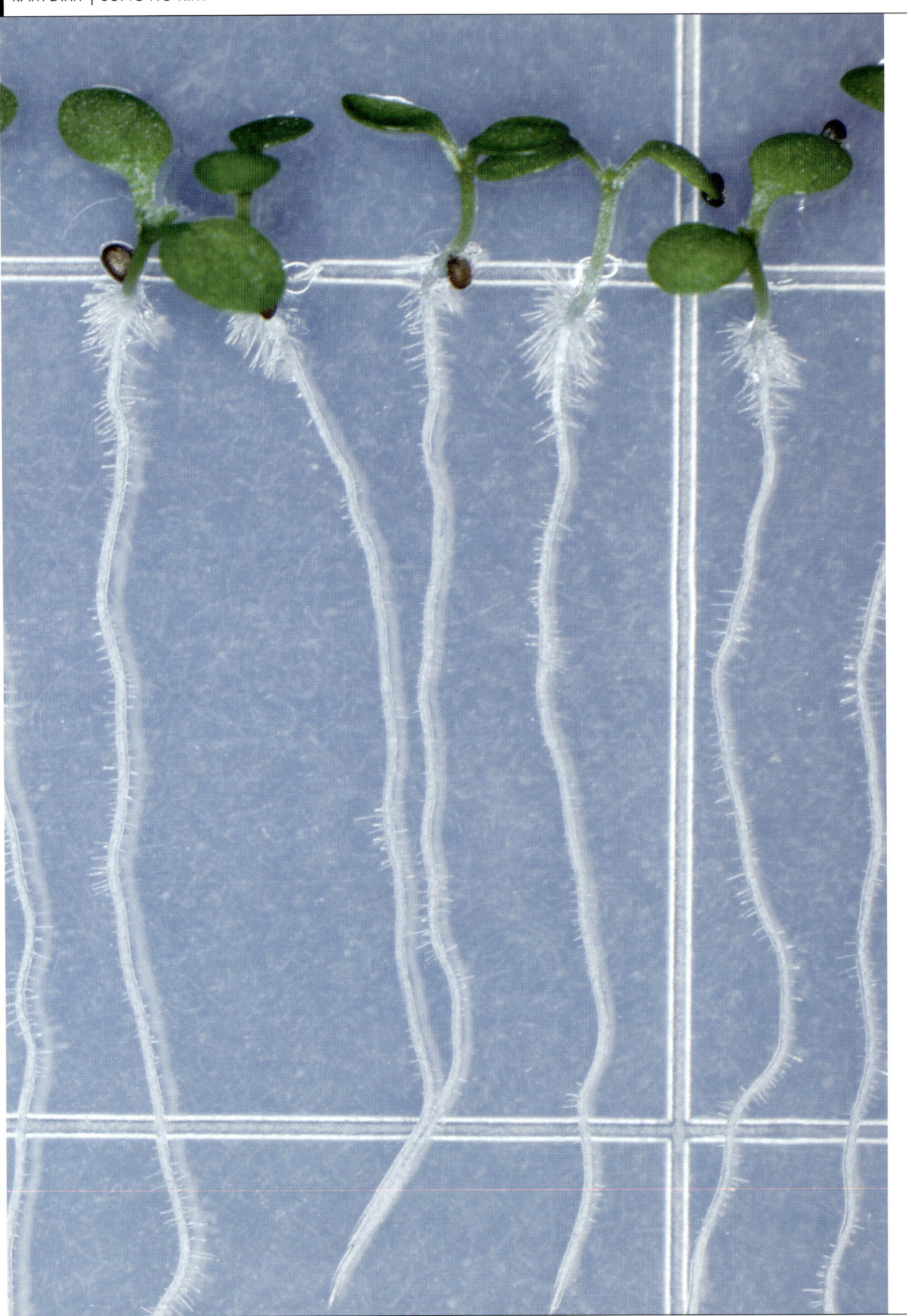

Countless environmental and sustainable advancements can be developed by working with biological organisms. This could translate into detecting and mitigating environmental issues by transforming the building blocks of cities with less energy and low carbon footprints. Employing biological systems and integrating biology as part of a design repertoire allows architecture to become less as singular, static, solitary objects and more as dynamic infrastructure composed of multiple interactive systems. Biological research can also expand the notion of lifespan of architecture by regenerating and healing the environment it engages in. This is the new beginning we envision by acknowledging biology and our built environment as a "symbiotic partnership" with the humanity that dwells on Earth.

Cellular Transformations is not just a simple imitation or simulation of biological form, but a total alteration of its properties to become something radically different from existing state based on necessities in the contemporary built environment.

In *Cellular Transformations,* we want to explore how principles underlying cellular architecture can be used to design and build new kinds of human-made structures. In this course, students actively investigate and apply the basics of biological organization, focusing on concepts such as self-assembly, dynamics, self-organization, and self-repair. They are exposed to different research areas and methodologies in biology through guest lectures and visits to research facilities. Students then develop their own projects and through abstract thinking, digital design, 3D modeling and scanning of biological structures, they develop a transformation process that analyzes the performative aspects of a new emerging design. We believe that multidisciplinary training through integration of Science and Arts will promote innovative ideas and applications to address the many challenges facing humanity.

Ram Dixit and Sung Ho Kim 12.24.2020

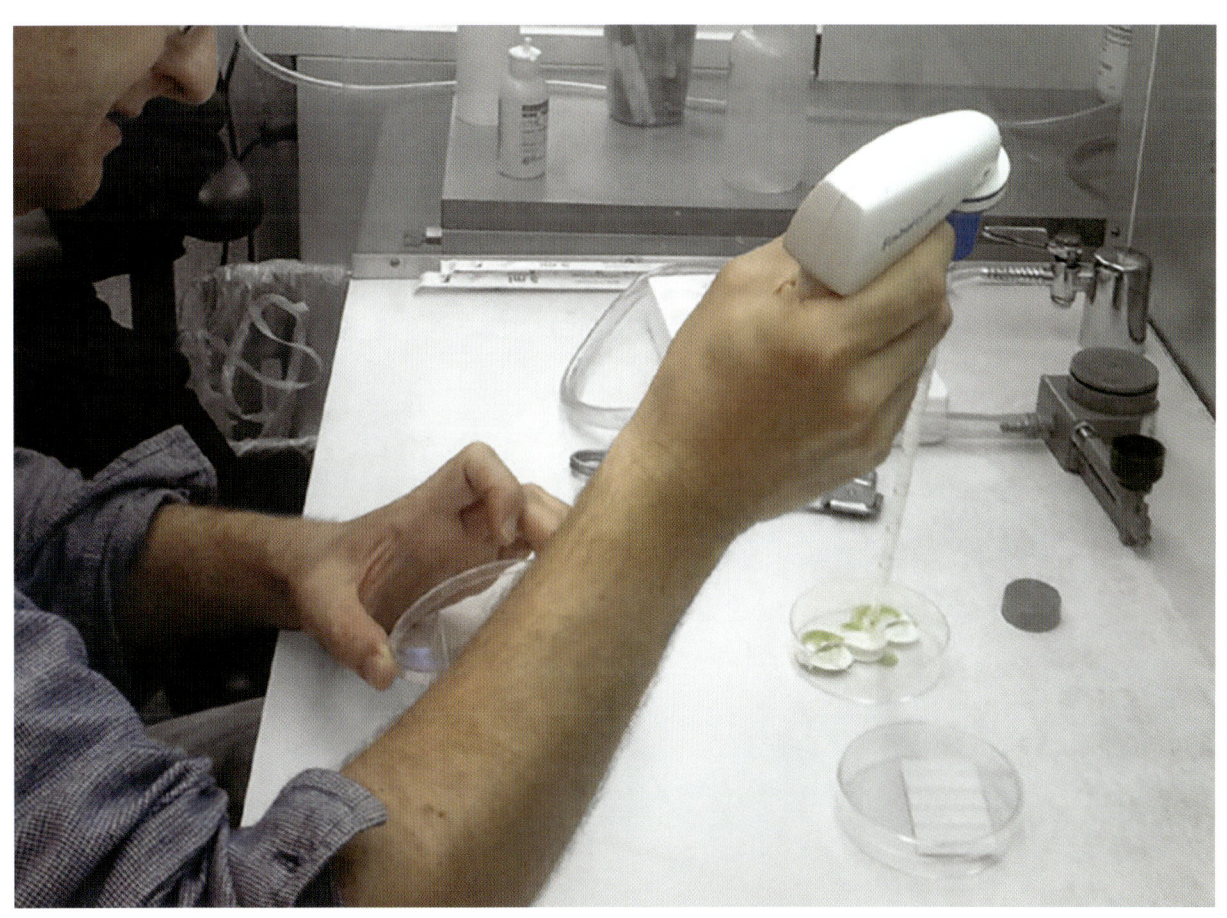

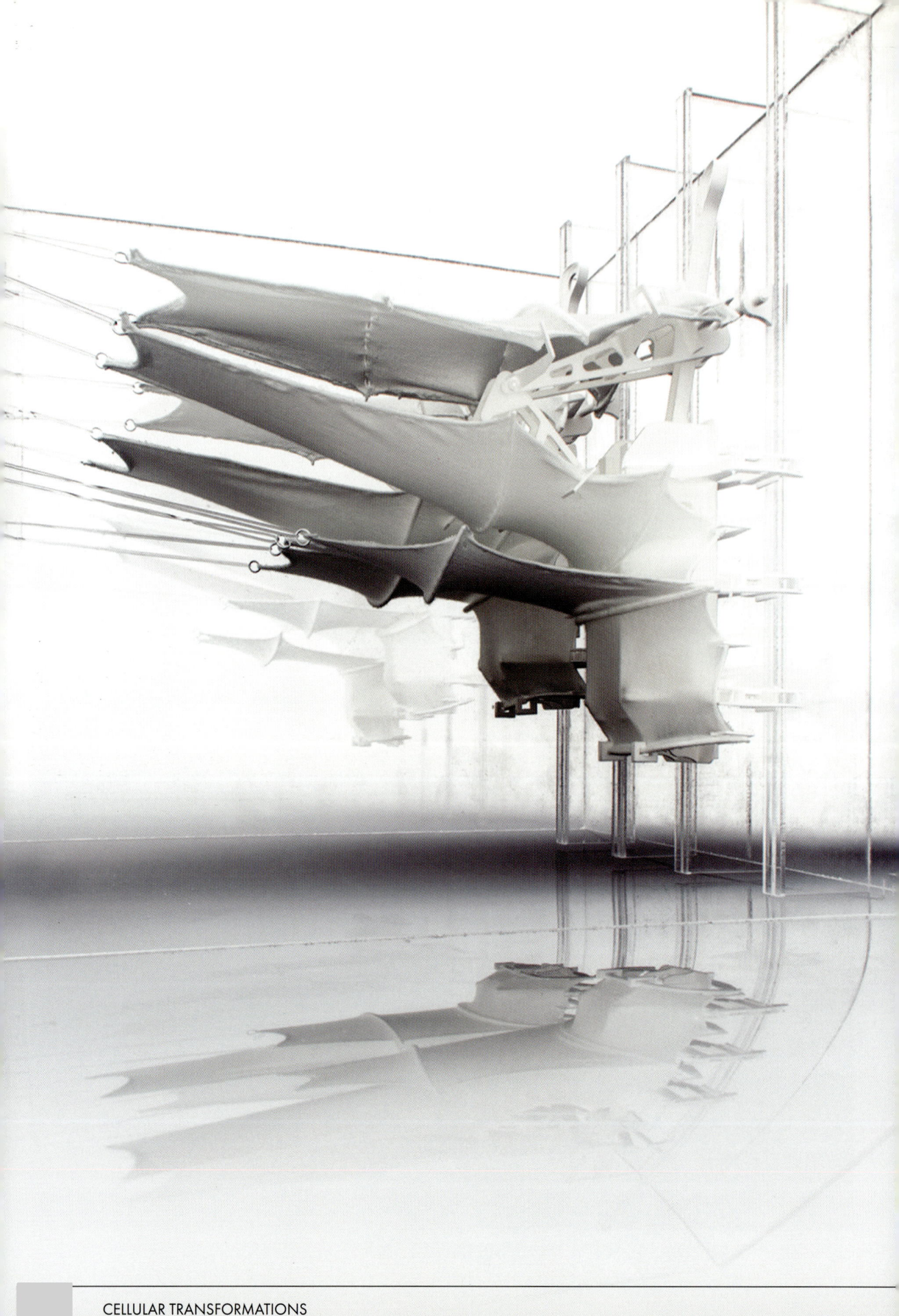

CELLULAR TRANSFORMATIONS

FOREWORD
BUILT FOR BIOTA

Ram Dixit and Sung Ho Kim have vividly fashioned a comprehensive and revealing fusion of architecture and biological sciences. The vast importance of these scholarly techniques, designs, and methods reverberates on a global scale. Their combined work is defined by its elegant use of precise organic materials, especially inside facades. The many salient projects contained within this volume are ethereal, tranquil, and extraordinarily geometric. By pairing unconventional methods of architecture with sophisticated cellular systems, they've shaped unforeseen alignments that magnificently bridge the gap between evolving architecture and the natural world.

In the perplexing context of hastening climate dynamics, the core emphasis of architectural thought is in uniting and advancing new formal strategic processes that revitalize the declining biosphere. Dixit and Kim have established a distinctive design agency that investigates projects through the regenerative use of animate materials, biological techniques, and the emergent field of synthetic life-based systems. This thoughtful approach and instrumentality strive to deploy actual living organisms in the realization of functional architectonic elements and viable programmatic spaces.

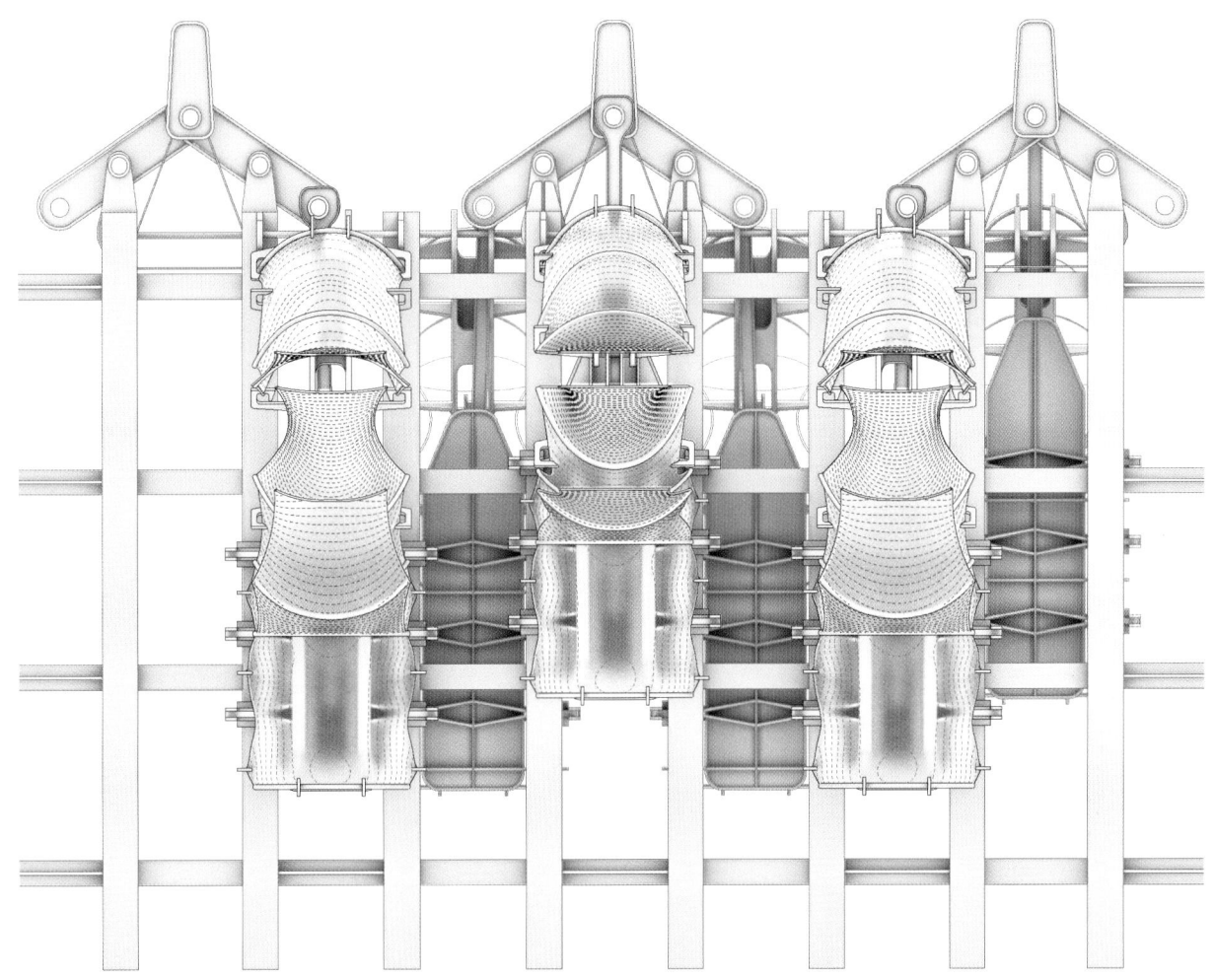

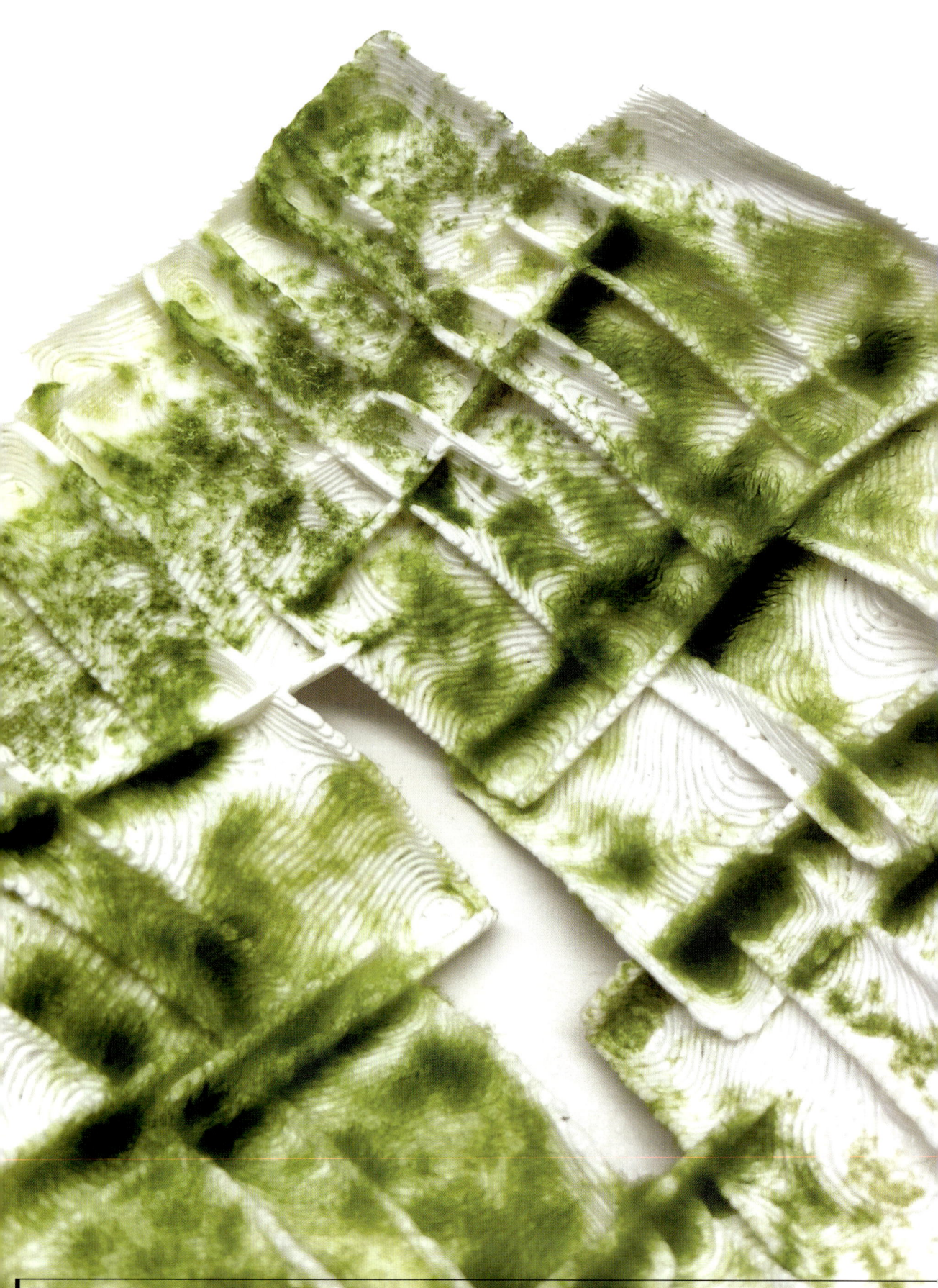

It is essential to underscore their principal exertions in this relatively unmapped territory. They are not making abstracted imitations of nature nor mere decoration, but striking formulas towards a living, breathing architecture. Perhaps this is humankind's primary path forward to achieve complete sustainability in the disconcerting age of the Anthropocene. Often in the past, architects have historically developed schemes that mimic forms in nature. While this former approach is noteworthy, it is highly derivative, vestigial, and ornamental. For instance, organic architecture under Frank Lloyd Wright was fashioned out of mechanized steel, carbon heavy concrete, and industrialized glass. These components are hardly associated with authentic living entities and are purely industrial in nature. The work Dixit and Kim have completed is a new order of organic architecture that supersedes the preceding ornamental and fabricated variants.

In summation, Dixit and Kim are a true heterodox authority. These anti-establishment schemes and structures within their profound oeuvre are undeniably invigorating. Their multifaceted programmatic actions are not only grounded in biological life on a wide range of scales but are also far-reaching in their application of digital prototyping, material tectonics, and micro-manufacturing culture. They are here to confront exigent environmental problems through the integrated use of pertinent living materials and explicit organic lifeforms. Without this technological and biologically centered approach, our days on the planet are severely numbered. Now, it is time for an architecture that makes no distinction between built and biota.

Mitchell Joachim 02.06.2021

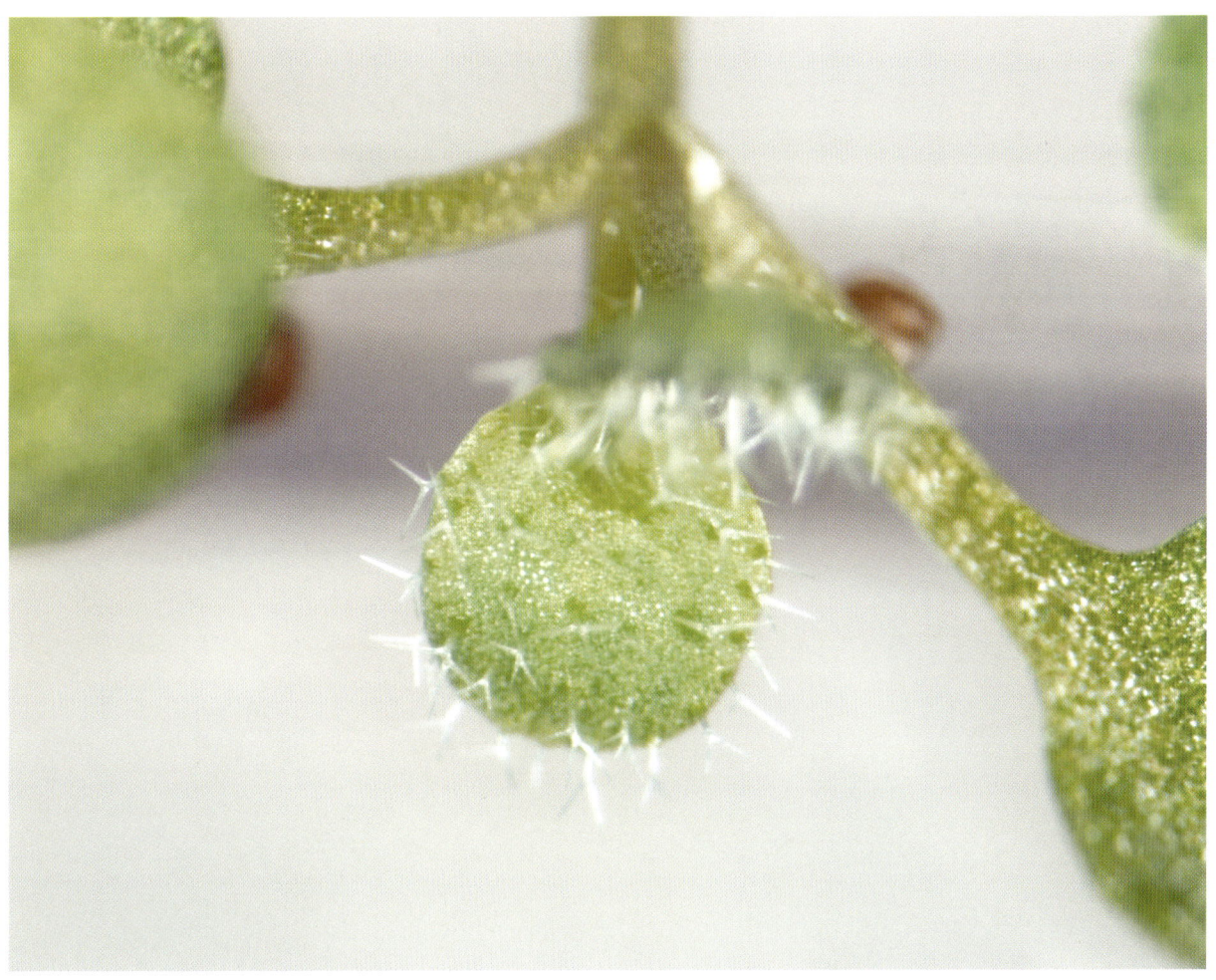

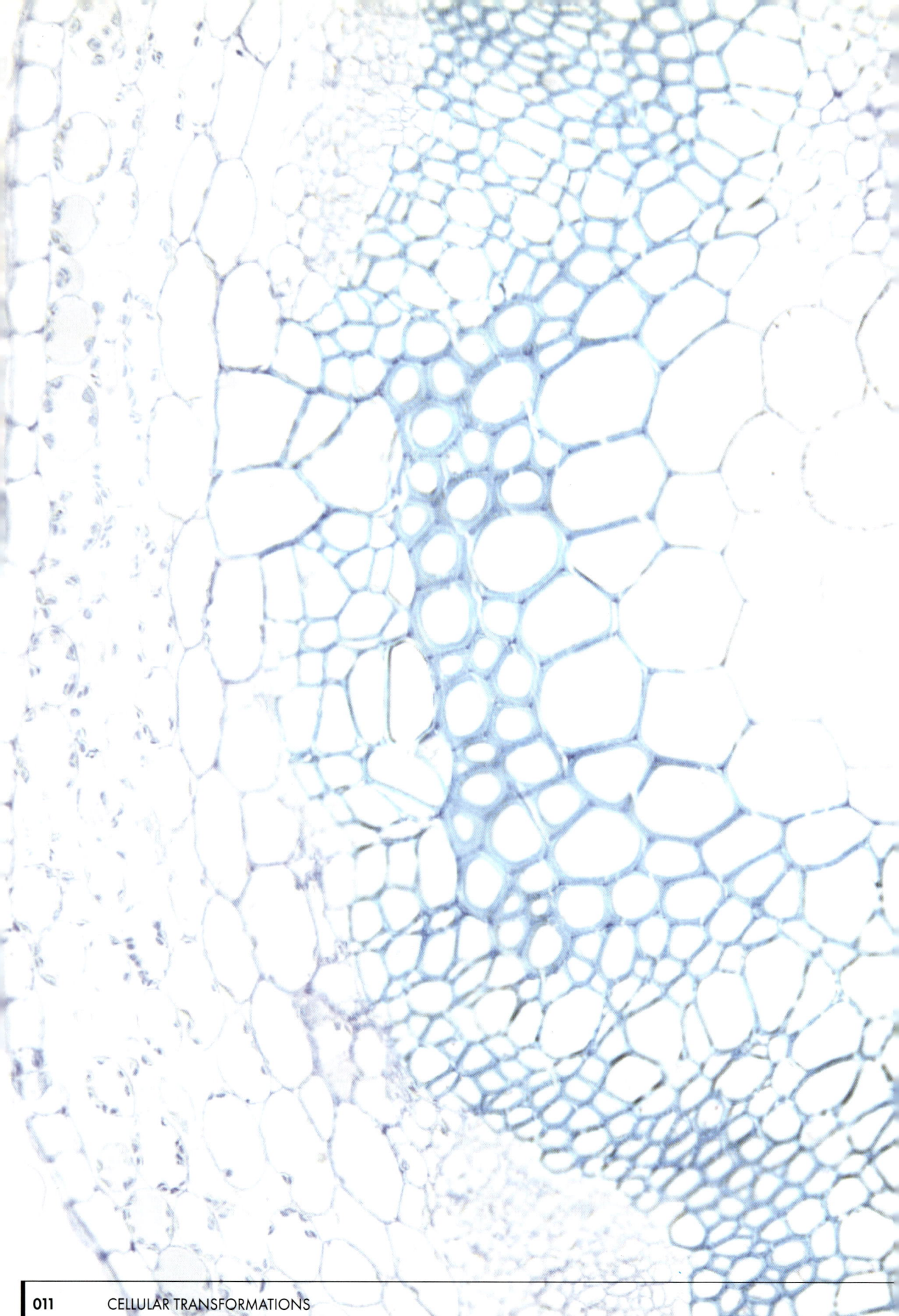

RAM DIXIT
BIOLOGY RESEARCH

PLANT CELL MORPHOGENESIS

Control of cell shape is a fundamental property of life, essential to the form and function of all organisms. Cell shape is determined primarily by an internal scaffolding structure called the cytoskeleton. Unlike human-made scaffolding structures, the cytoskeleton is highly dynamic and can change its configuration in response to developmental and environmental signals, allowing cells to adapt to prevailing conditions. Thus, the cytoskeleton is like an ever-changing "diagram" for cell morphogenesis, and the goal of my research group is to understand how these diagrams are generated and how they produce cell shape. My lab uses the cortical microtubule cytoskeleton of the model plant *Arabidopsis thaliana* as the experimental system of choice. Despite intensive research, it is still unclear how cortical microtubules form wonderfully complex ordered arrays in the absence of a centralized organizing structure like the centrosome of animal cells. The pattern of the cortical microtubule cytoskeleton imparts cell shape by directing the assembly of the rigid cell wall that determines the axis of cell expansion. We use an interdisciplinary and multi-scale approach to understand how activities at the molecular level drive the assembly of microtubule polymers into cellular-scale functional arrays. Our research is of fundamental and practical importance since noncentrosomal microtubule organization has long posed a conundrum in fungi, plants and humans and because understanding cortical microtubule organization has the potential for engineering plants to increase yield, produce new biomaterials from cell walls and make lignocellulosic biomass more conducive for biofuel production.

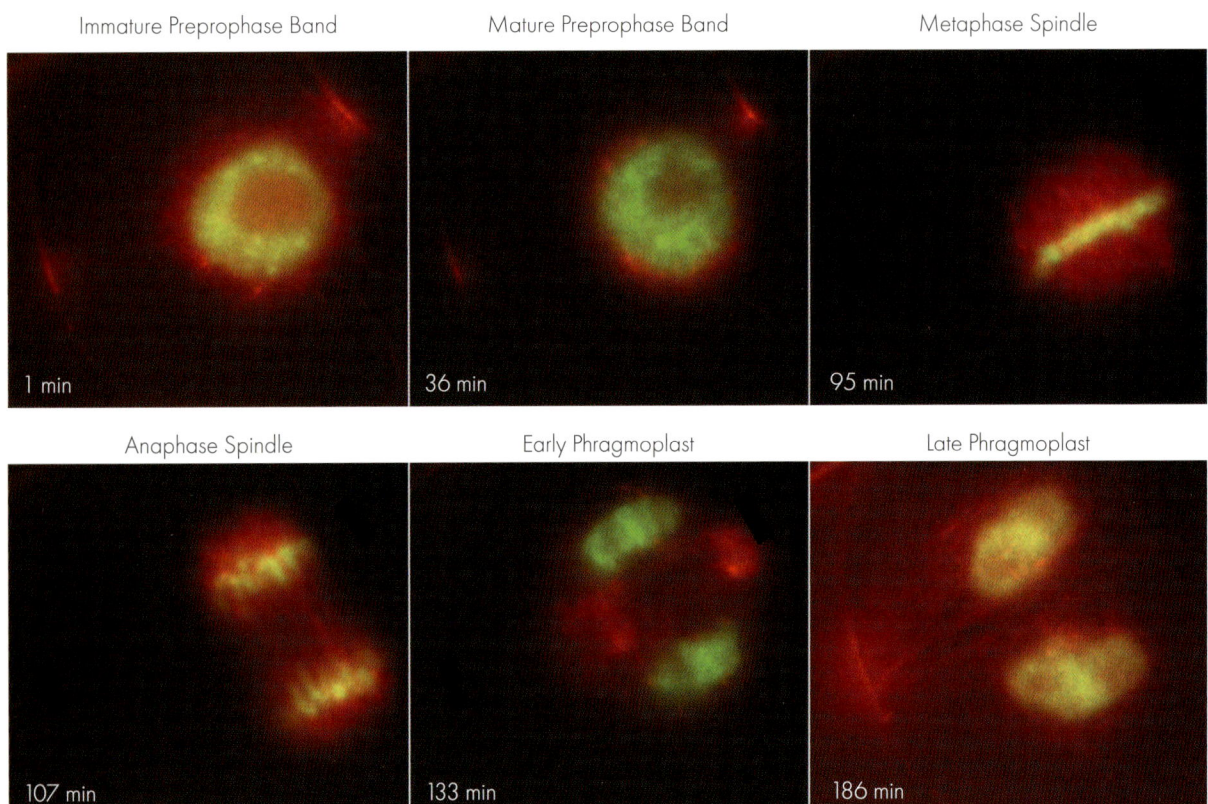

Figure 1: Fluorescence microscopy images of microtubule arrays in a dividing tobacco Bright Yellow-2 cultured cell. Microtubules were visualized using a red fluorescent protein-labeled microtubule binding protein and chromosomes were visualized using a yellow fluorescent protein-labeled histone protein. Note the dramatic changes in microtubule array structure at different stages of cell division.

Cells—the fundamental unit of life on Earth—have much in common with modern cities. Both are crowded and busy environments but contain recognizable hubs that are dedicated to specific tasks such as governance, energy production, manufacturing, delivery and recycling. Both need an elaborate transportation system to move materials to desired locations and a sophisticated communication network to send, receive and respond to information. And both depend on an extensive infrastructure for the reliable operation of these complex tasks.

In cells, one of the major infrastructures is the cytoskeleton, which consists of filamentous protein polymers arranged into specific three-dimensional arrays. Unlike the infrastructure of cities, the cytoskeleton is highly dynamic and is able to rapidly change configuration. The dynamic nature of the cytoskeleton enables cells to adapt to changing conditions and to perform different functions such as the ones needed at distinct stages of the cell division cycle (Figure 1). A major objective of my research group is to understand how cells construct specific cytoskeletal architectures and dynamically alter them in response to information from their internal and external environment. My lab uses plants as a model system to study how tubular cytoskeletal elements called microtubules are assembled into specific patterns to confer cell shape.

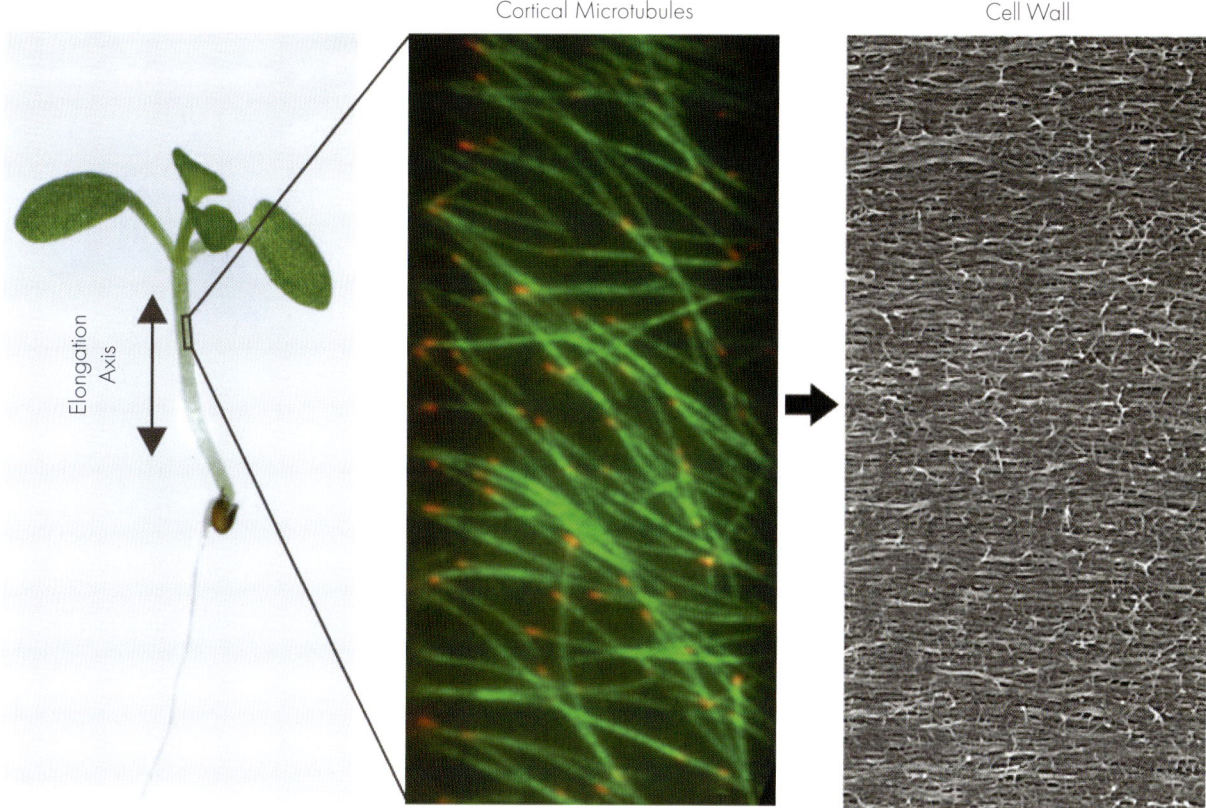

Figure 2: Plant cortical microtubules determine cell shape by patterning the cell wall. Cortical microtubules spatially pattern the deposition of cell wall material. In rapidly growing epidermal cells of an *Arabidopsis thaliana* seedling, transversely arranged cortical microtubules lead to strengthening of the cell wall like hoops around a barrel causing cells to elongate vertically.

Multicellular organisms consist of many different cell types that are distinguished by their shape and function. New cells arise by division of existing cells. In plants and animals, stem cells at specific locations serve as cradles of cell division that give rise to new cells that grow and differentiate to produce the beautiful diversity of plant and animal forms found in nature. Cell division is typically a cookie cutter process, resulting in new cells that are unremarkable in size and shape. Depending on their lineage and position in tissues, cells go on to adopt different identities which often involves acquisition of specialized cell morphology.

The microtubule cytoskeleton is the morphogenetic engine of plant cells. It performs this function by serving as a scaffolding structure for the deposition of cell wall material (Figure 2). Enzyme complexes that synthesize cellulose physically interact with and move along these microtubules as they extrude cellulose outside the cell. In addition, these microtubules serve as tracks for molecular motor proteins that are thought to transport membrane-bound compartments containing noncellulosic cell wall material for secretion. In this manner, microtubules influence the arrangement of cell wall components in the extracellular environment. The spatial organization of the cell wall determines its mechanical property that in turn defines the axis of cell expansion to produce cell shape. We can conceptualize microtubule array organization and cell wall construction as the cellular equivalents of civil engineering projects that shape cities. But while we understand how complex building projects are planned and executed in cities, how this occurs in cells remains poorly understood.

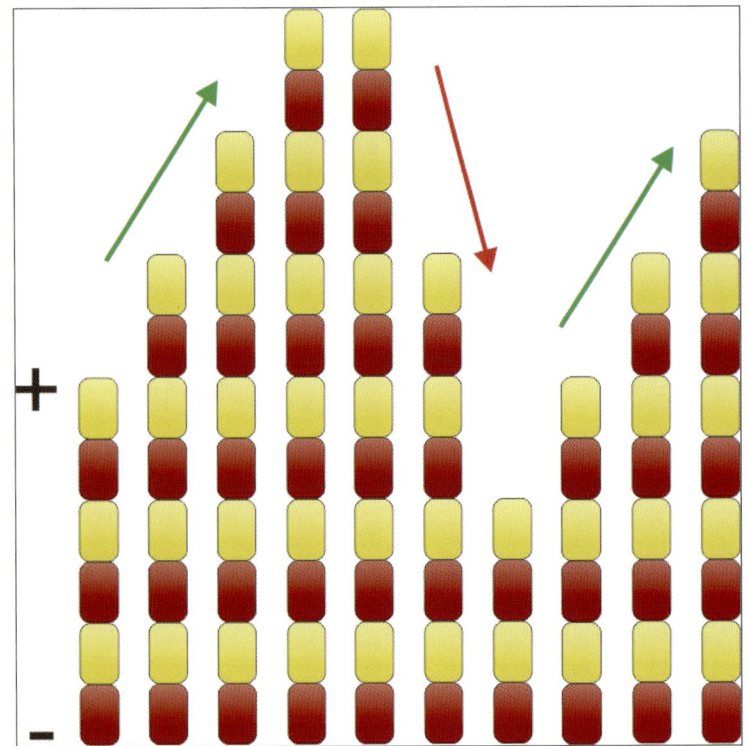

Figure 3: Dynamics of microtubules. Microtubules are tubular structures consisting of 13 linear strands called protofilaments. Here a single protofilament is shown for simplicity. Microtubules alternate between periods of growth, when αβ-tubulin subunits (red and yellow subunits) add at the tips, and shortening, when αβ-tubulin subunits dissociate from the tips. Microtubules have polarity due to head-to-tail binding of the subunits. The more dynamic end is called the plus-end and the less dynamic end is called the minus-end.

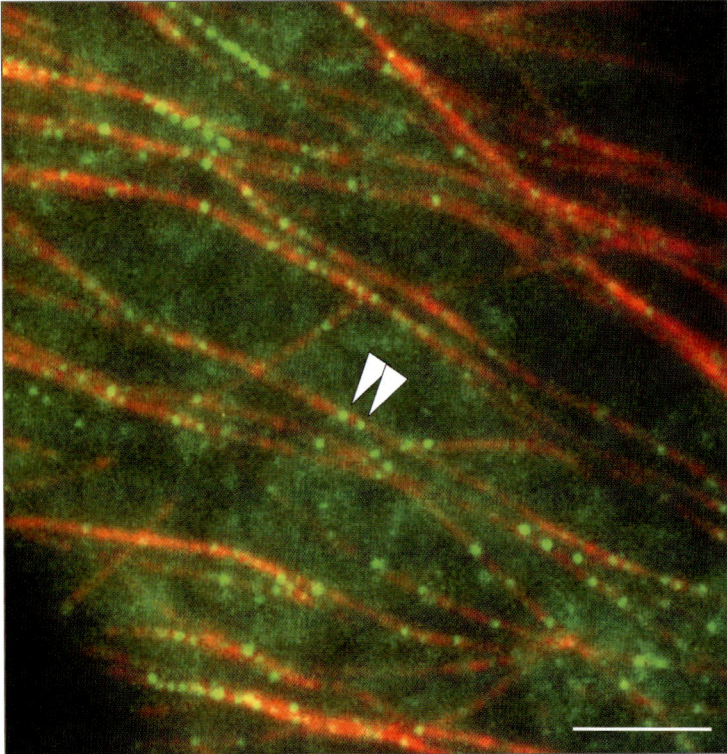

Figure 4: Visualization of the FRA1 motor protein in living cells. Fluoresence microscopy image of green fluorescent protein-labeled FRA1 motor proteins (green) moving along cortical microtubules (red). Arrow heads point to two FRA1 particles on a cortical microtubule.

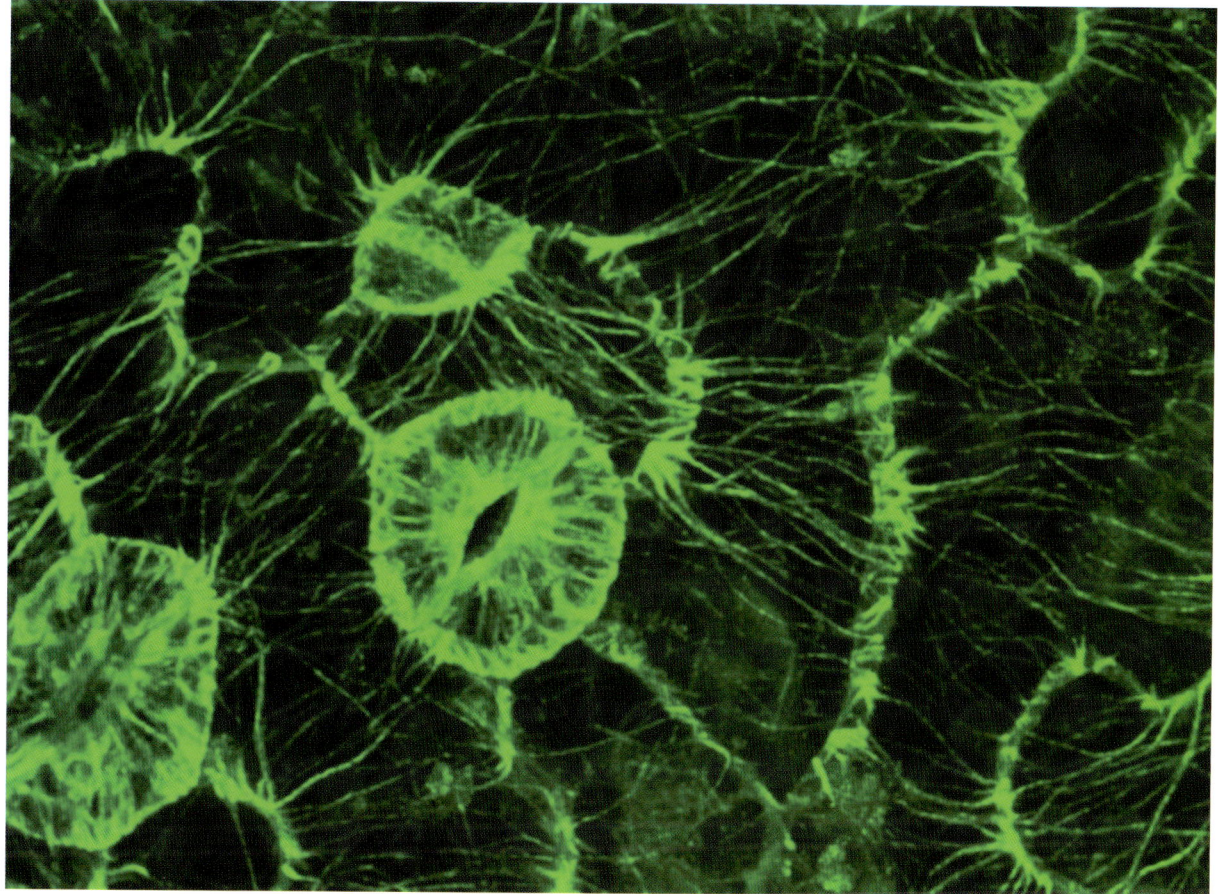

Figure 5: Cortical microtubules are arranged into distinct configurations in different cell types. In the leaf epidermis, the kidney bean-shaped guard cells contain radial microtubule arrays while the jigsaw puzzle-piece-shaped pavement cells contain net-like microtubule arrays.

Microtubules are inherently dynamic polymers that randomly alternate between periods of growth and shortening by the addition and removal of subunits, respectively (Figure 3). Nonetheless, cells are able to construct elaborate microtubule structures of defined shape and size whose overall shape can persist over time even though individual elements remain dynamic. Cells achieve this complex task through a host of regulatory proteins called microtubule-associated proteins. Some of these proteins bind to microtubule tips to regulate subunit addition and removal, while other regulatory proteins bind to the sides of microtubules to either stabilize, destabilize or crosslink microtubules. Together, the various microtubule regulatory proteins function as a molecular toolkit that allows cells to precisely control number, length, and lifetime of microtubules. Much of my research focuses on studying the mechanism of action of specific microtubule regulatory proteins and how cells control the location, timing and activity of these proteins to pattern microtubules.

Construction of the cell wall requires that its various constituents be secreted at the right place, at the right time and in the right amounts. To investigate how cells tackle this supply chain problem, we have focused on a particular motor protein called FRA1 that was implicated in cell wall assembly. Motor proteins are nanoscale engines that transport cellular cargo in a directional manner. We showed that FRA1 moves on microtubules over long distances and likely transports vesicles containing cell wall polysaccharides such as pectin (Figure 4). Similar to increased traffic volume during rush hours in cities, the abundance and motility of this motor protein increases when the demand for cell wall deposition is high. In addition, this motor protein helps to anchor its own tracks in place to stabilize the sites of cell wall deposition during times of high activity.

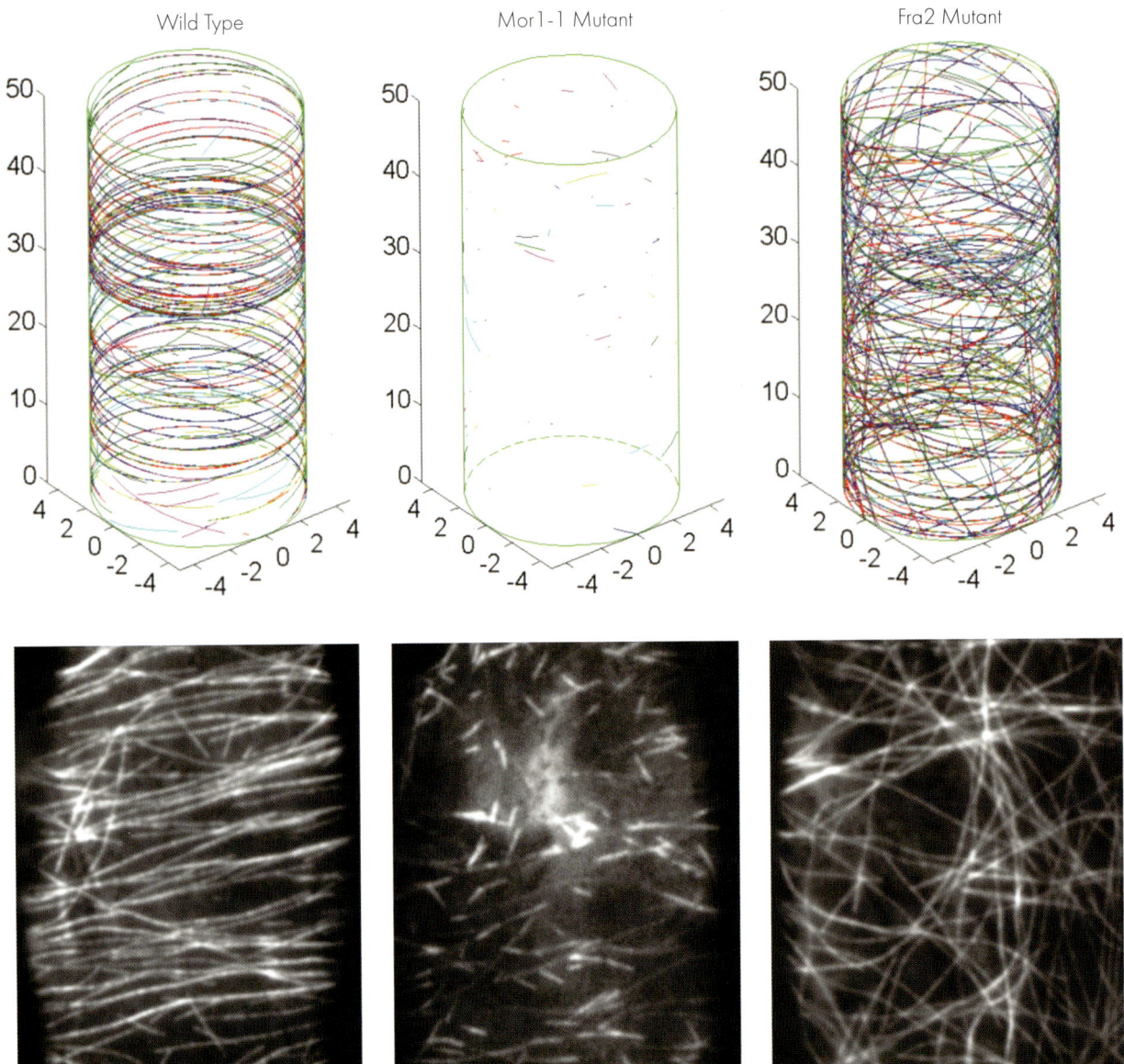

Figure 6: Computational models of cortical microtubule organization. Computer models were developed based on the dynamic behavior of plant cortical microtubules to study the mechanisms for array organization. The models accurately recreate ordered microtubule arrays seen in wild-type plants and different types of aberrant arrays seen in mutant *Arabidopsis thaliana* plants in which specific microtubule regulatory proteins are either non-functional (*mor1-1* mutant) or lacking (*fra2* mutant).

Our work uses a combination of fluorescence microscopy to visualize microtubule dynamics and motor protein motility in living cells (Figures 4 and 5), genetics to study the effect of mutants that either lack or overproduce proteins of interest, biochemistry to measure the activity of specific proteins, and computer simulations to explore the self-organizing properties and mechanism of transition between different organizational states of microtubules (Figure 6).

Recently, we have embarked on a project to recreate realistic plant tissues on fibrous scaffolds that resemble the cell wall to study how plants sense and respond to their mechanical environment under controlled conditions (Figure 7). This project is in collaboration with engineering colleagues within an NSF-funded multi-institution Science and Technology Center for Engineering Mechanobiology.

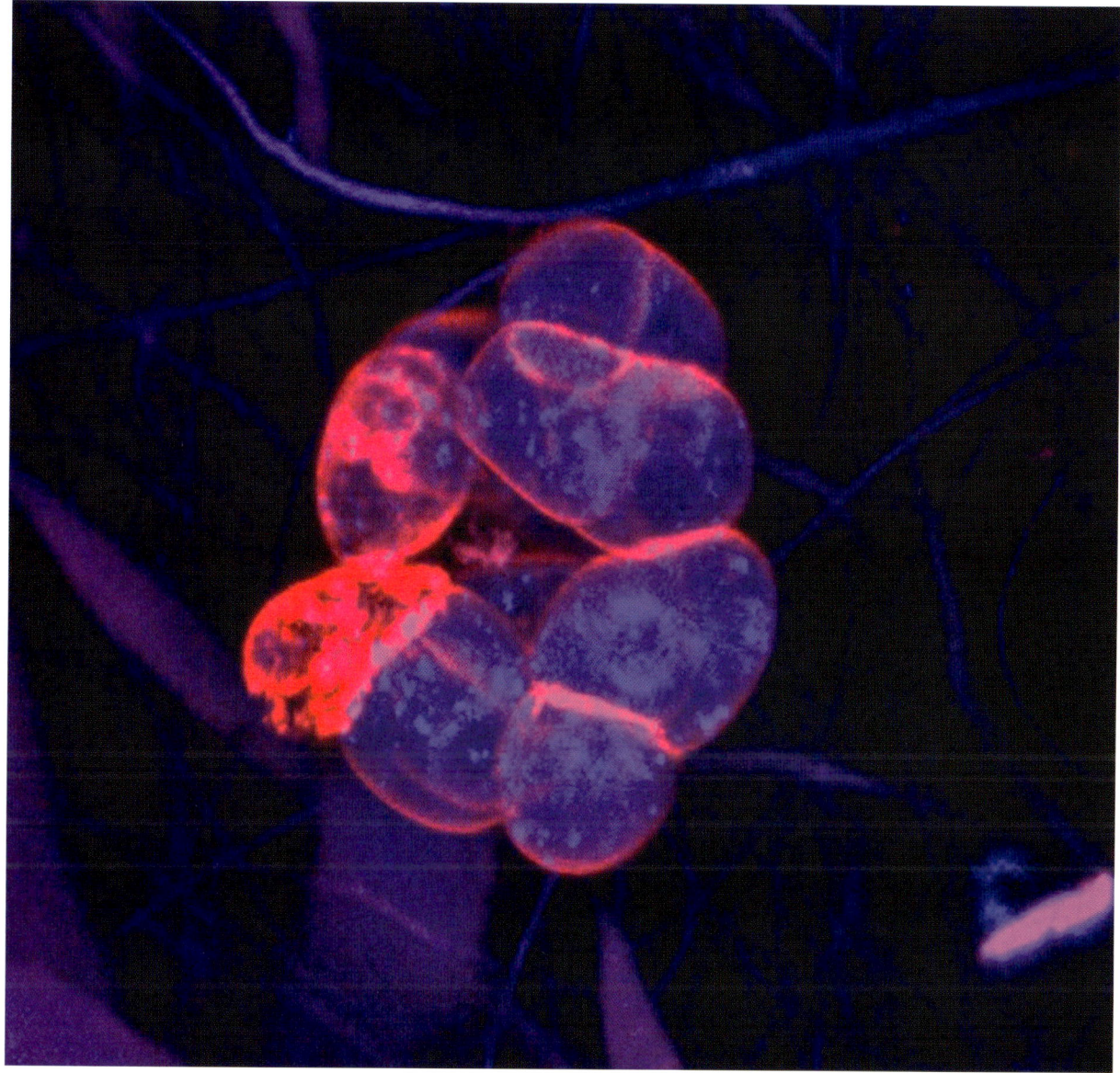

Figure 7: Development of biomimetic scaffolds for plant cell research. Fluorescence microscopy image of cultured tobacco cells bound to an artificial fibrous scaffold.

The goal of this interdisciplinary center is to decipher how mechanical forces influence biological systems to sculpt morphogenesis of plants and animals, to enable cells to migrate, proliferate, or differentiate, and to modulate the function of single molecules.

Since the microtubule cytoskeleton and much of its regulatory machinery is conserved between plants and animals, our research can provide insights into how malfunction of microtubule dynamics and organization can cause diseases such as cancer and neurological disorders in humans. In addition, the information gained from our work has the potential to be used to engineer plants to enhance food, fiber and biofuel production.

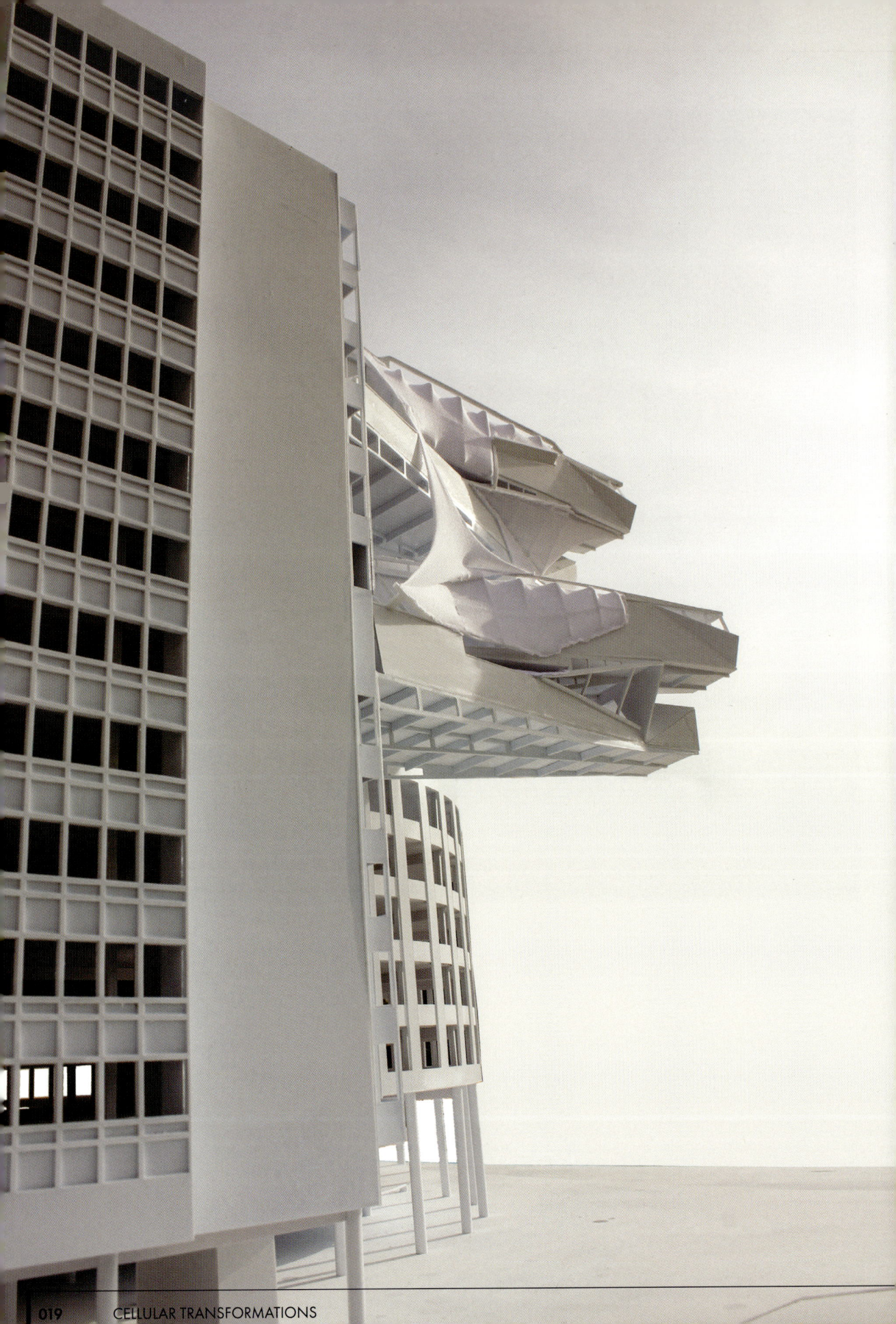

SUNG HO KIM and ANDREW YOO
ARCHITECTURE RESEARCH

ARCHITECTURE OF SKIN

Throughout the last 200 years, architecture has depended on a basic material palette that consists of masonry (concrete, brick, stone and ceramics), metals (alloys and steel), timber, glass and plastics. The emerging development of material research in the building industry has expedited the urgency of inventing ecologically responsive array of materials. To this end, sustainable and environmental material research has crossed into the territory of biology to explore possibilities in entropic and dynamic material spectrums. This new research embraces the emergent phenomenon of organic matters blending with natural elements. At its core is the biophilia hypothesis, the innate necessity for humans to connect with flora and fauna on this planet. The important factor of life is that all living matter is interconnected through energy and unseen dynamic forces demonstrated in the likes of biofeedback and biomechanics. All these phenomena are interwoven into the infrastructural network and mapping of the cellular structures of all life on earth.

The Research Architecture Graduate Studio: ARCHITECTURE of SKIN_REDEFINING the SURGICAL PRACTICE is an experimentation into new organic materials in architecture and into the innovation of future medical procedures. The clinical processes in health sciences have not been reimagined in over 100 years. This research studio allows a glimpse into the future of healthcare where technology and environments are assimilated with human bodies. Building with innovative organic skin protects environments from microbes and elements, assists in regulating temperature by sweating and secreting moisture, allows the sensation of touch and energy, and absorbs liquids with controlling factors. The skin, through its vessel infrastructure, can administer medications and read vital signs without any invasive procedures.

SKIN AS ARCHITECTURAL ORGAN

During development, gene activations lead to molecular processes and pathways that specify stem cells' differentiation to a particular cell type. The differentiated state is usually "locked-in" by epigenetic mechanisms that prevent the transition of one cell type to another. Recent advances in biomedical research have challenged this view, such that a somatic cell type, for example, skin cells, can be altered to another cell type by genetic perturbations. One famous example is the fate reprogramming of a skin cell type, dermal fibroblasts, to embryonic stem cell-like pluripotent stem cells, providing tremendous regenerative medicine implications. Recent studies also demonstrated the feasibility of turning skin fibroblasts directly to nerve cells via direct fate conversion. Such experimental techniques now allow the generation of human nerve cells from skin fibroblasts to model neurological disorders.

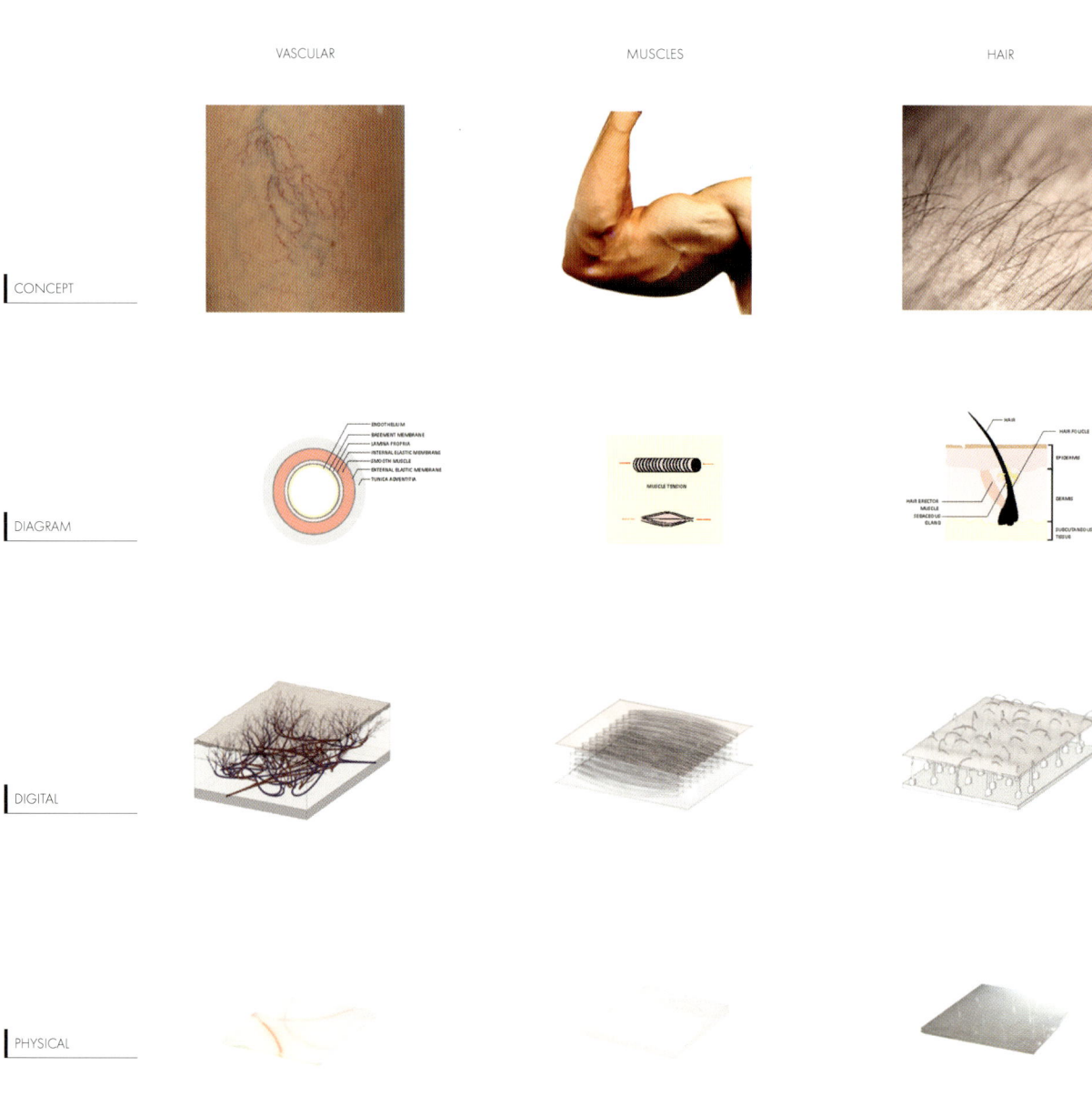

The skin is the largest organ in the human body. Skin is made up of three layers, the epidermis, dermis and the hypodermis layer. The epidermis is the outer layer of skin that keeps vital fluids in and harmful bacteria out of the body. The dermis is the inner layer of skin that contains blood vessels, nerves, hair follicles, oil, and sweat glands. The studio explores the possibility of inventing new forms of bioengineered artificial skins that is able to interface with architectural conditions. The current built environment does not have to be static and rigid. With the advancement in bioengineering, architecture can respond fluidly to transformative readings in temperature and moisture level and healing itself through regeneration.

| CARTILAGE | BIOLUMINOUS | SWEATING | TATTOOS |

A recent development in the synthetic skin technique has been made by imparting the color changing properties of the skin. By tuning the wavelength of light, the color transforms and senses any irregularity in the system. This technology can be used in color-shifting camouflages and sensors that can detect otherwise imperceptible defects in buildings and structures. The bioengineering design practice with material research develops new conditions in architecture that can alter the properties to changing environmental conditions. Living materials provokes the possibility that buildings can make a positive impact on the environment by performing remedial operations that can heal a stressed environment by removing toxins or filtering greenhouse gases.

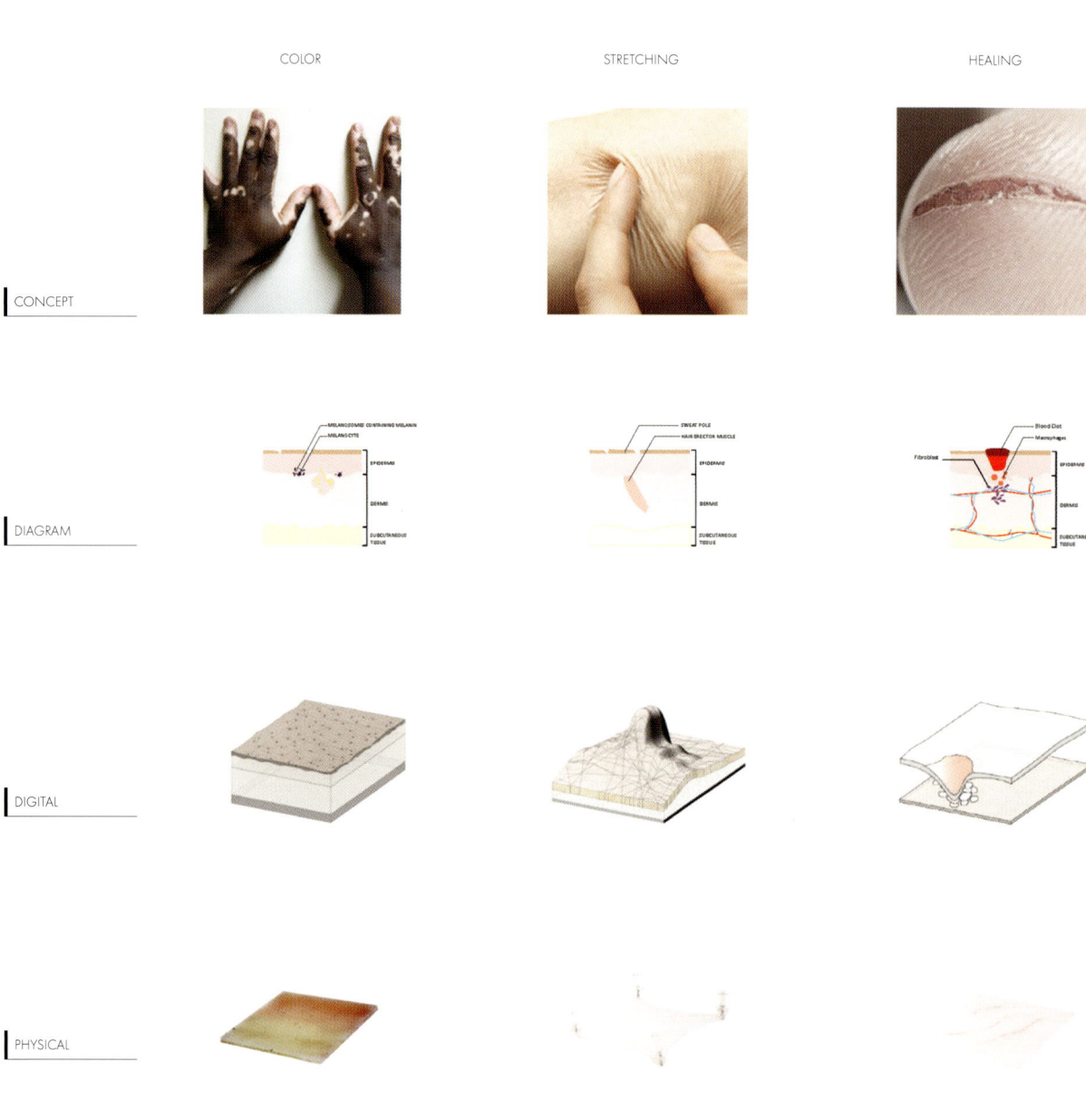

Living technologies may ultimately have the ability to change the fundamental relationship between human development and the environment. This is a major shift in our architectural practices that could contribute to our continued survival rather than the destruction of our environment. We may think of our buildings as synthetic skin that offers robust protection against the consequences of climatic and natural disturbances.

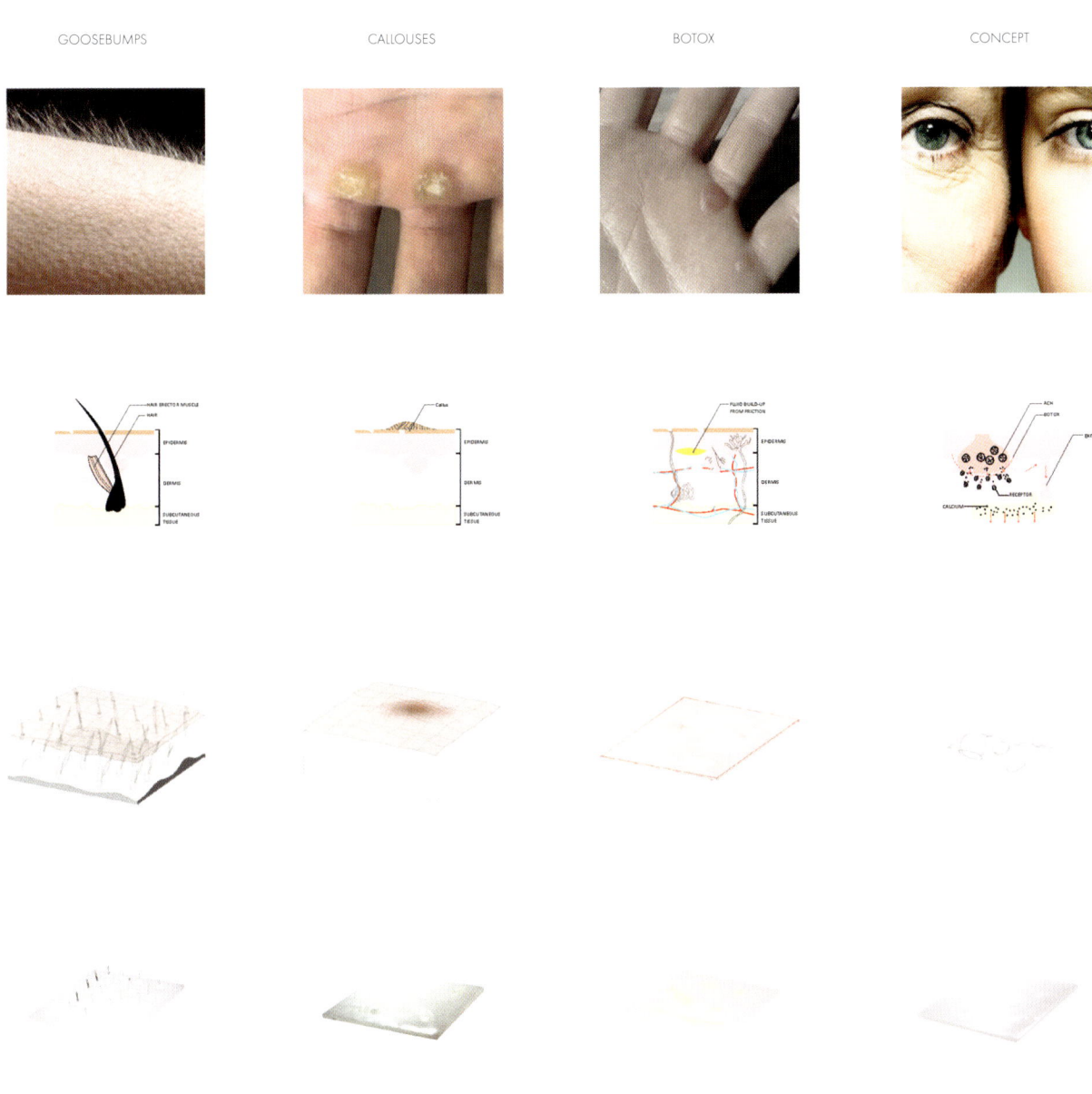

REDEFINING THE SURGICAL PRACTICE

The history of operating theaters as a significant site of modern surgical practice and analysis of sociology, science and technology is the focus of the program. The studio research is to explore the transformations within spaces used for surgery and surgeons' strategy to achieve more control over their working conditions and thus over the bodies they sought to manipulate. Operating theaters are rooms in a hospital equipped for the performance of surgical operations that are spacious, easy to disinfect, and organized with visual connection to the operation and the audience. Operating theaters need to control temperature and humidity for suppressing infections. Special air handlers filter the air and maintain a slightly elevated pressure. Several operating theaters are part of the operating suite that forms a distinct section within a healthcare facility. The operating suite contains washrooms, personnel rooms and recovery rooms, storage, cleaning facilities, offices and laboratories for medical research.

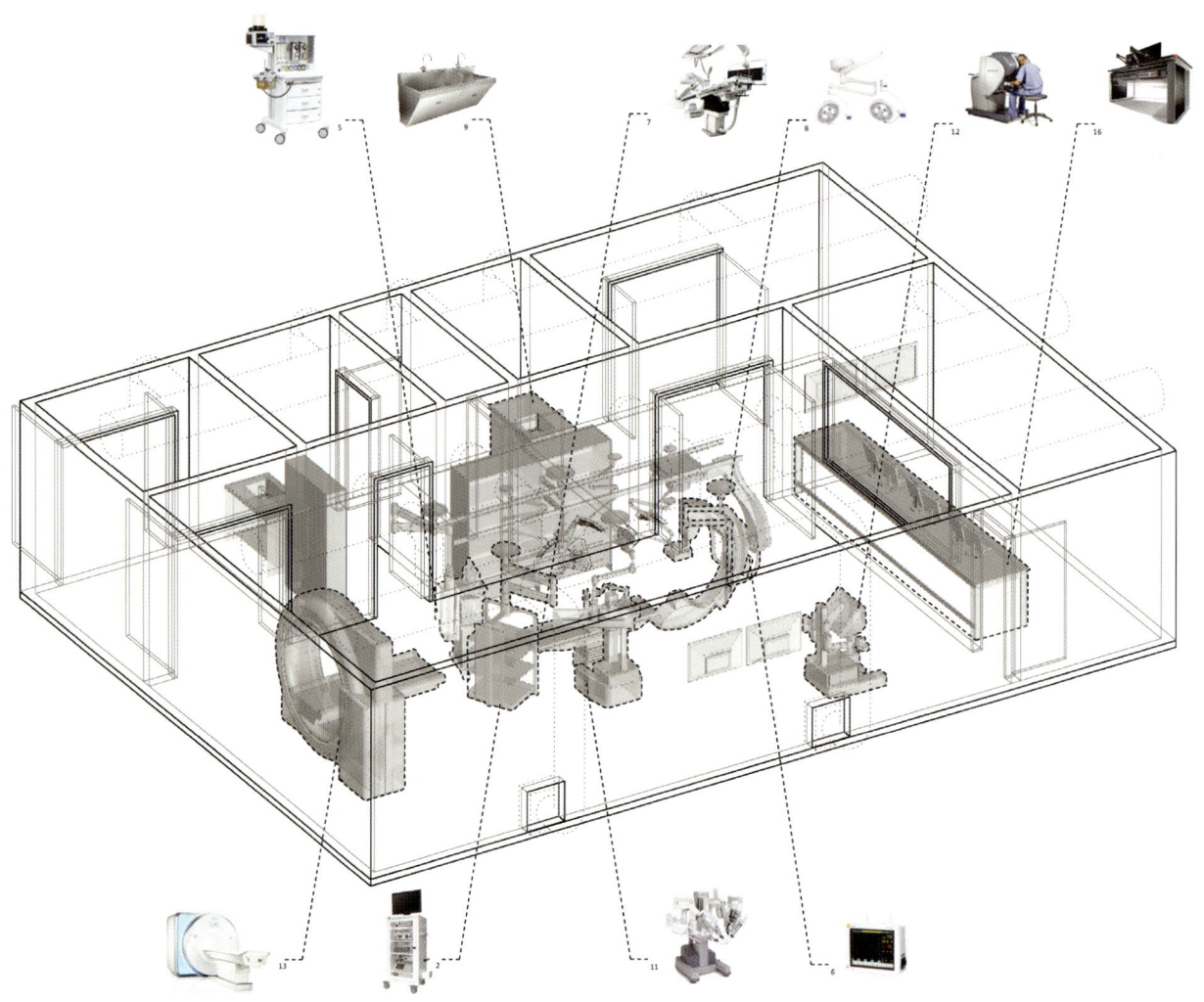

YAFENG LIU | TAOKAI MA | JOSEPH VIZURRAGA

Equipment List

 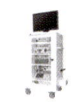   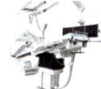

1. Microscope 2. Endoscopy Tower 3. Electro Surgical Generator 4. Suction Pumps 5. Anesthesia Equipment 6. Vital Signs Monitors 7. Hybrid Operating Tables 8. LED Surgery Light

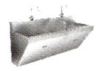   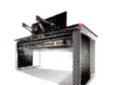

9. Scrub Sinks 10. Cabinet 11. Robotic Arms 12. Computer For Robotic Arms 13. MRI 14. Autoclaves and Sterilizers 15. Patient Warmers 16. Control Room Desk

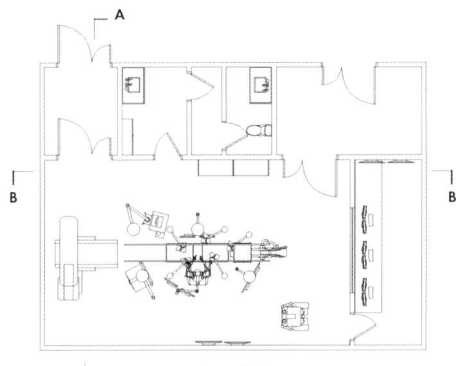

Clinical Plan

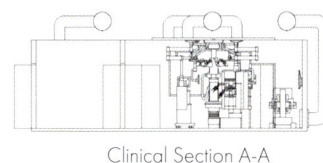

Clinical Section A-A

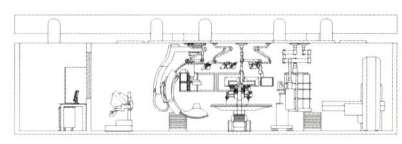

Clinical Section B-B

 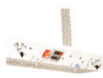

1. Sterilizer 2. Overhead Service Carrier 3. Exhaust Hood 4. Service Spine 5. Cold Storage 6. Blood Analyzer 7. Microscope

     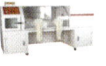

8. Centrifuge 9. Incubator 10. Distilled Water Plant 11. Homogeniser 12. Oven 13. Chamber 14. Autoclave

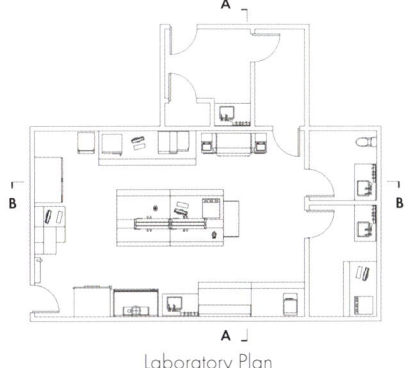

Laboratory Plan

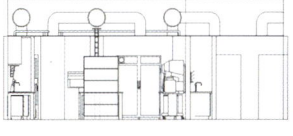

Laboratory Section A-A

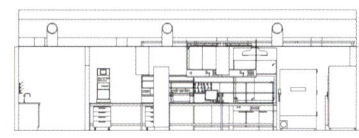

Laboratory Section B-B

ARCHITECTURE OF SKIN   026

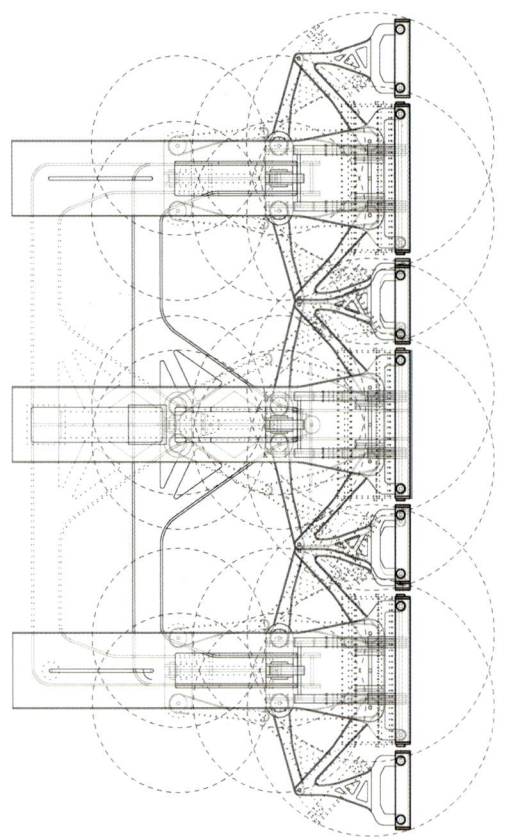

Cell Printing Machine Elevation

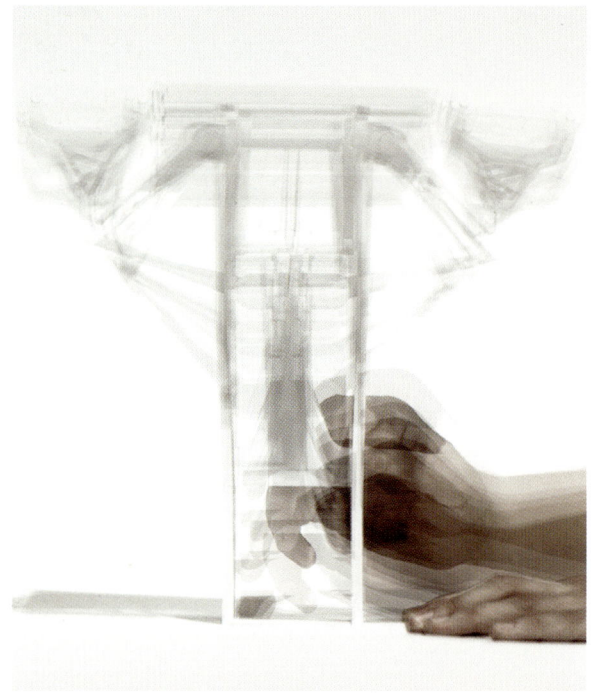

Cell Printing Machine Model

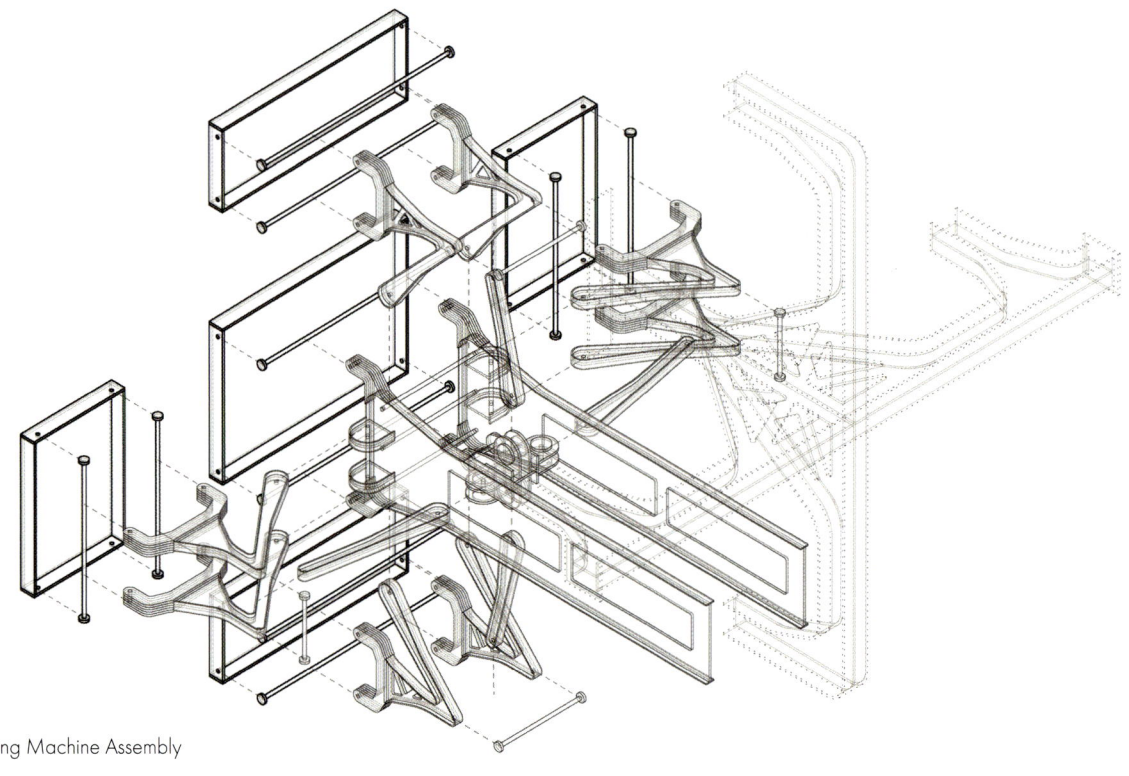

Cell Printing Machine Assembly

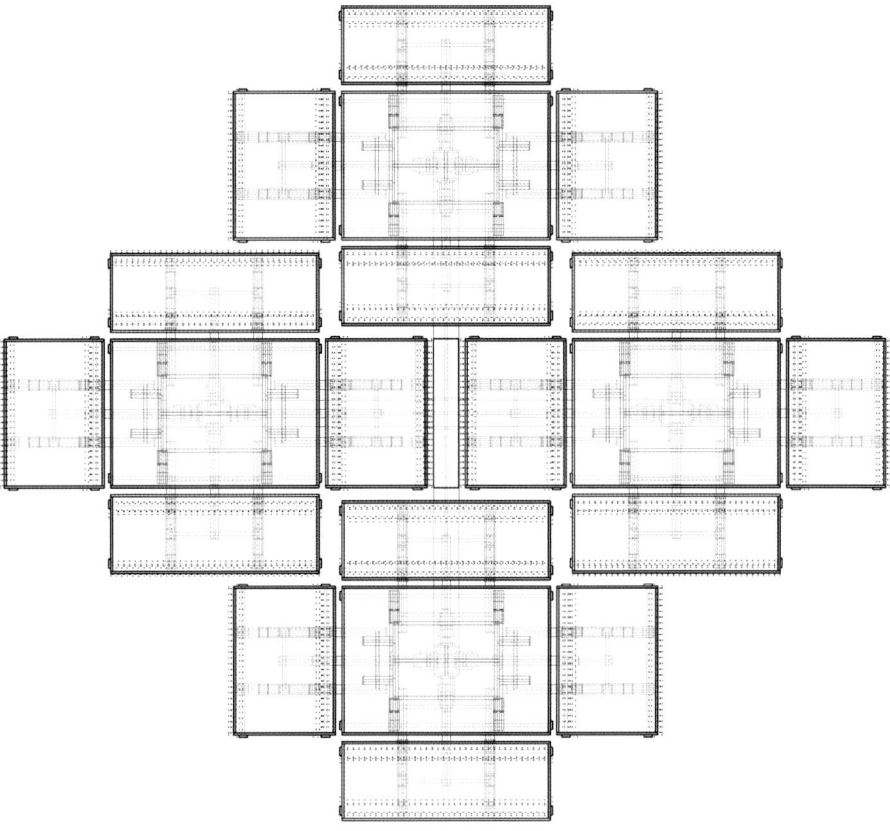

Cell Printing Machine Front Elevation

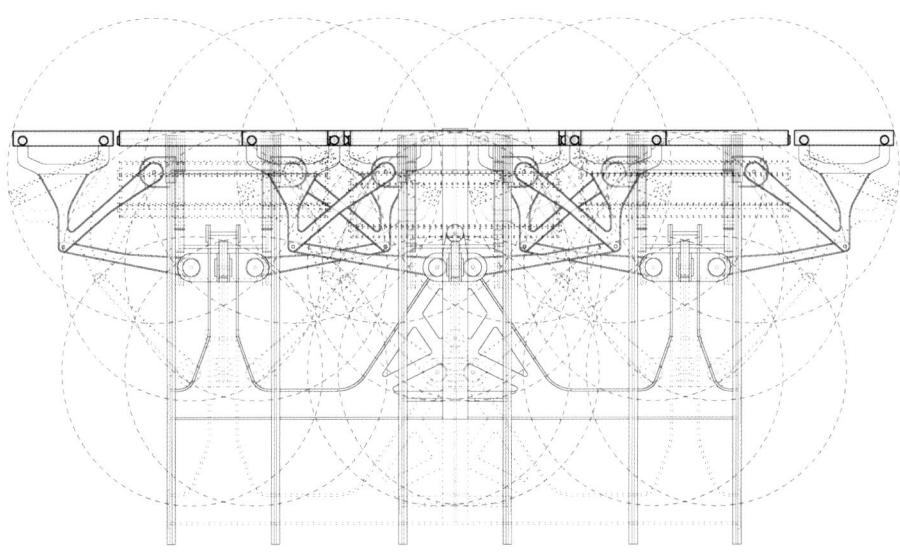

Cell Printing Machine Plan

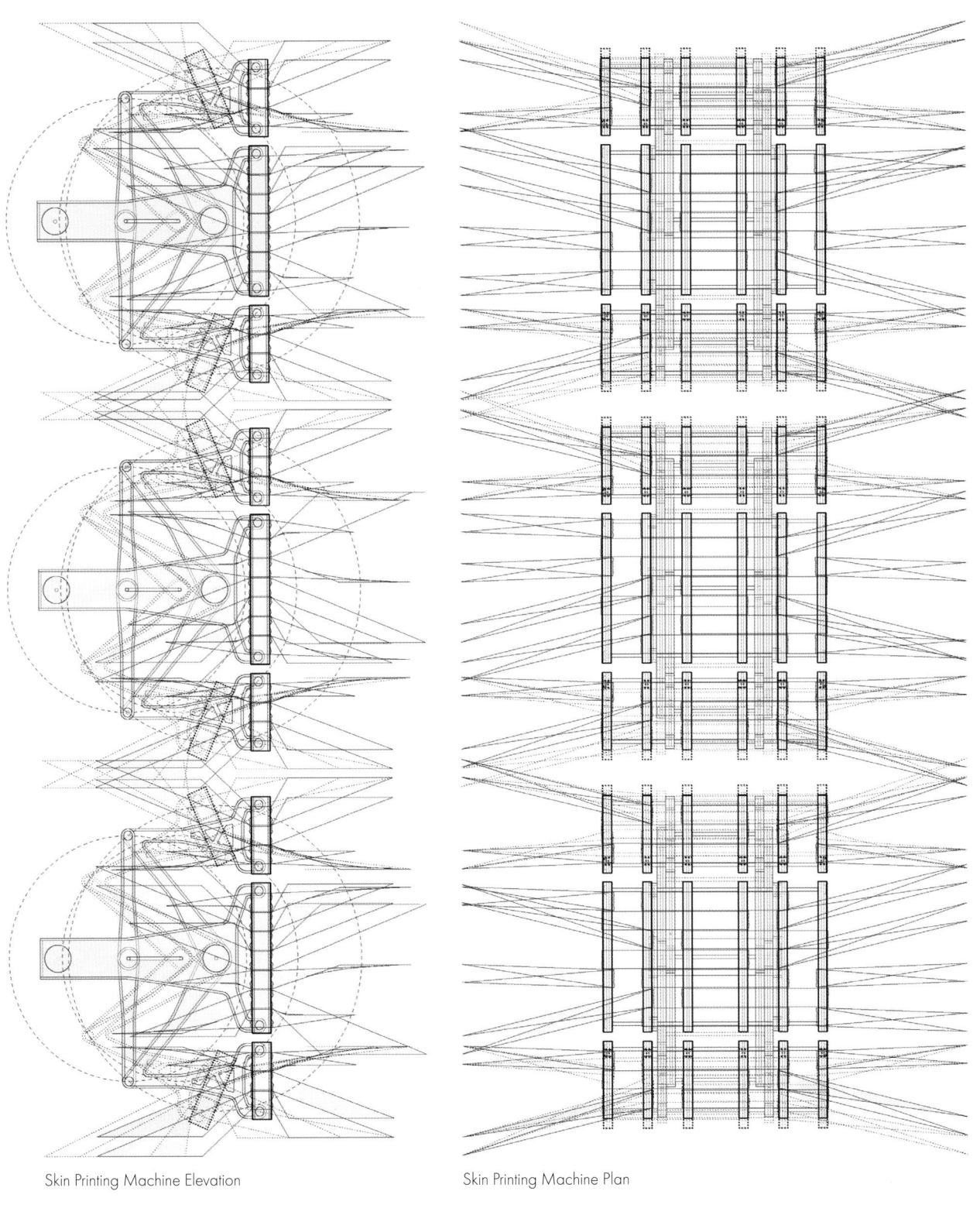

Skin Printing Machine Elevation

Skin Printing Machine Plan

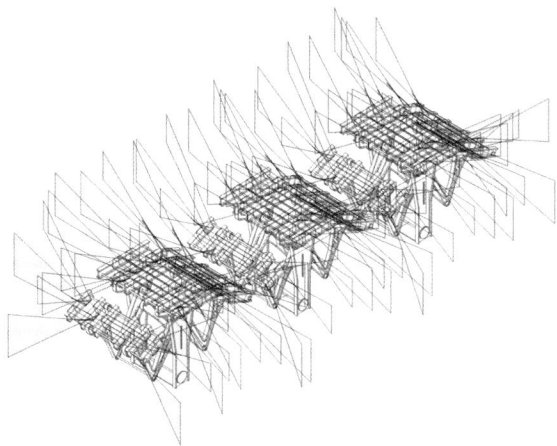

Skin Printing Machine Assembly Diagram (Active)

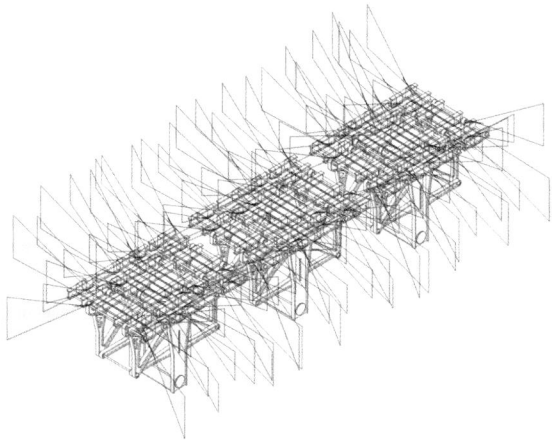

Skin Printing Machine Assembly Diagram (Non-Active)

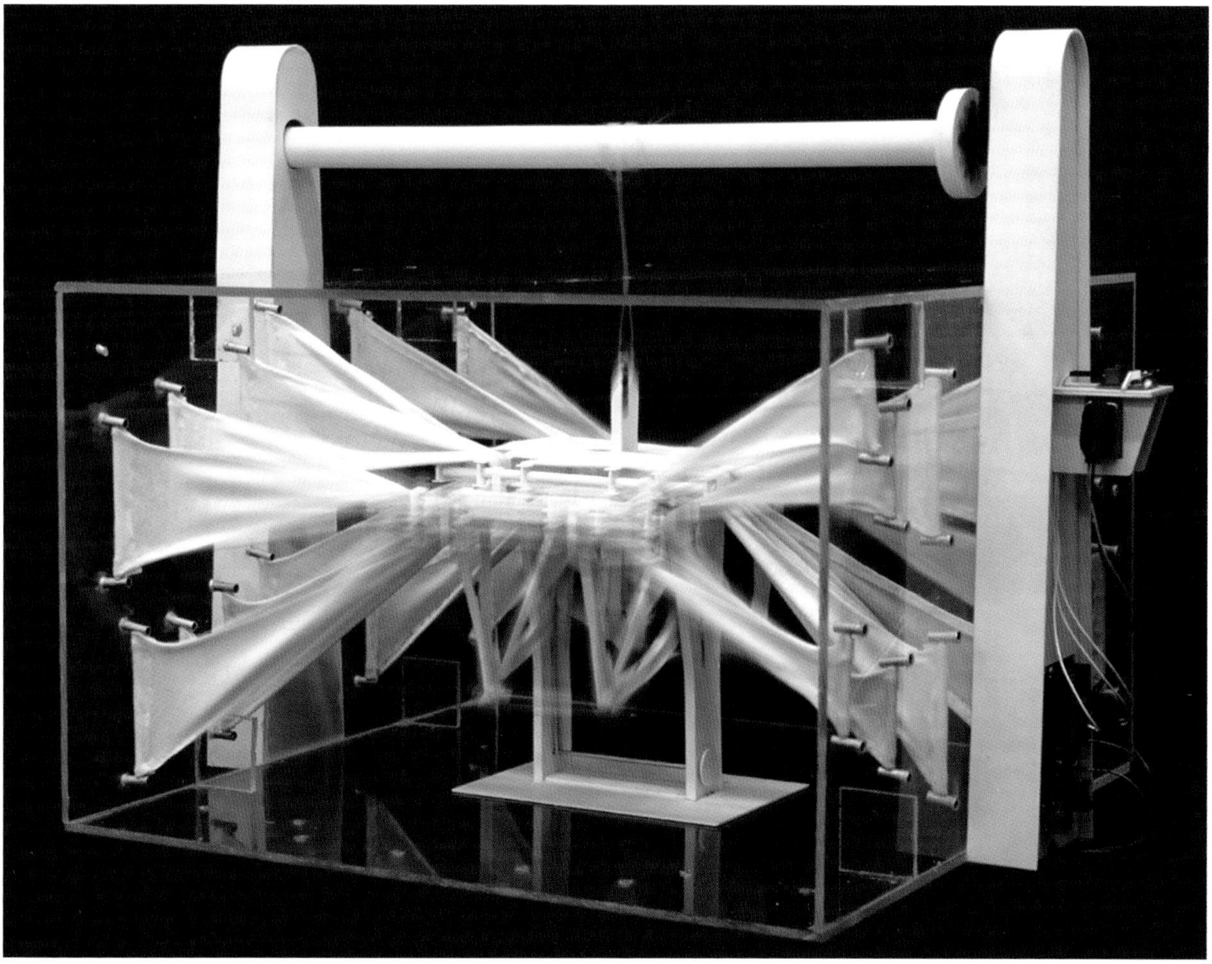

Skin Printing Machine Model

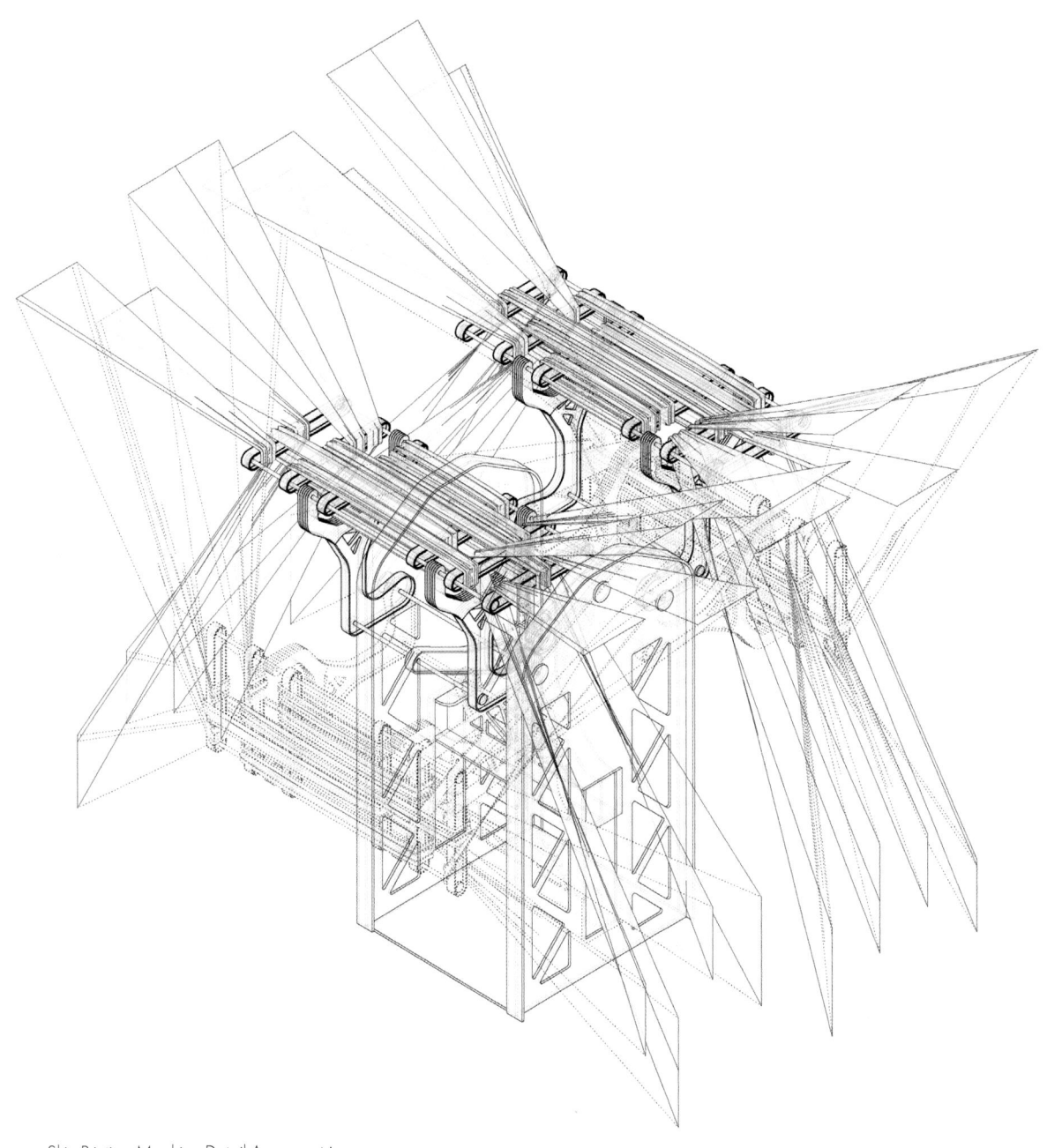

Skin Printing Machine Detail Axonometric

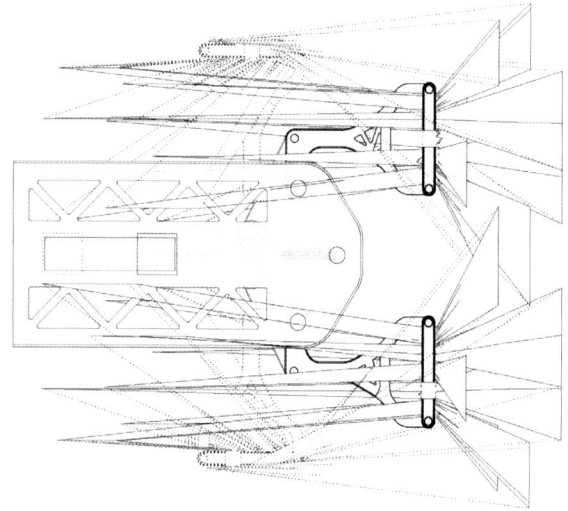
Skin Printing Machine Detail Section

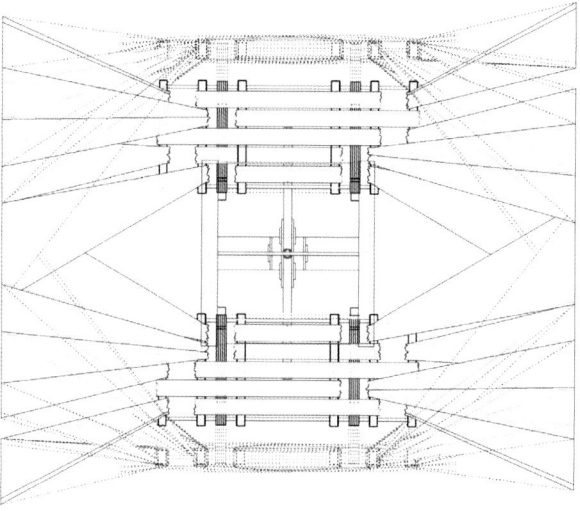
Skin Printing Machine Detail Plan

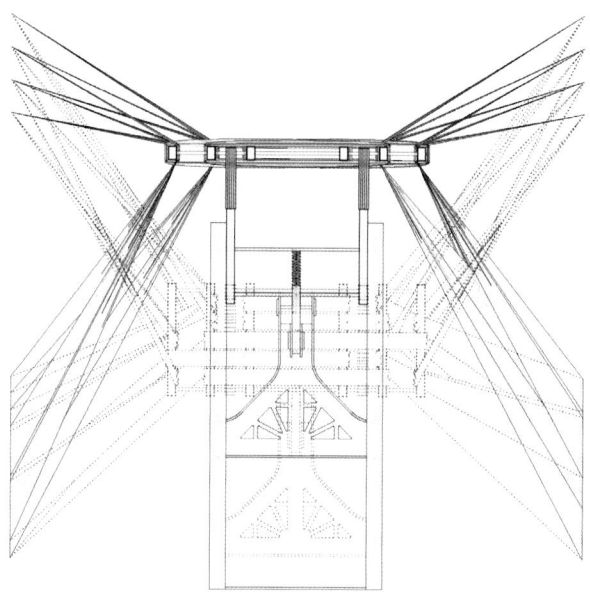
Skin Printing Machine Detail Elevation

JOSEPH VIZURRAGA

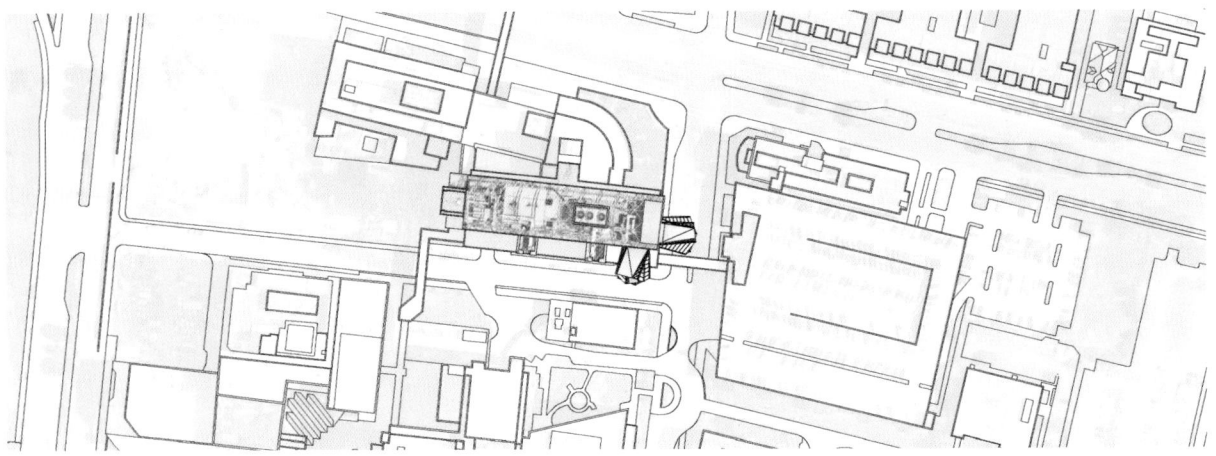

Site Plan

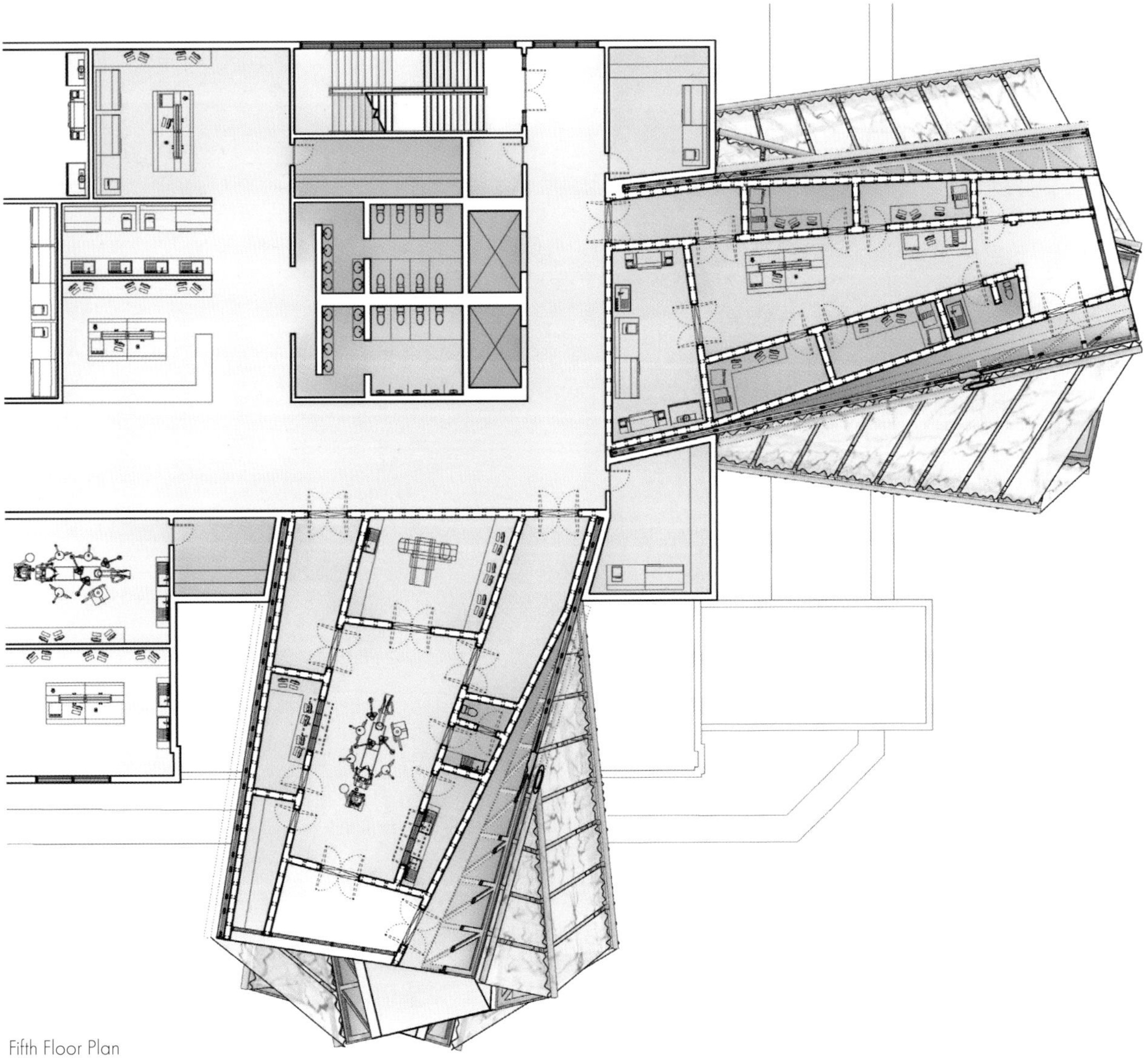

Fifth Floor Plan

033 CELLULAR TRANSFORMATIONS

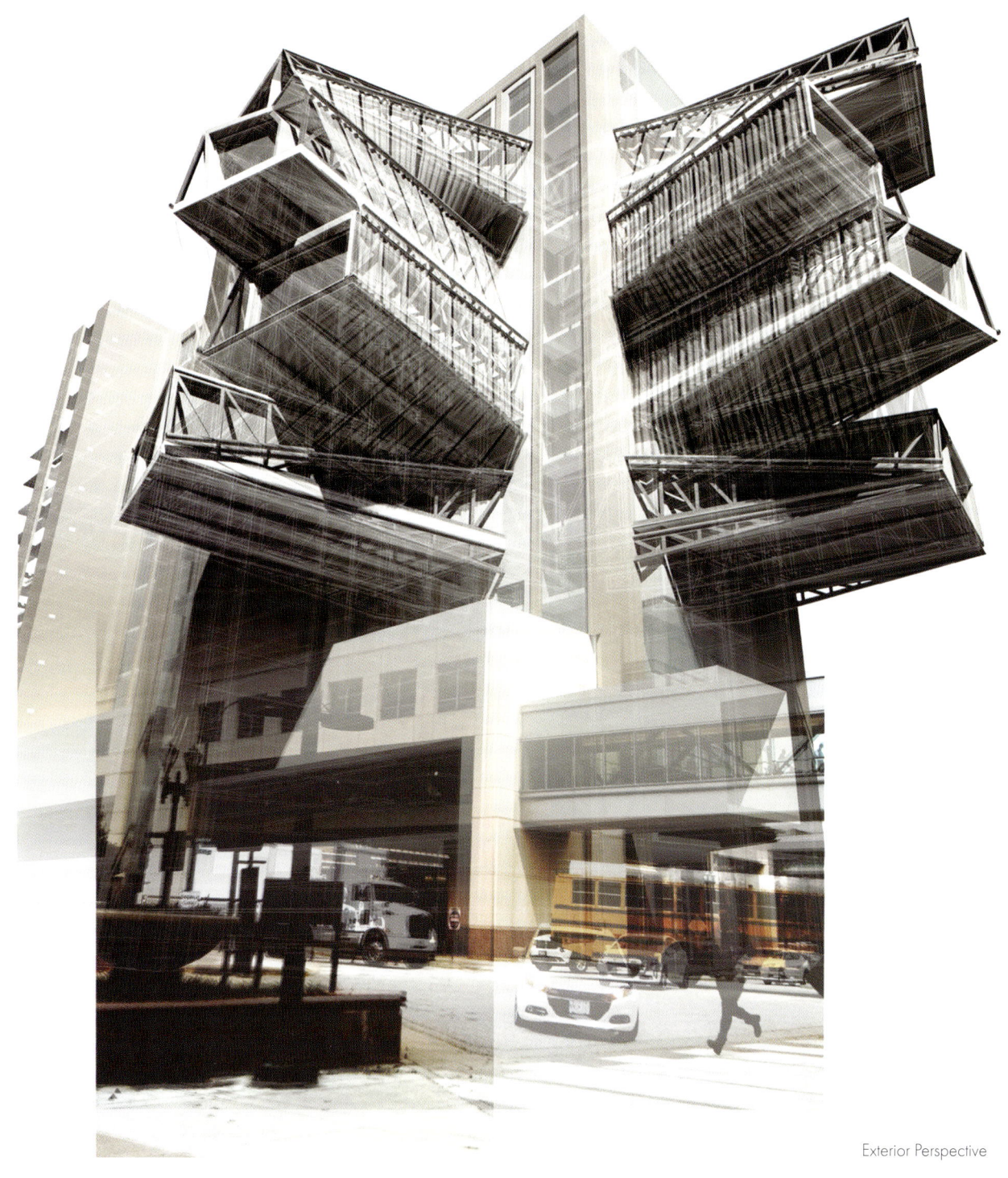

Exterior Perspective

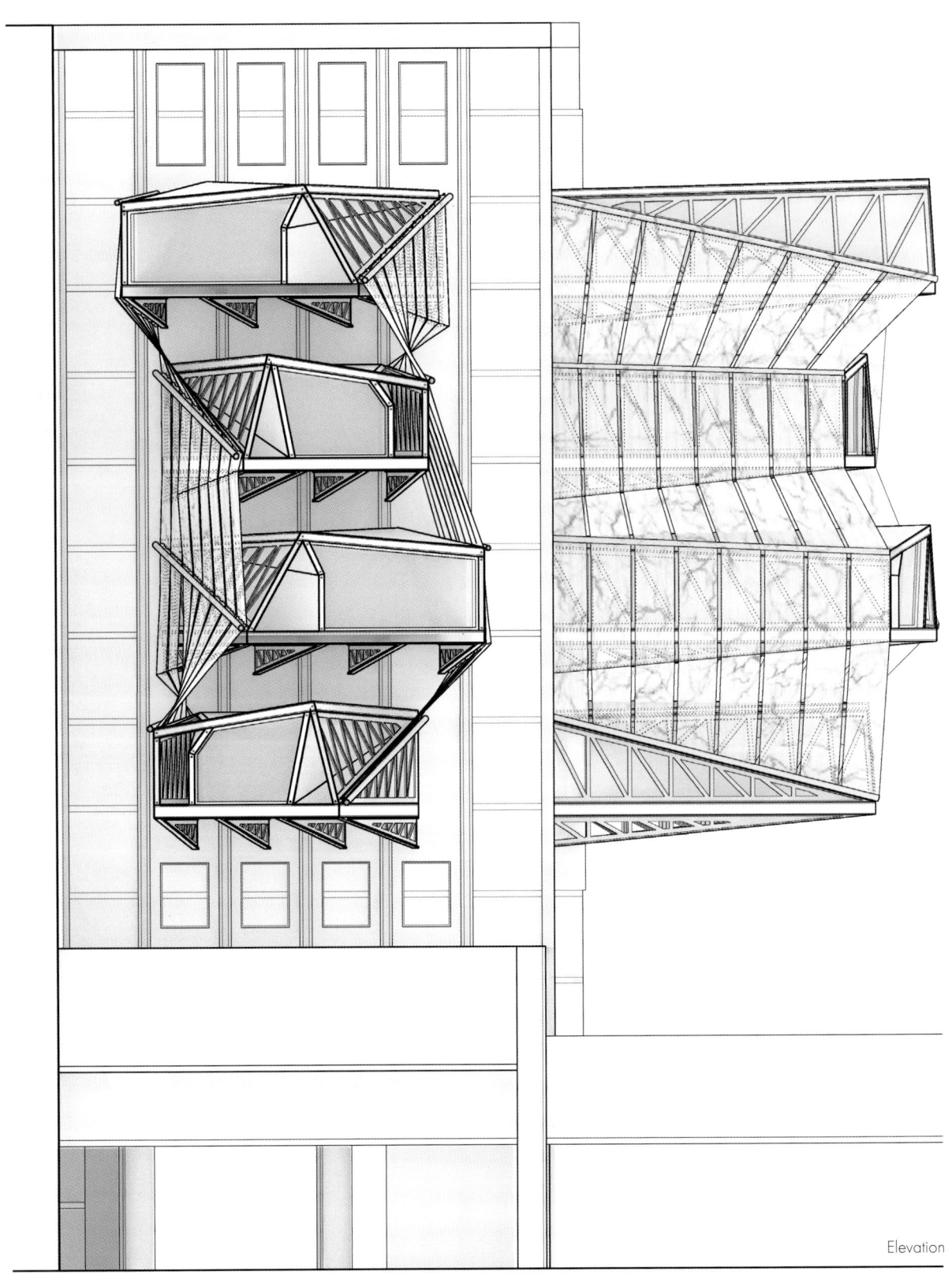

Elevation

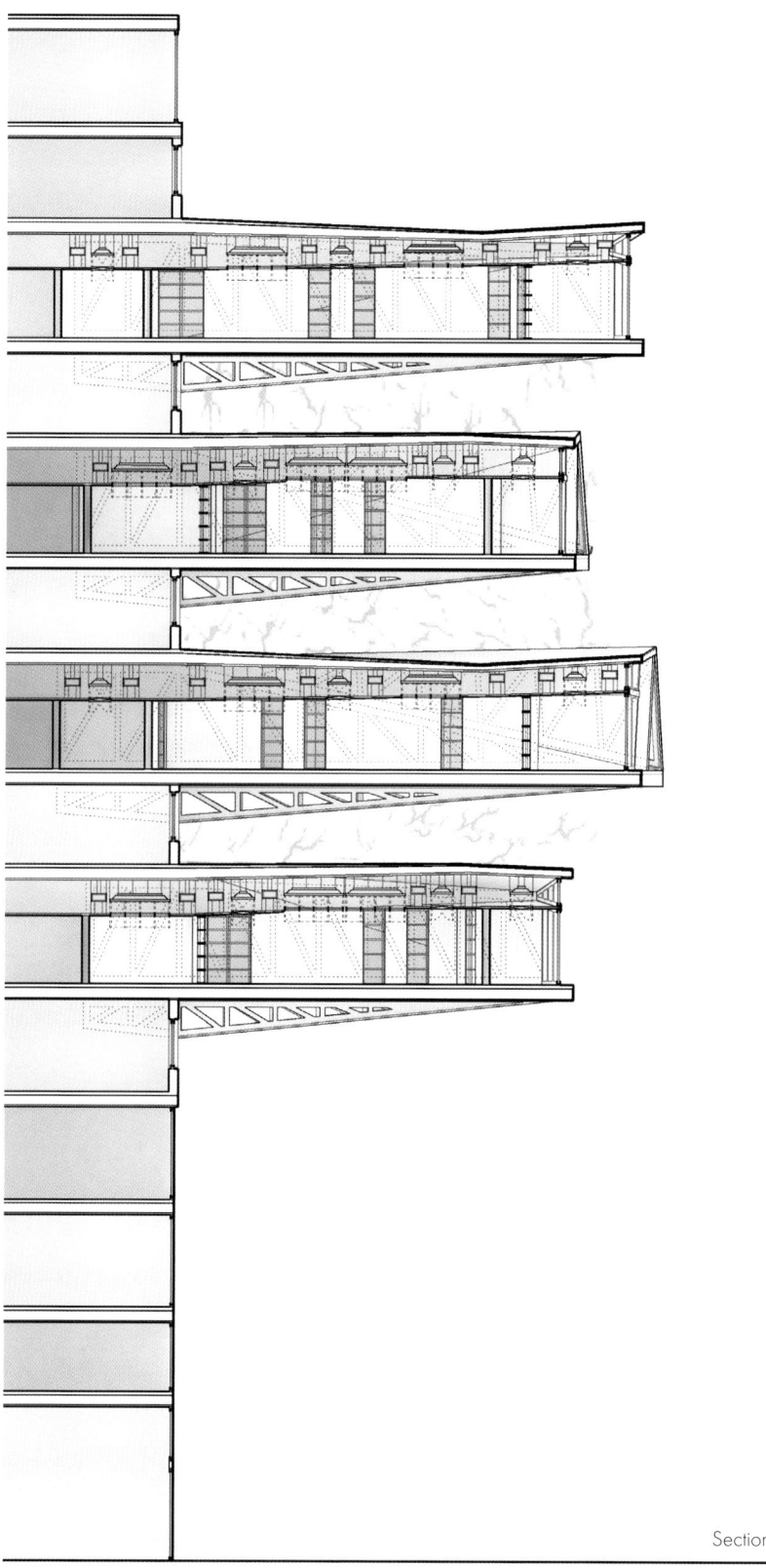

Section

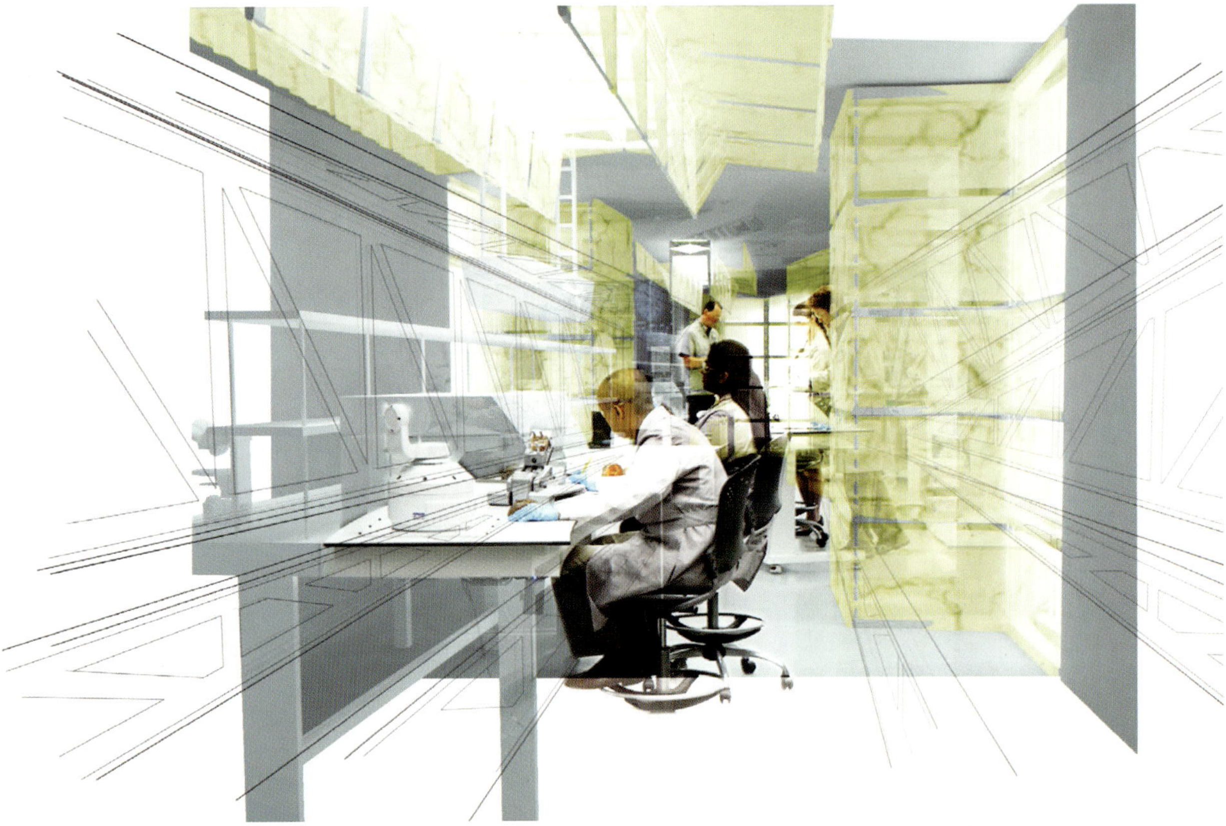

JOSEPH VIZURRAGA

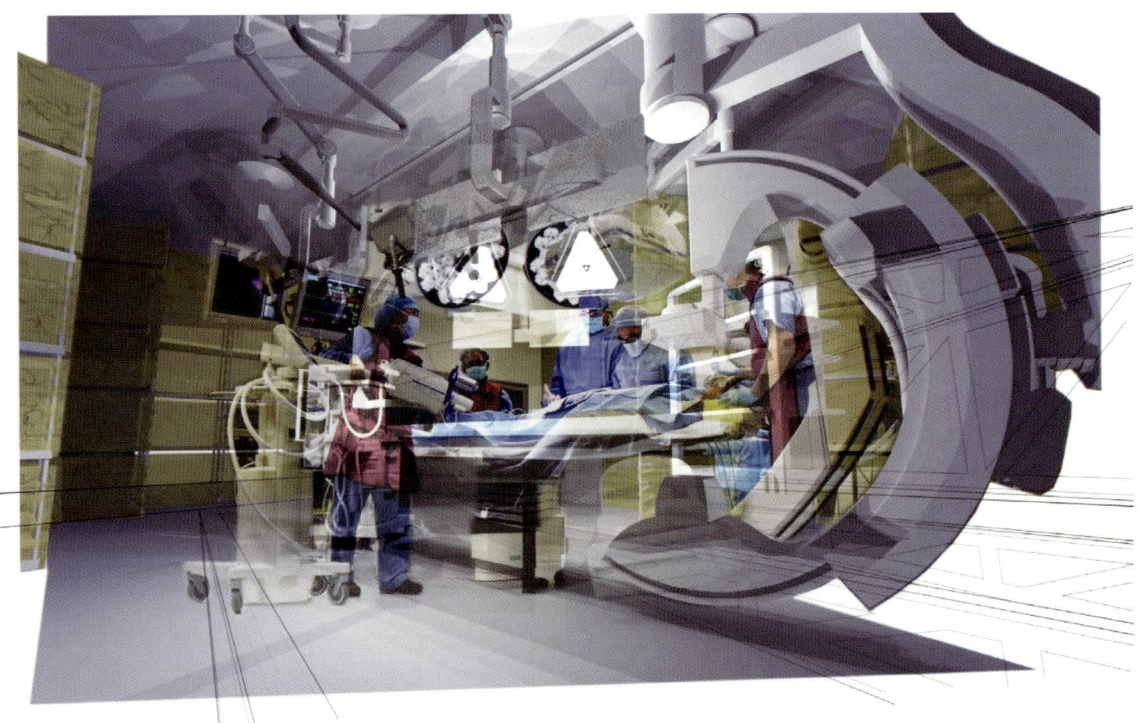

Interior Laboratory Perspective

Interior Operation Room Perspective

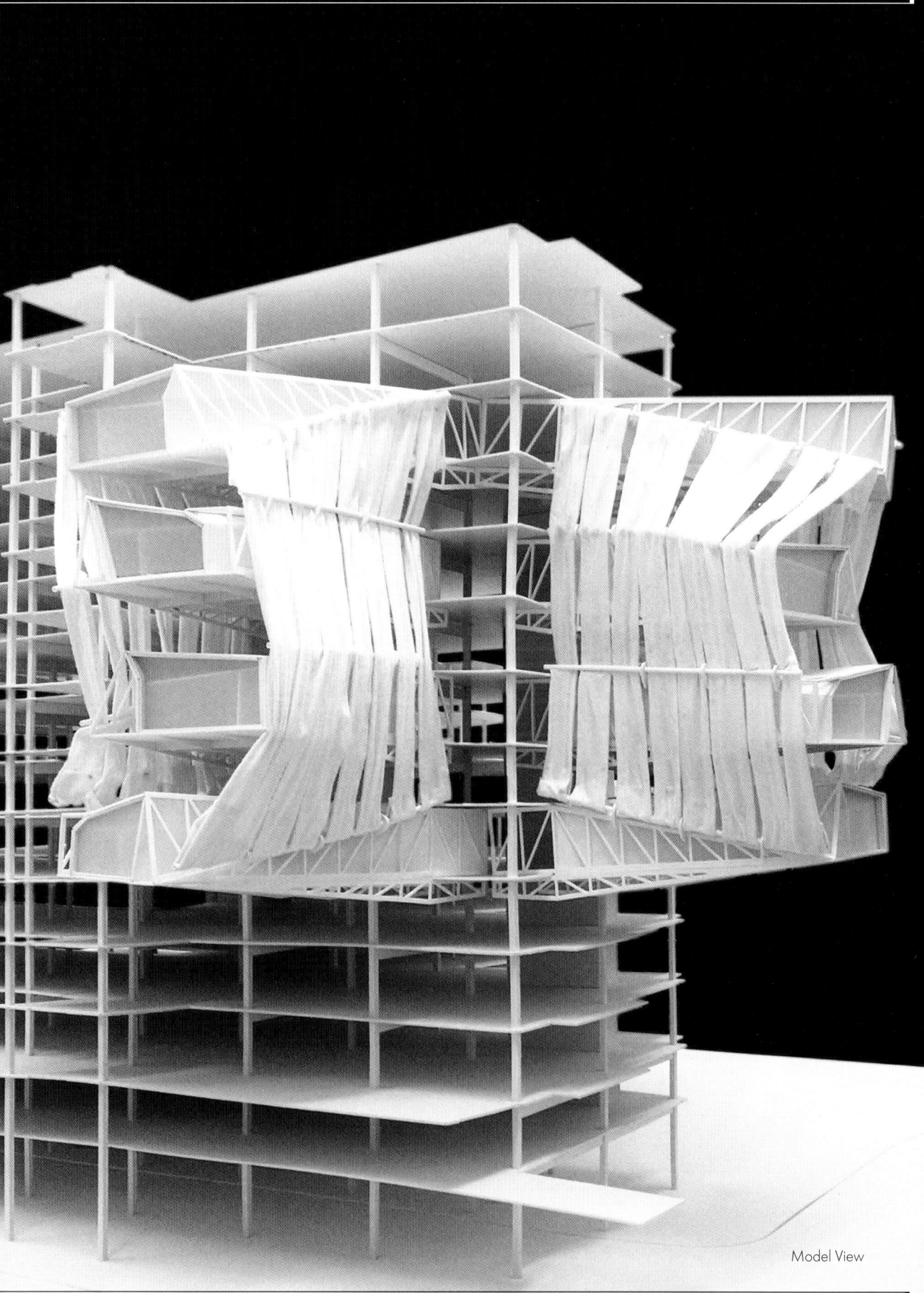
Model View

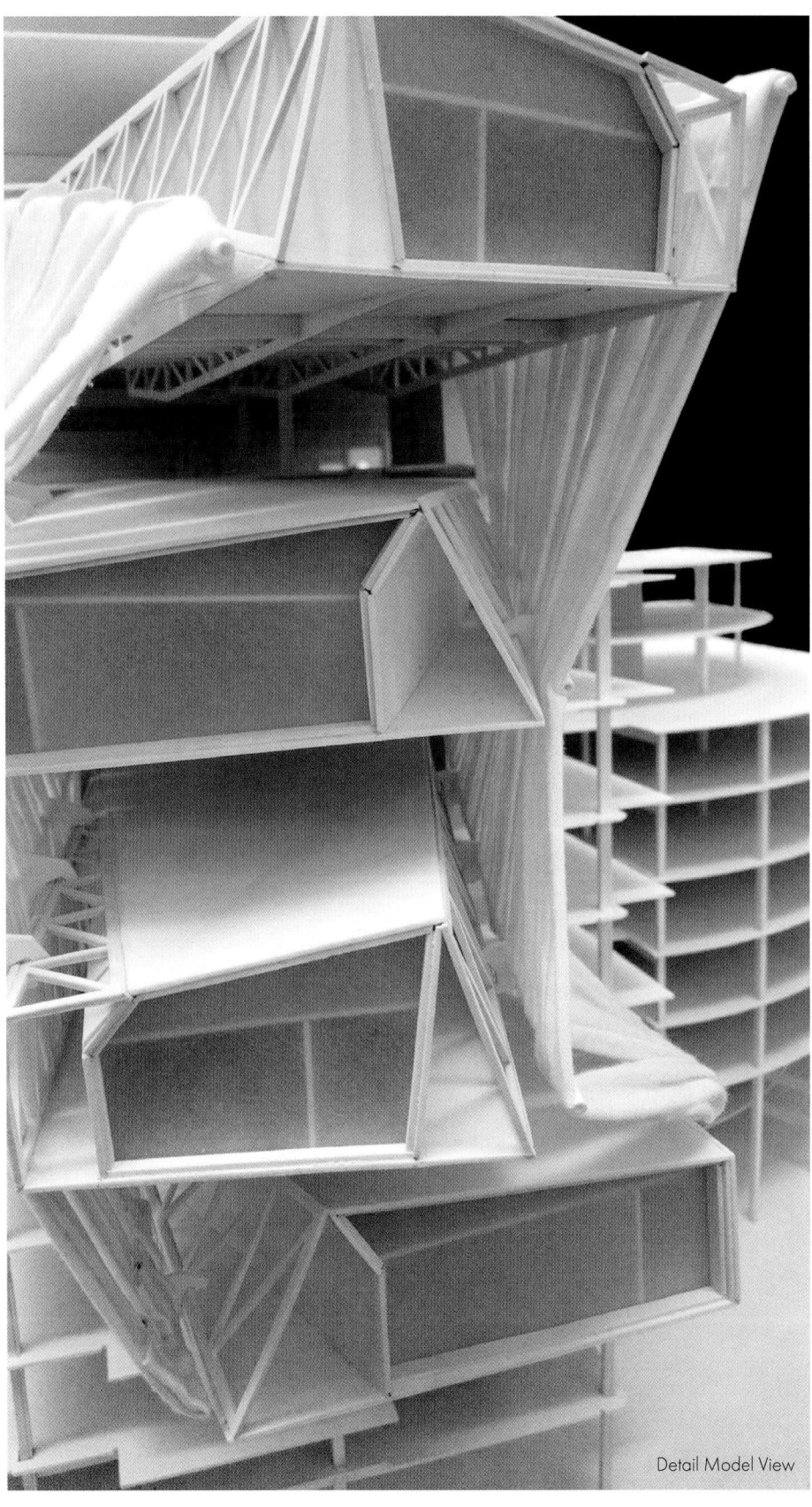
Detail Model View

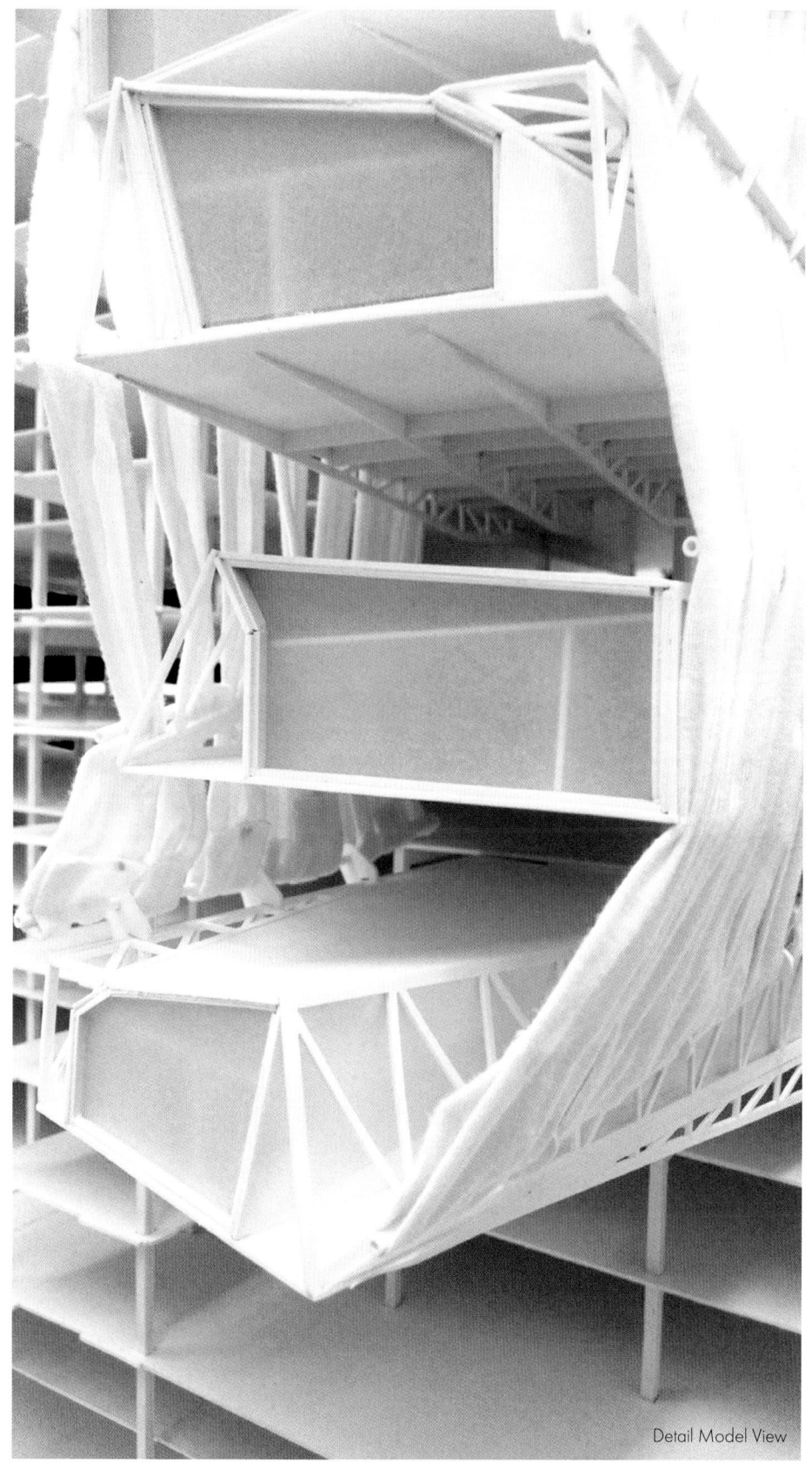
Detail Model View

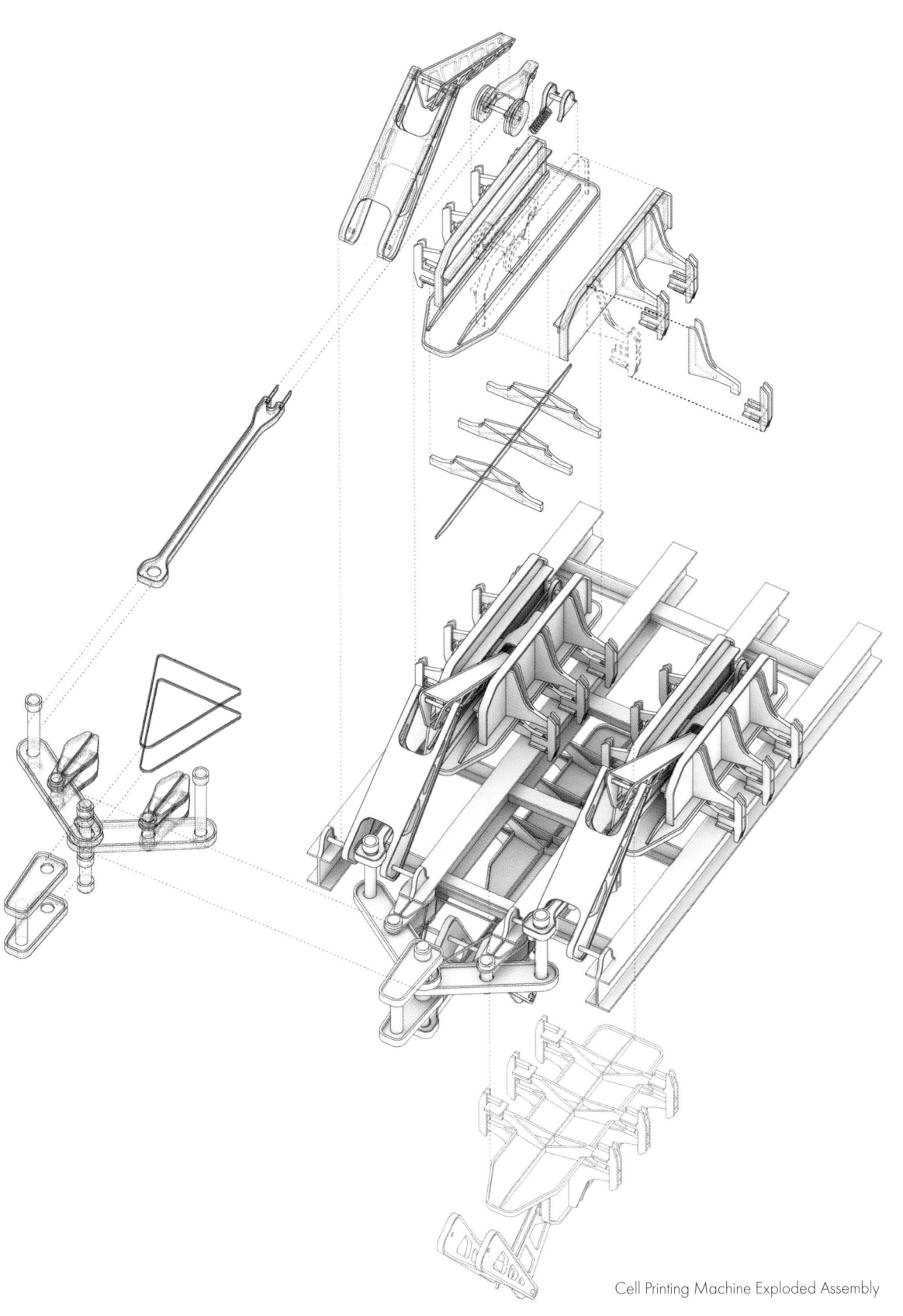

Cell Printing Machine Exploded Assembly

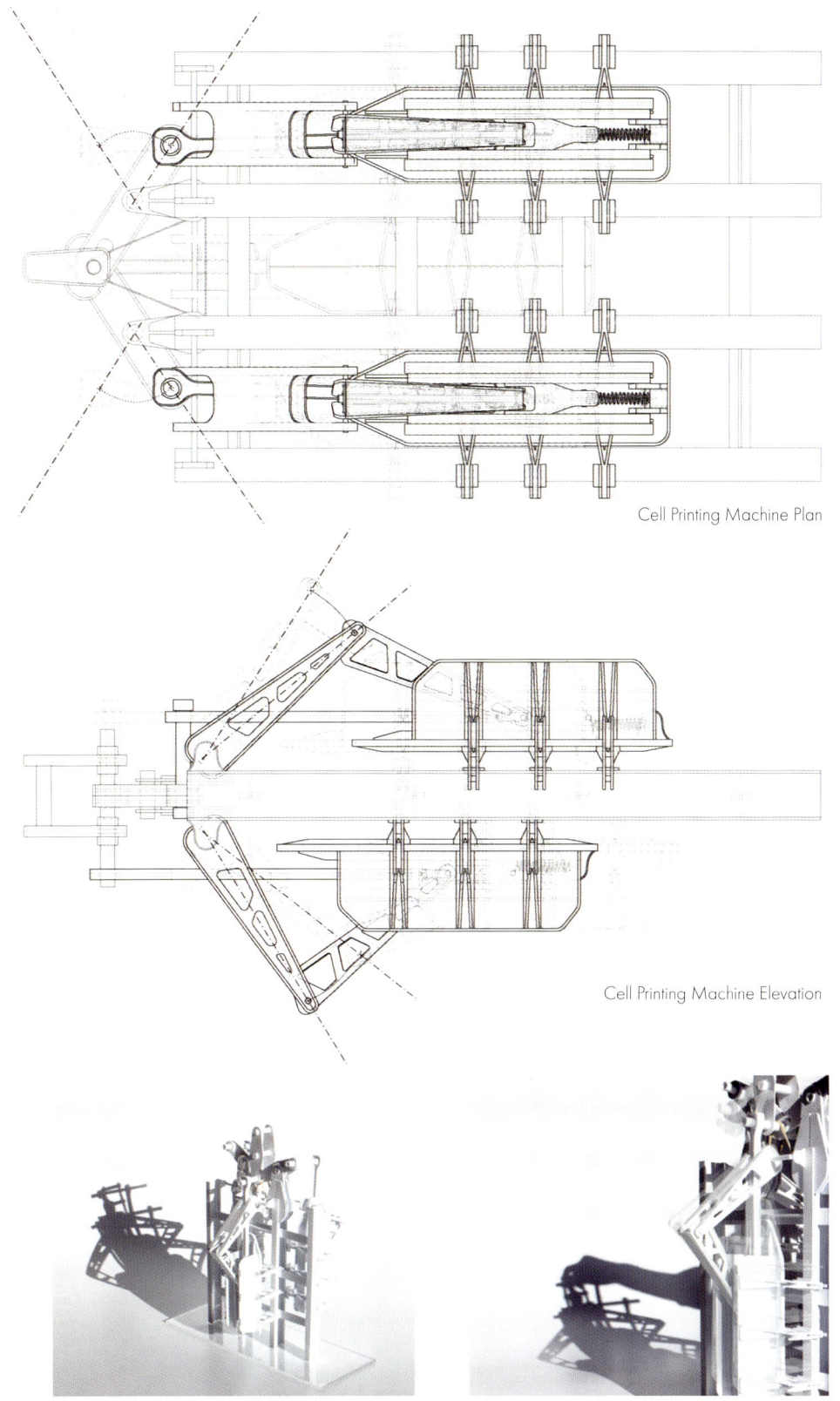

Cell Printing Machine Plan

Cell Printing Machine Elevation

Cell Printing Machine Model

Cell Printing Machine Detail Model

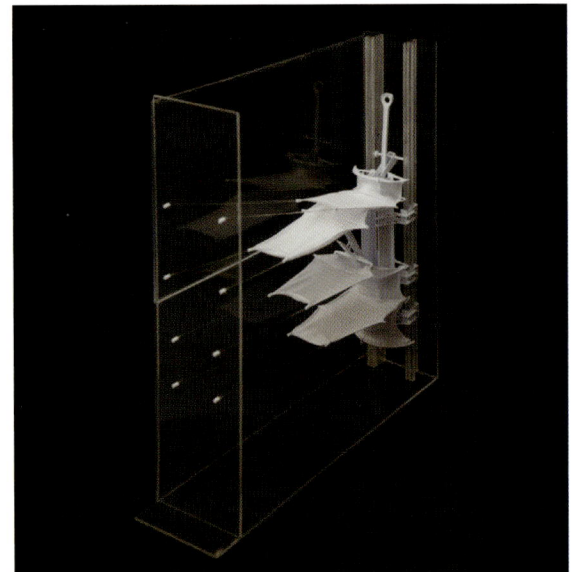

Skin Printing Machine Model

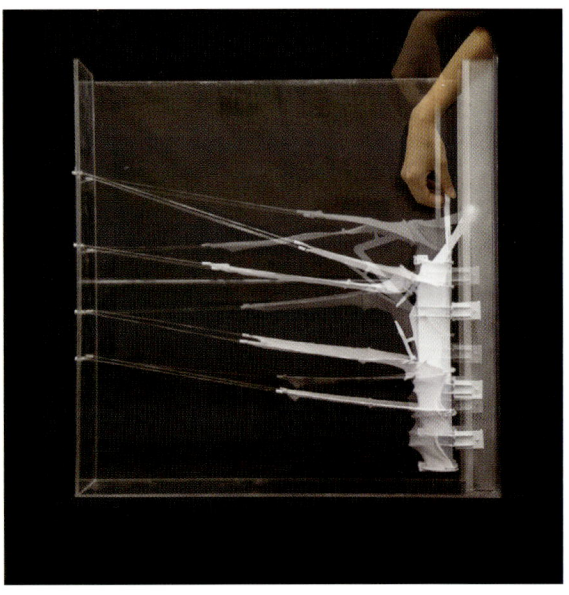

Skin Printing Machine Model (Active)

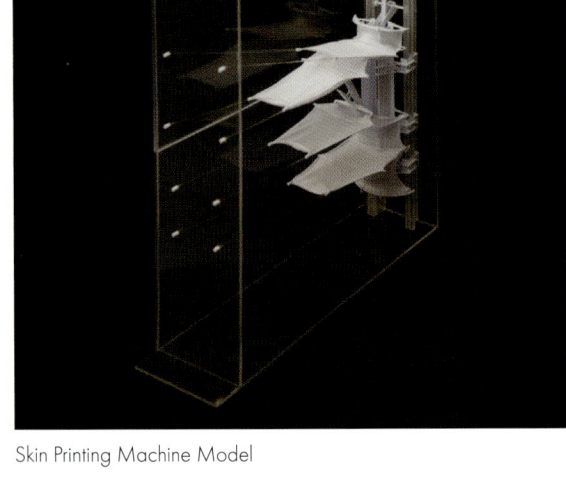

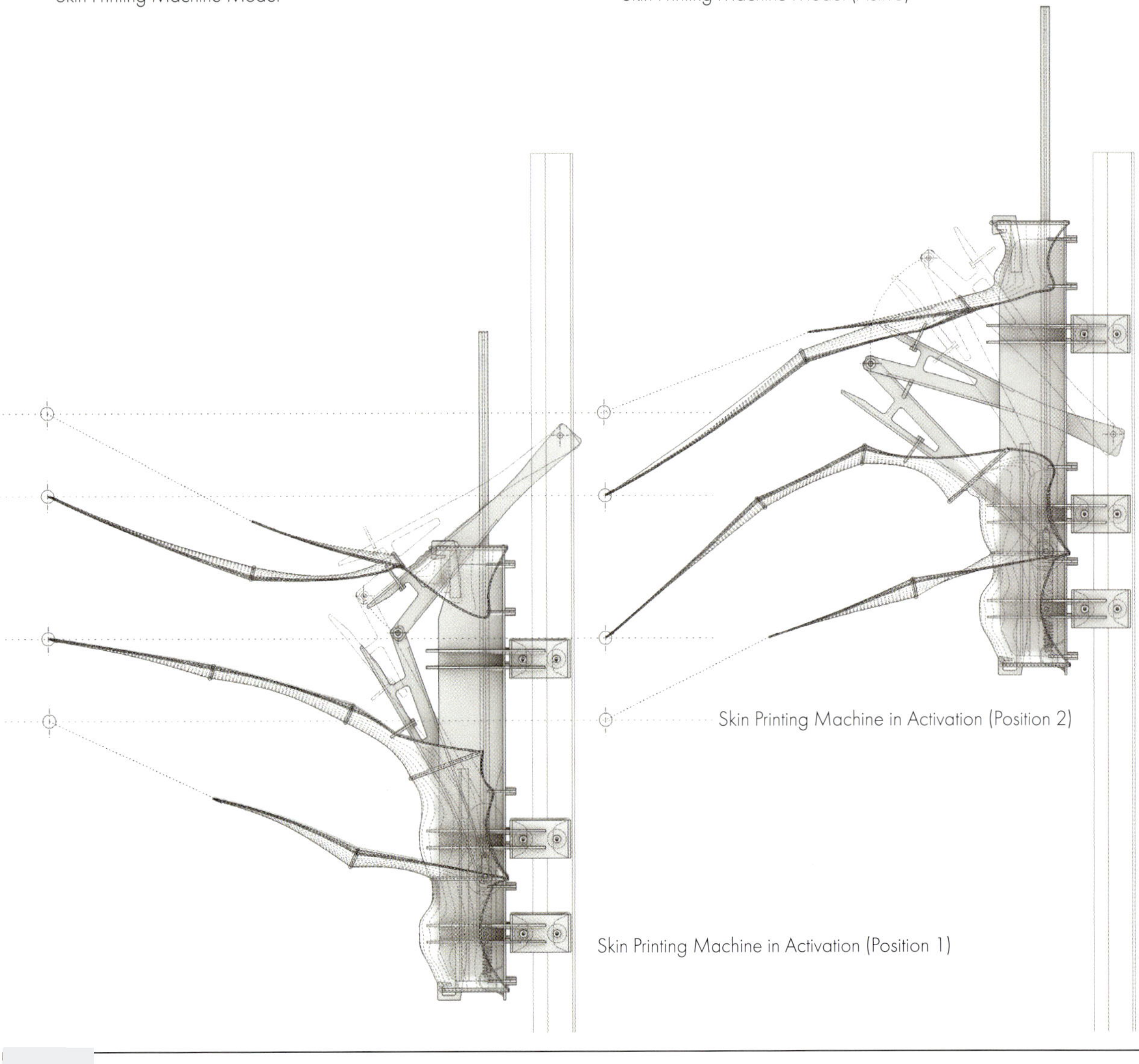

Skin Printing Machine in Activation (Position 2)

Skin Printing Machine in Activation (Position 1)

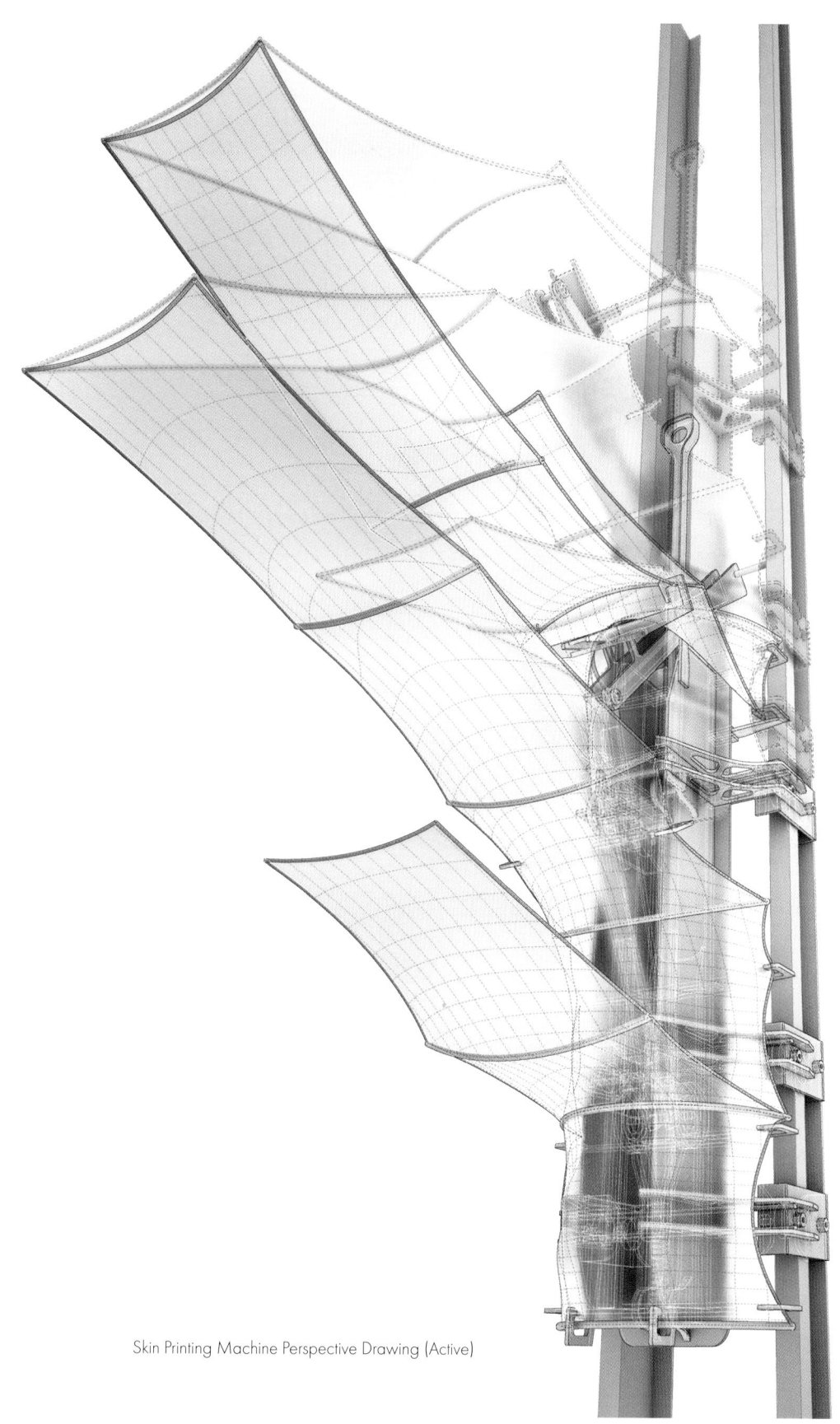

Skin Printing Machine Perspective Drawing (Active)

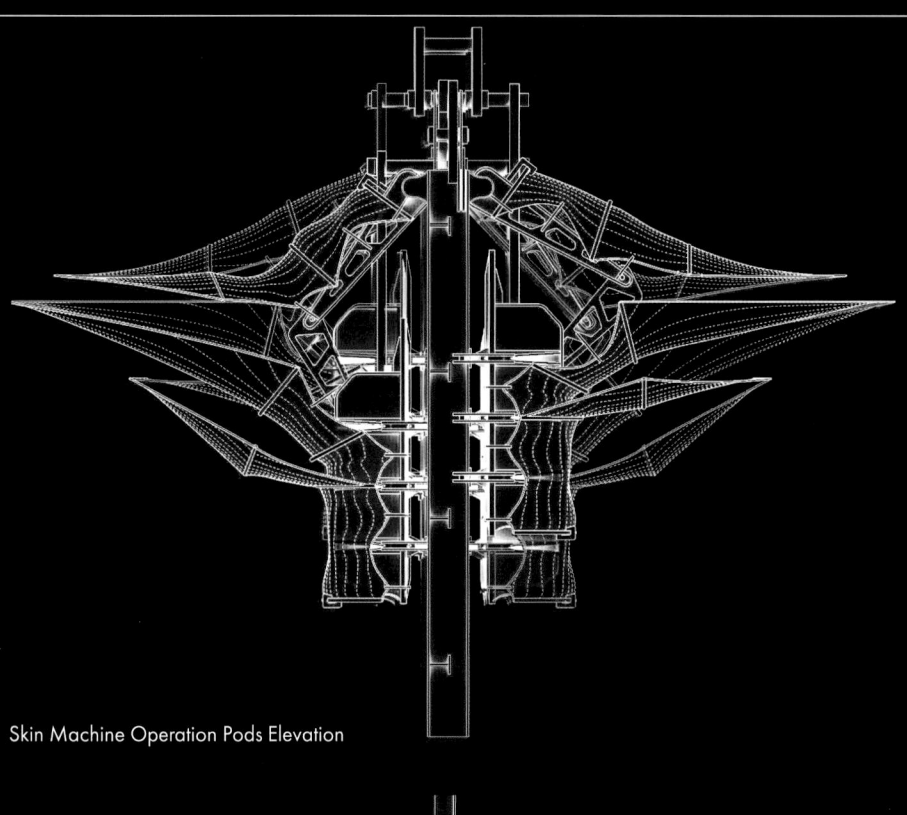

Skin Machine Operation Pods Elevation

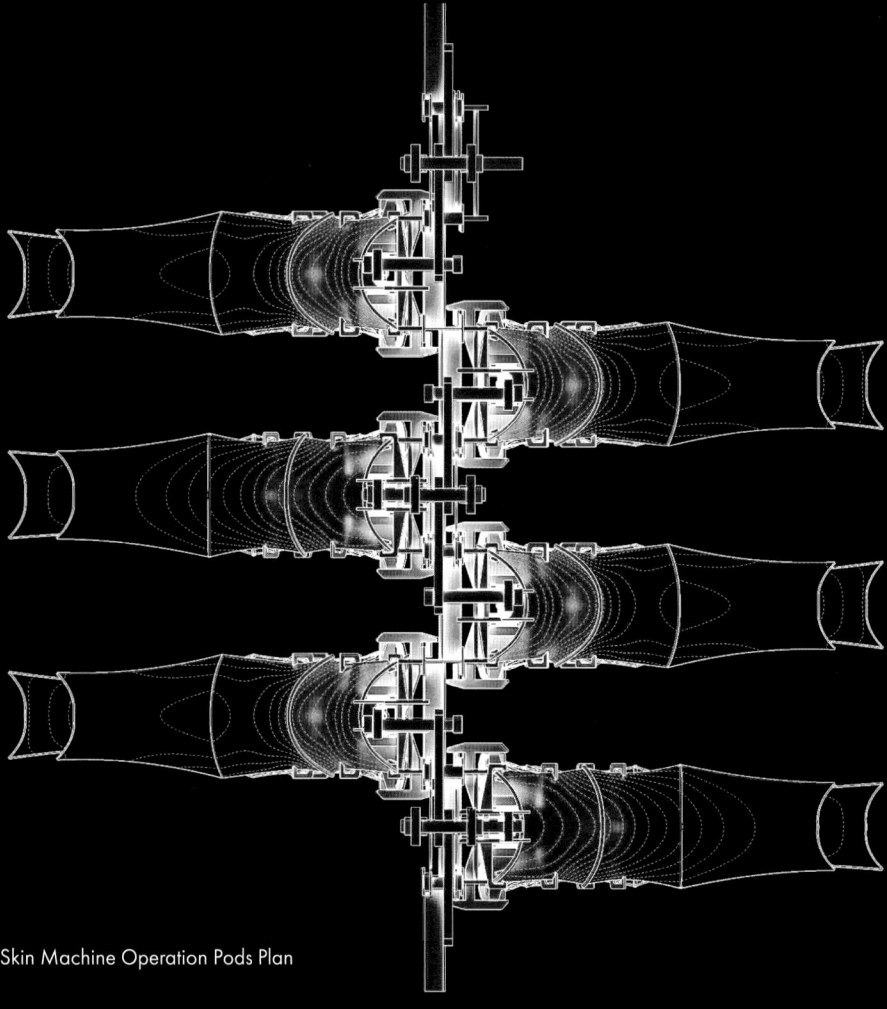

Skin Machine Operation Pods Plan

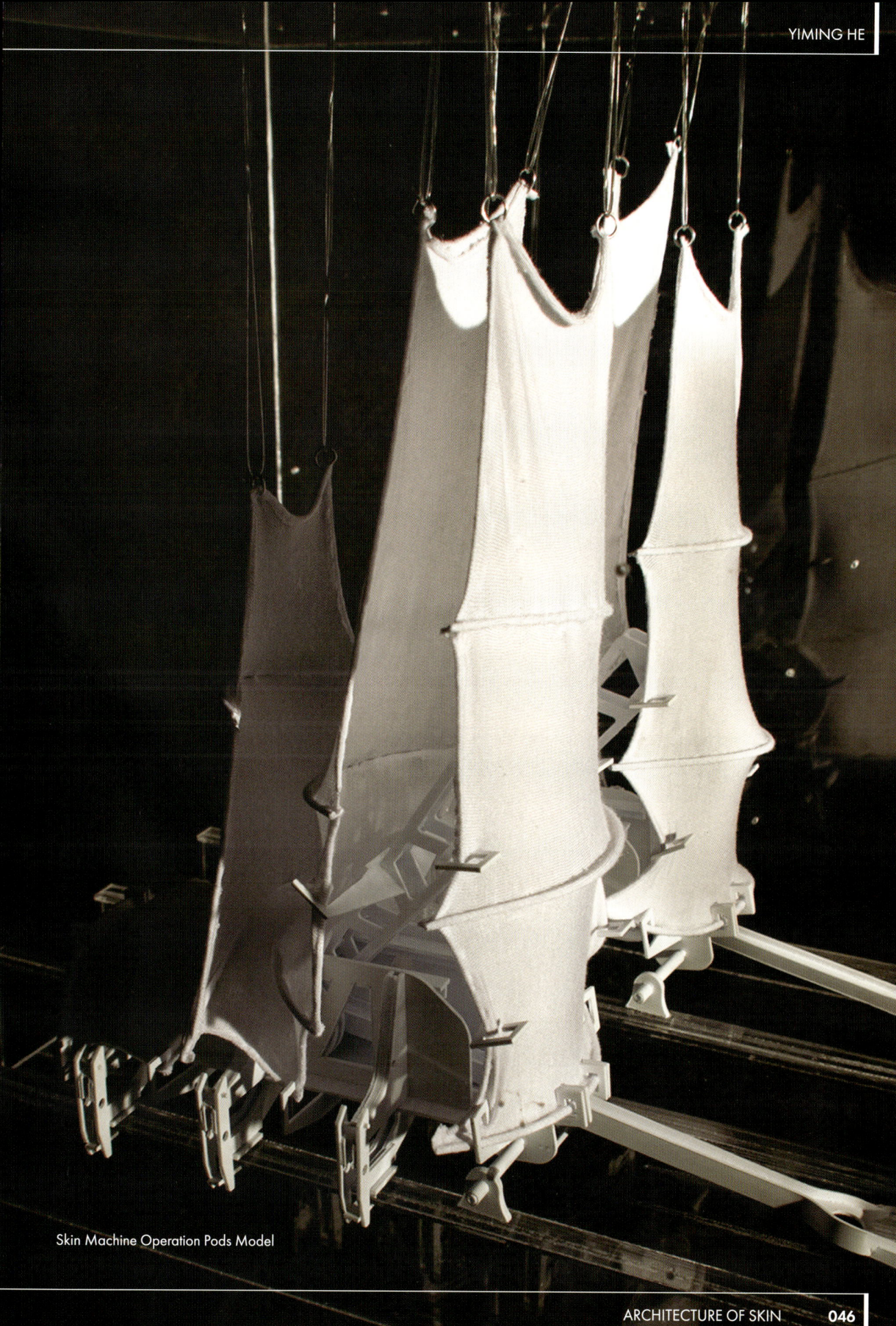
Skin Machine Operation Pods Model

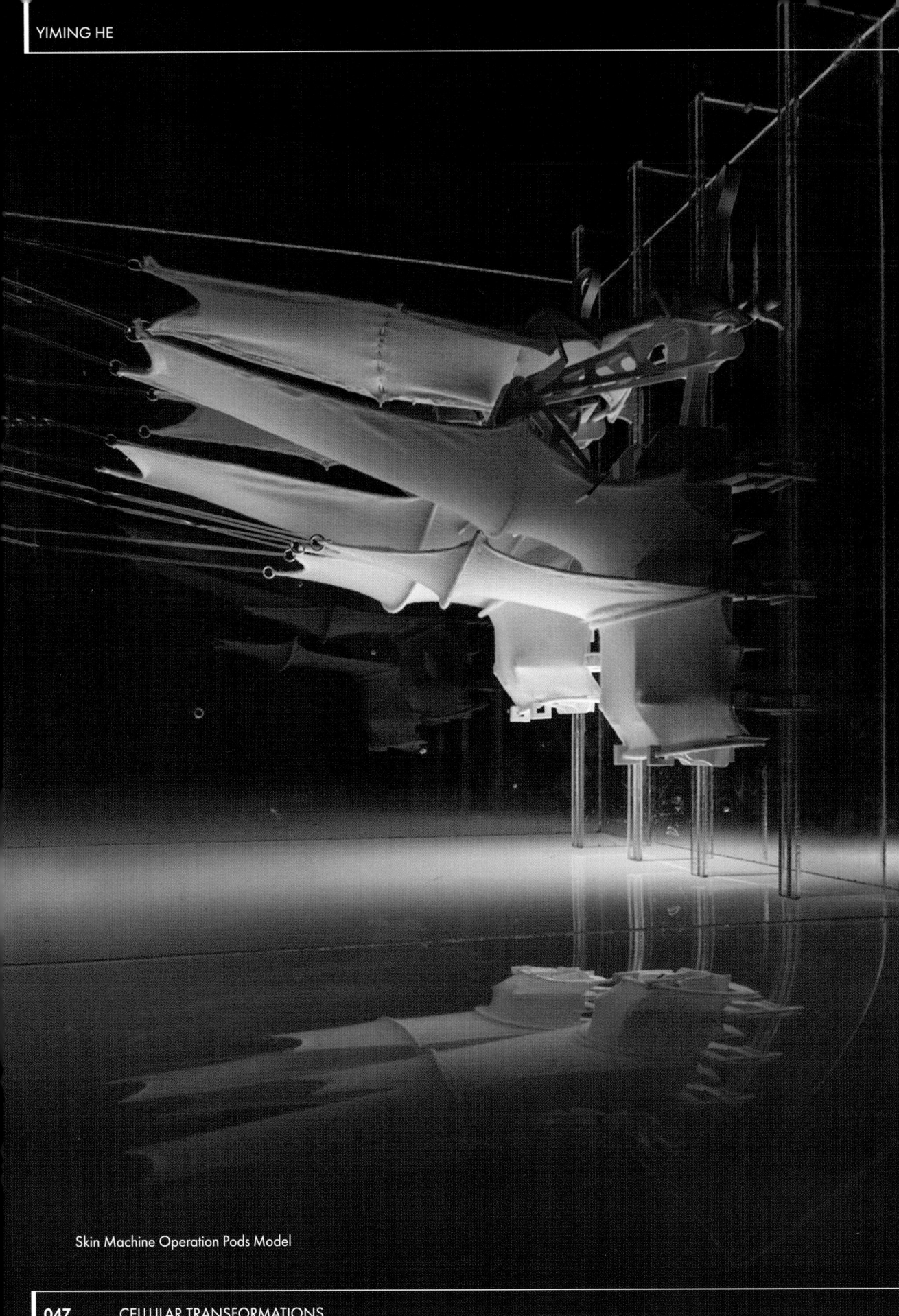

Skin Machine Operation Pods Model

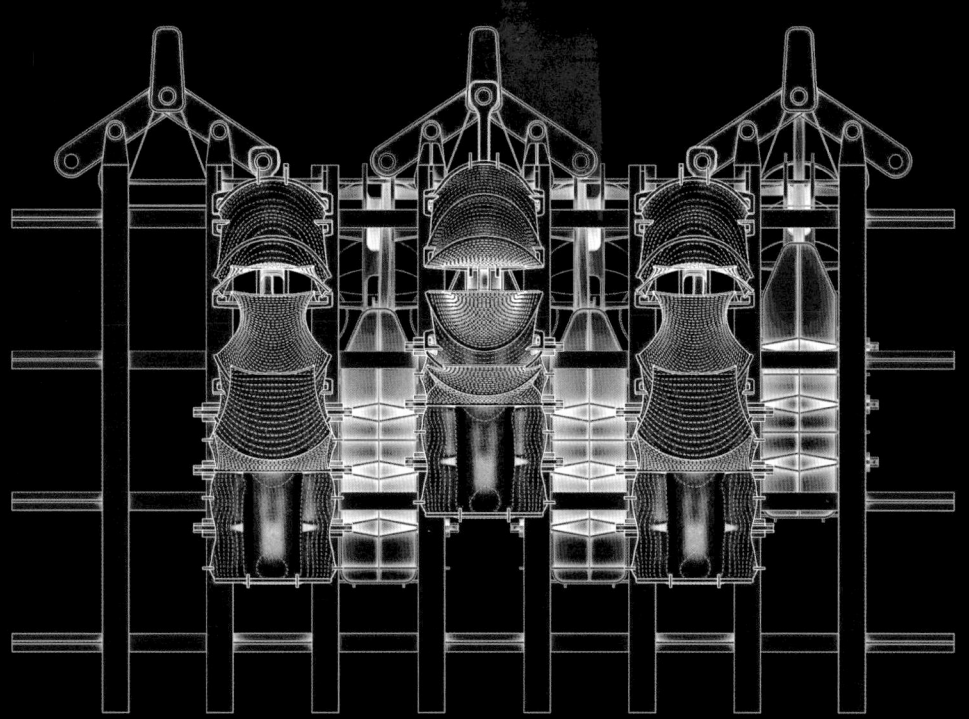

Skin Printed Operation Pod Units Plan

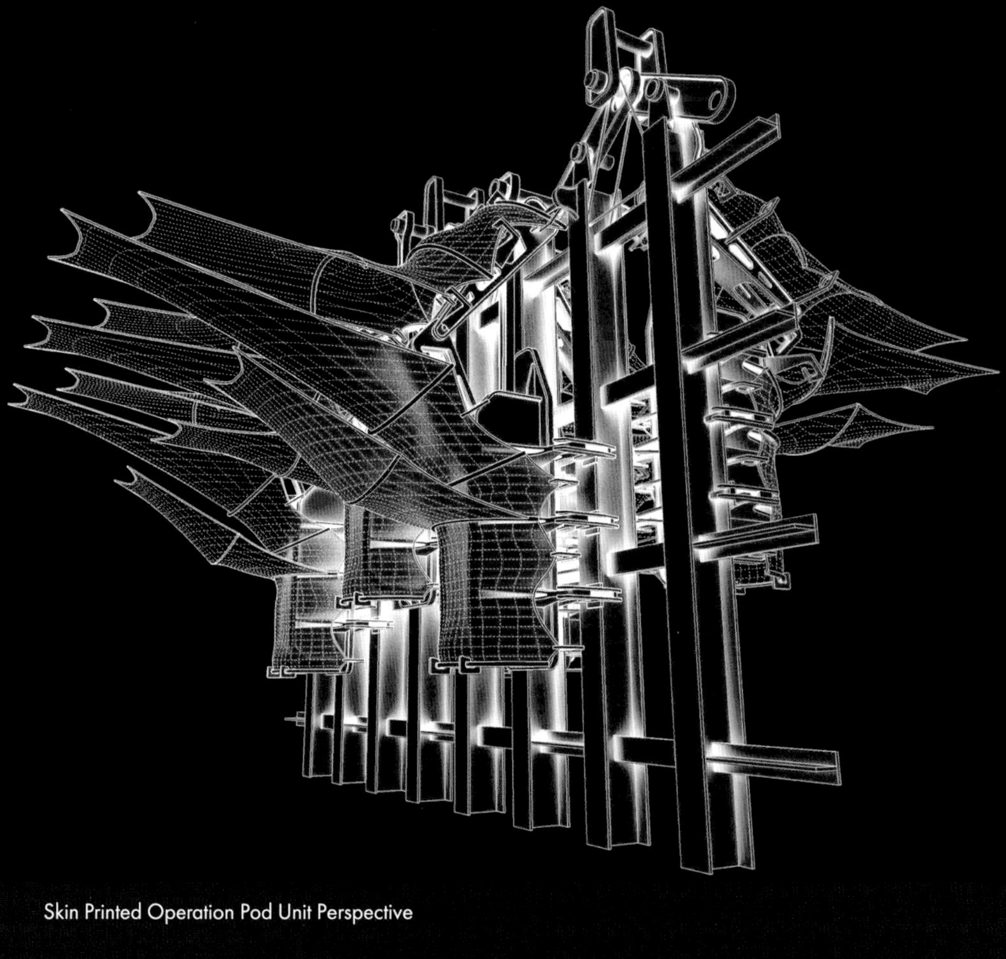

Skin Printed Operation Pod Unit Perspective

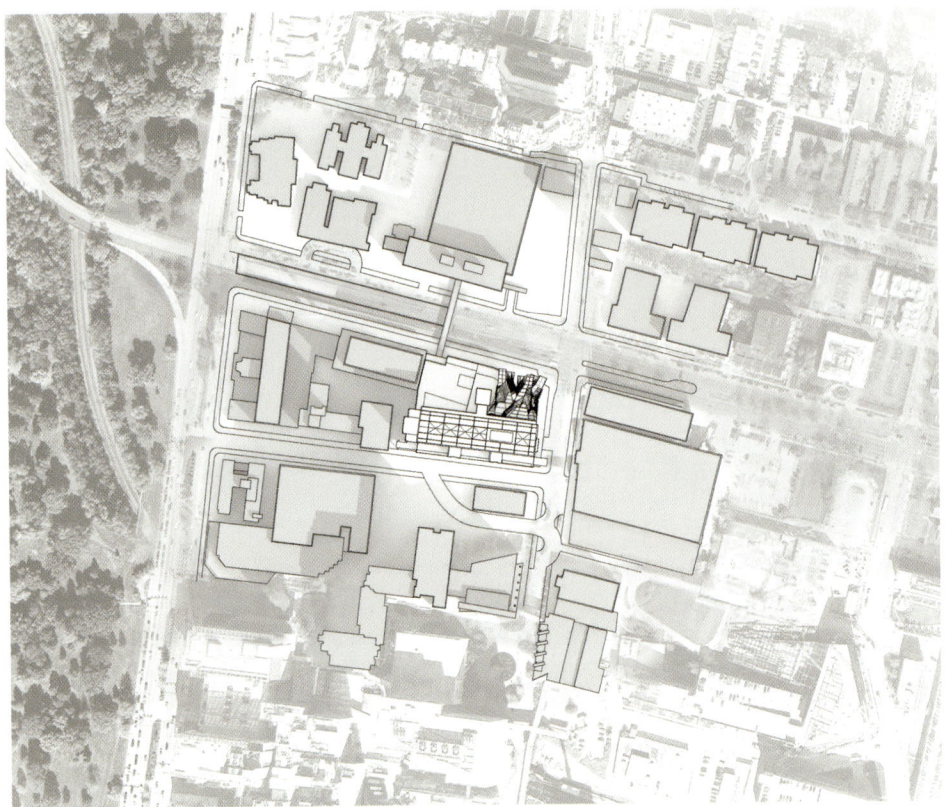
Site Plan

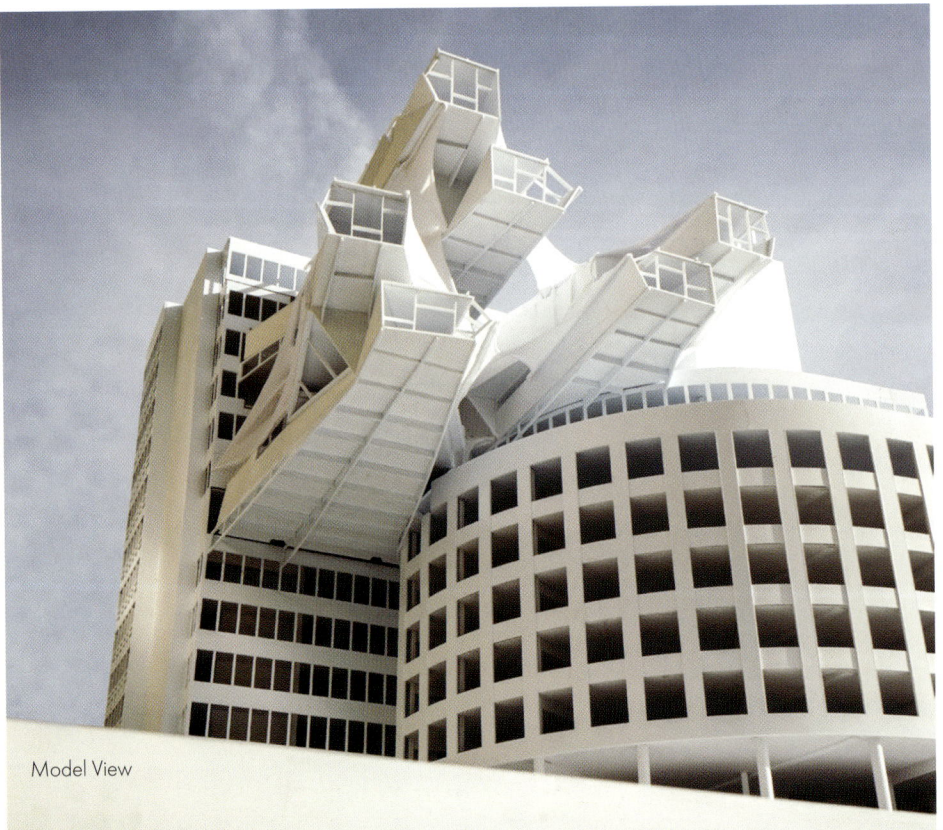
Model View

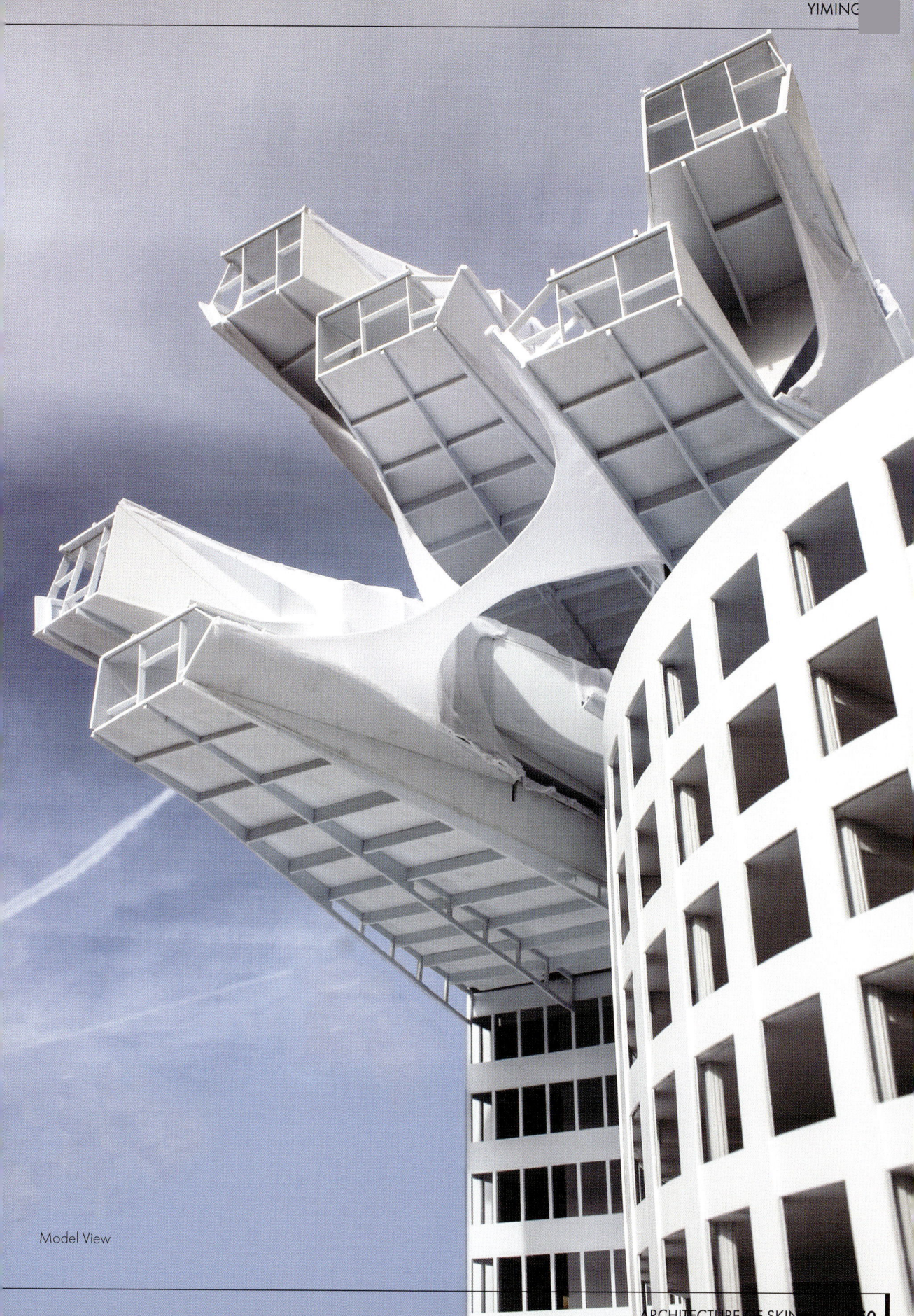

Model View

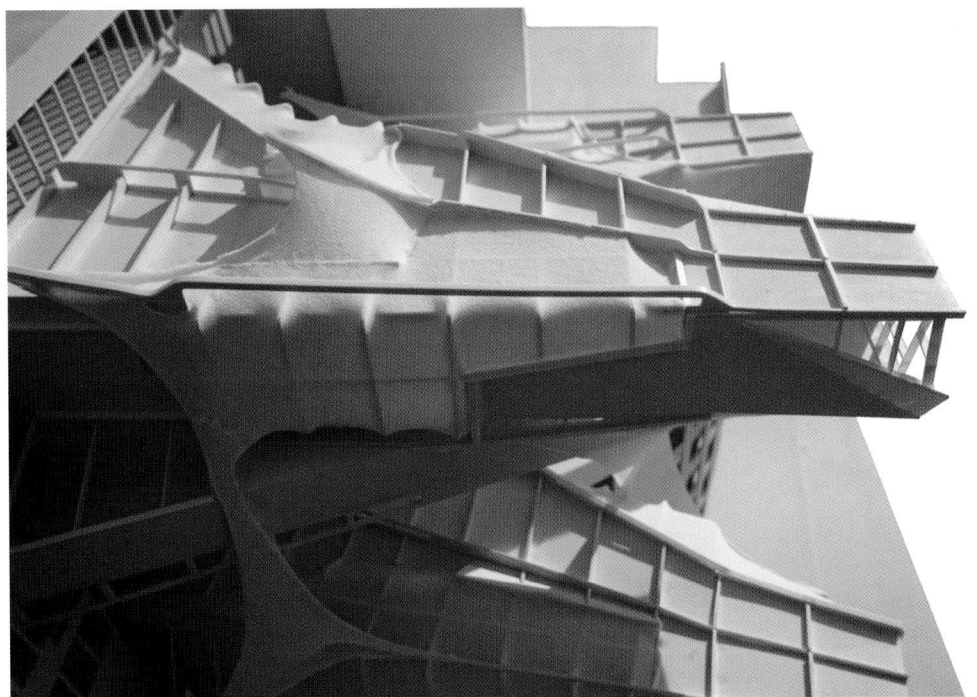
Model View

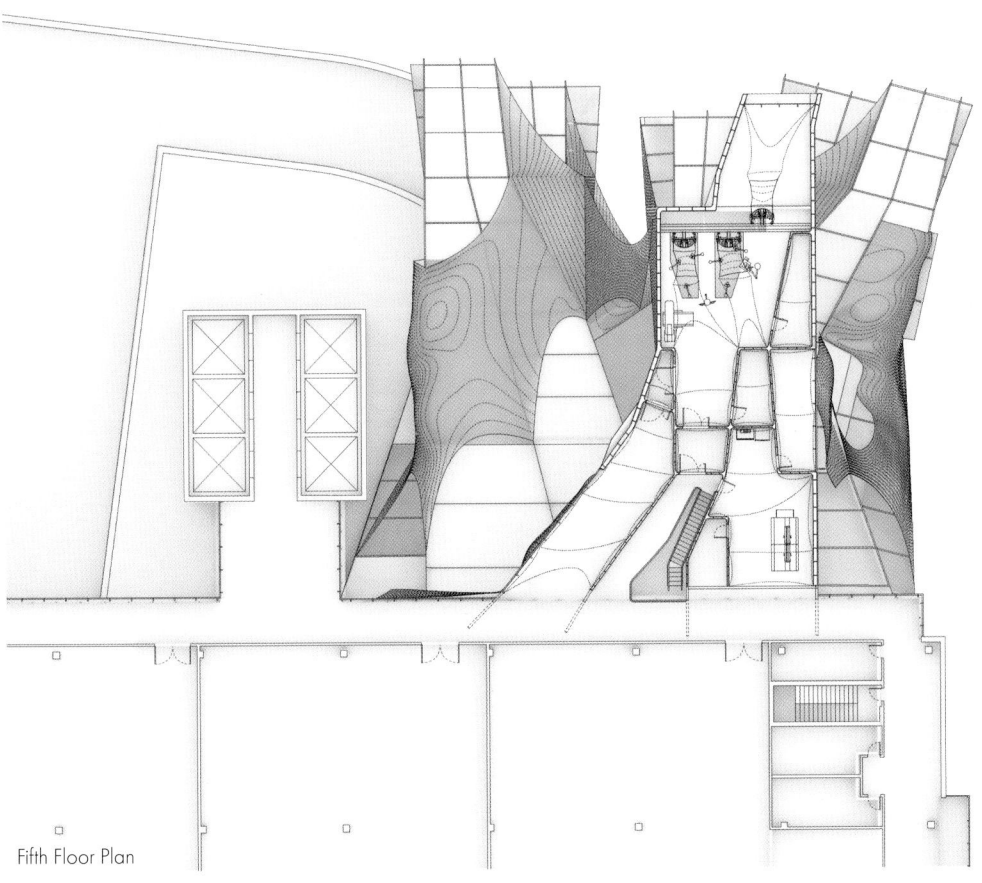
Fifth Floor Plan

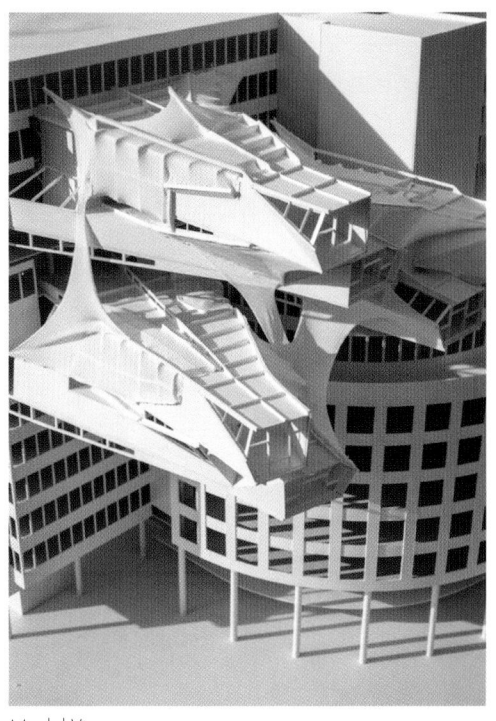
Model View

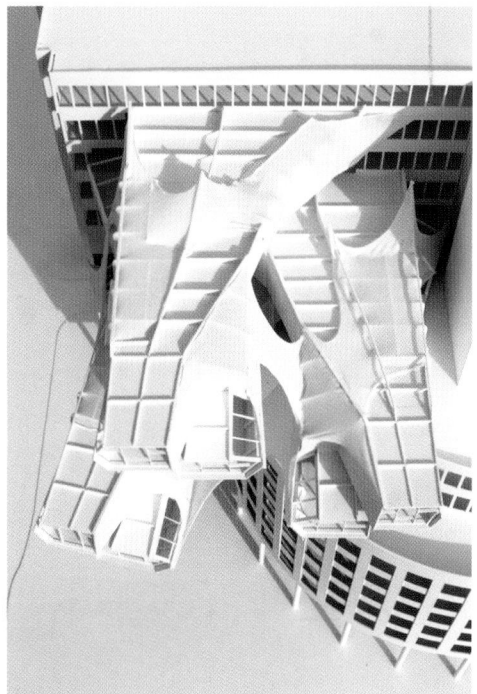
Model View

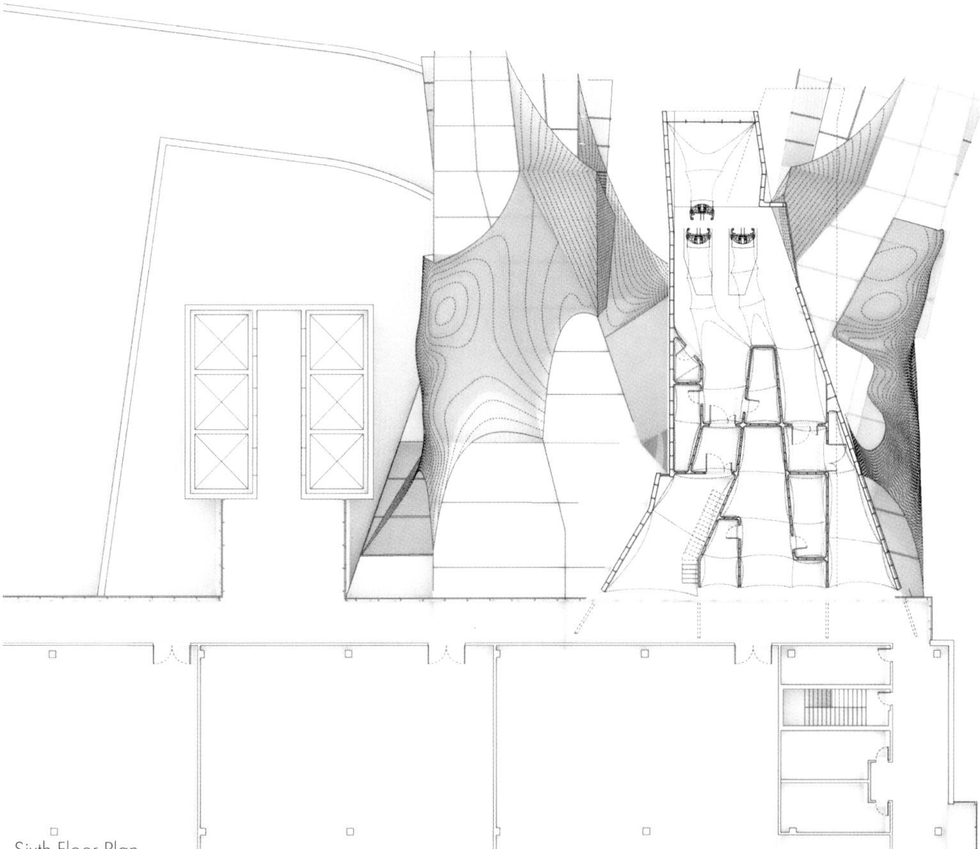

Sixth Floor Plan

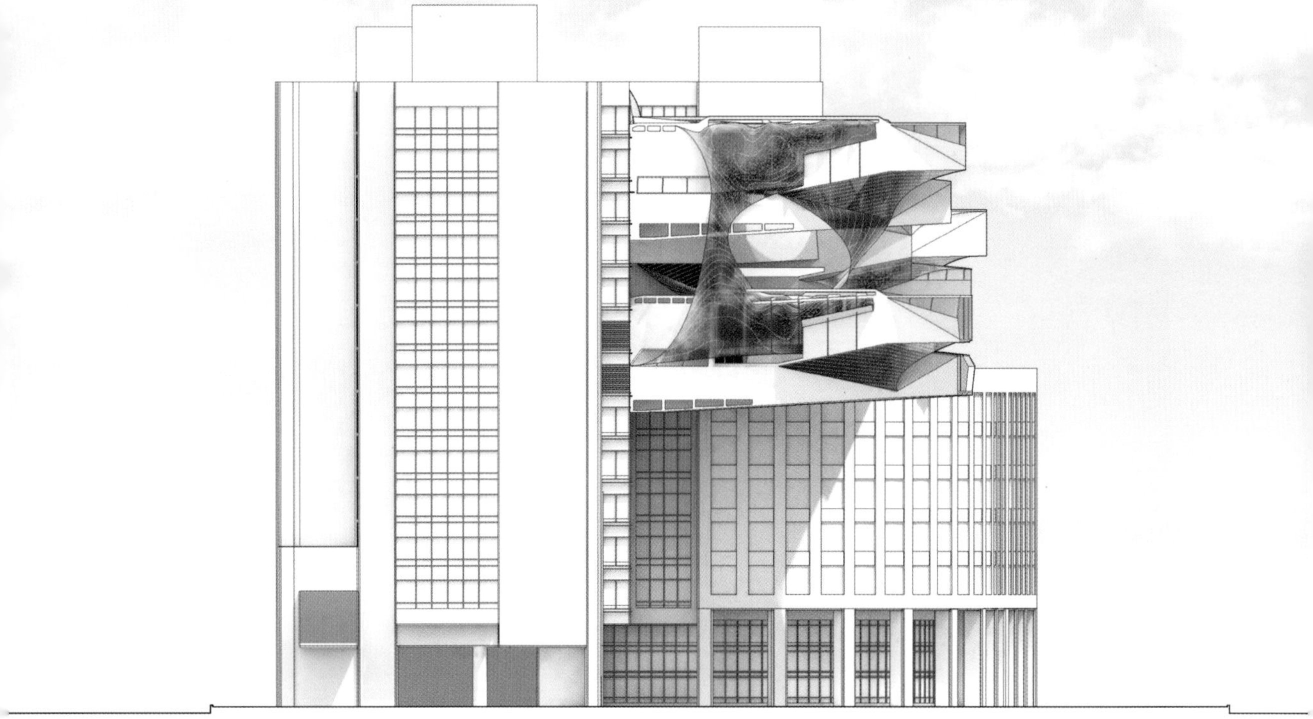

YIMING HE

Side Elevation

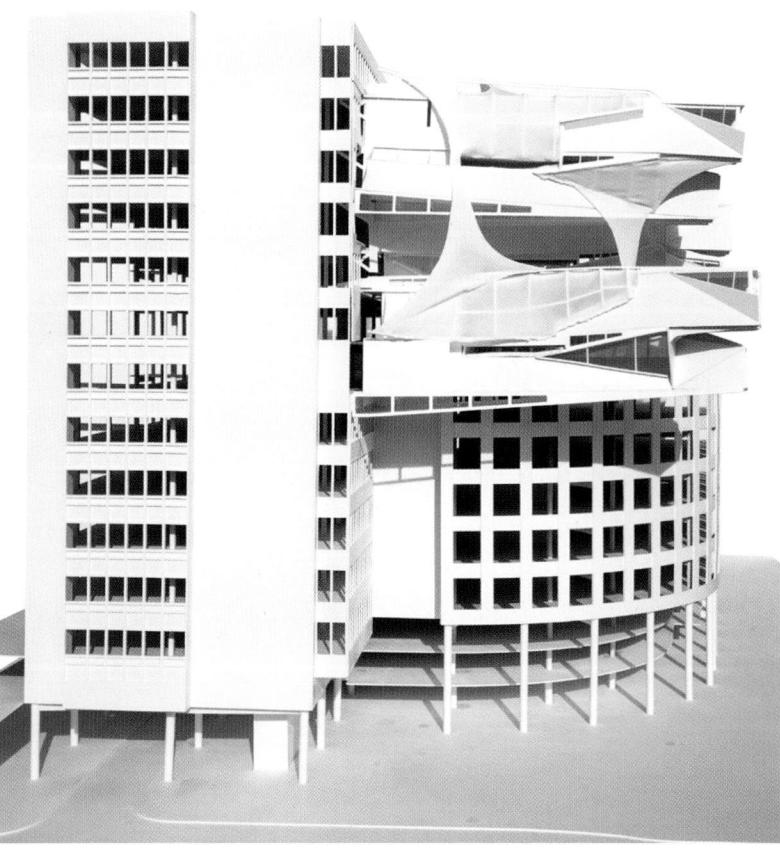

Model View

CELLULAR TRANSFORMATIONS

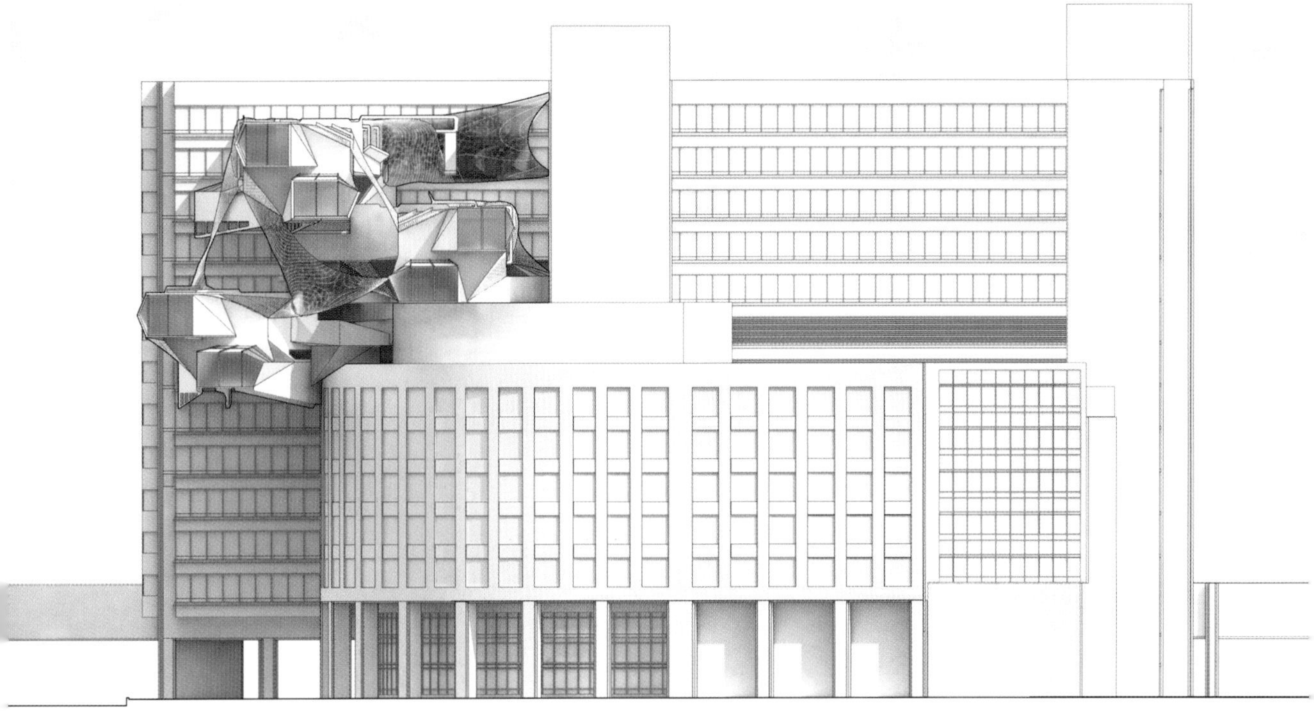

Front Elevation

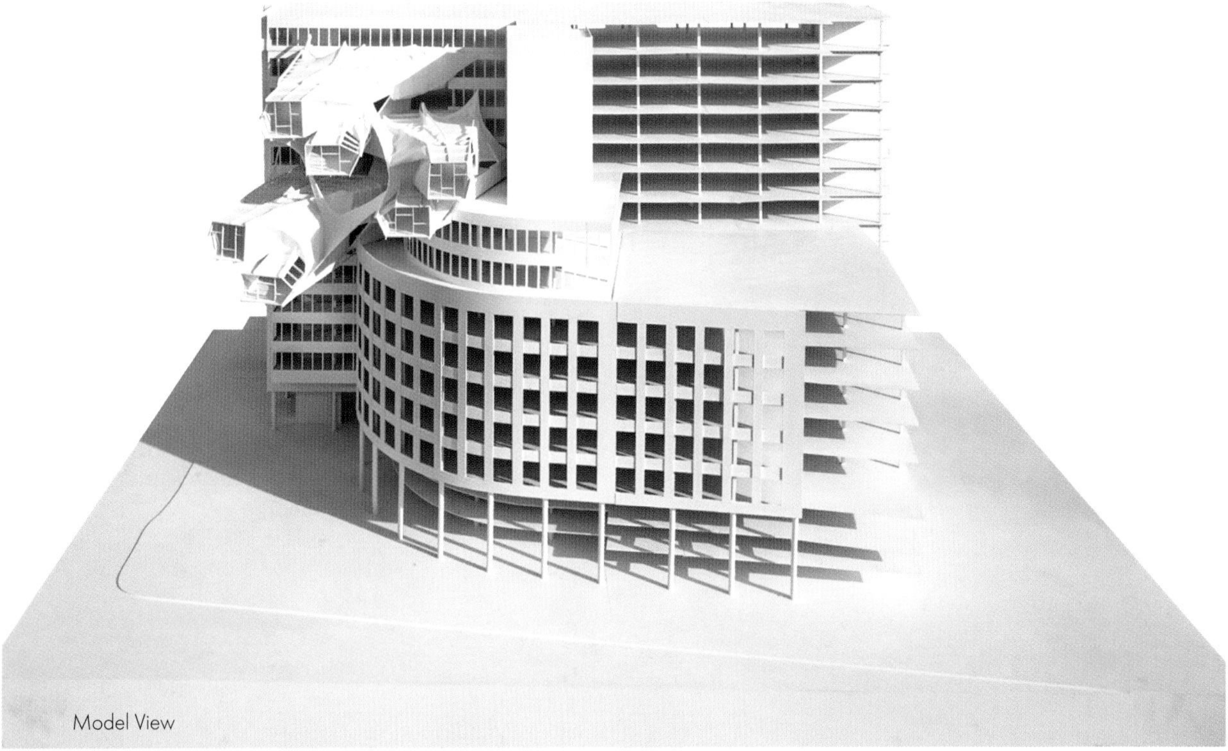

Model View

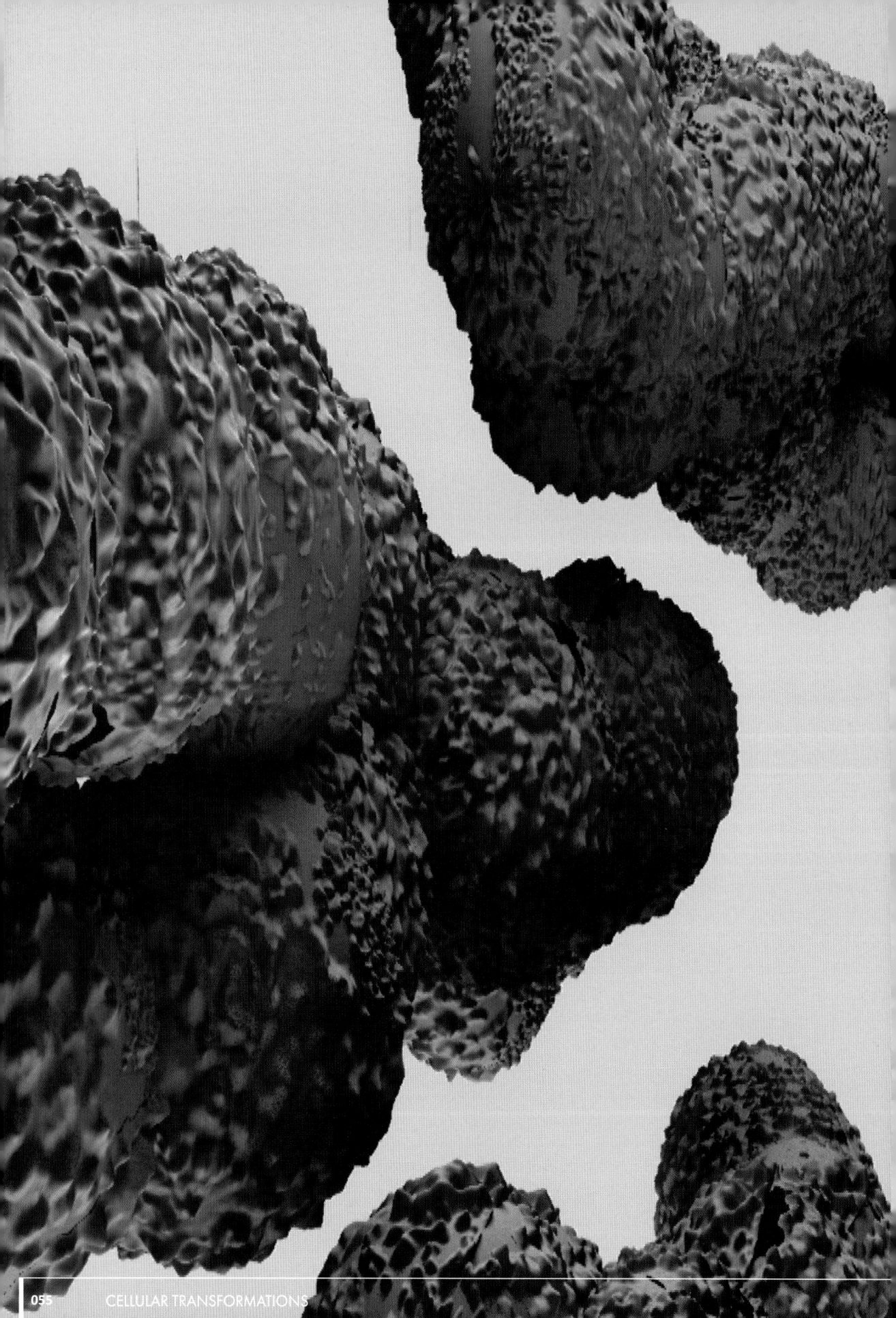

BEGINNINGS: 2011
MAPPING SOFT BODIES

Mapping Soft Bodies was the beginning of a collaborative course between architecture and biology to teach students to develop research projects based on visualization of cellular and sub-cellular structural systems. Student projects spanned multiple length scales, from molecular complexes to tissue architecture, and examined the principles underlying their assembly. These studies laid the groundwork for a design agenda that explored the dynamic and functional properties of cellular structures. The outcome for the course was detailed analytical drawings with digital models that emphasized the performative aspects of cellular structures through physical prototyping. The dynamics of the prototypes enables the cellular structures to be remodeled and repurposed into various design projects.

YT OH

ACTIN PROTEIN IN THE MUSCLE

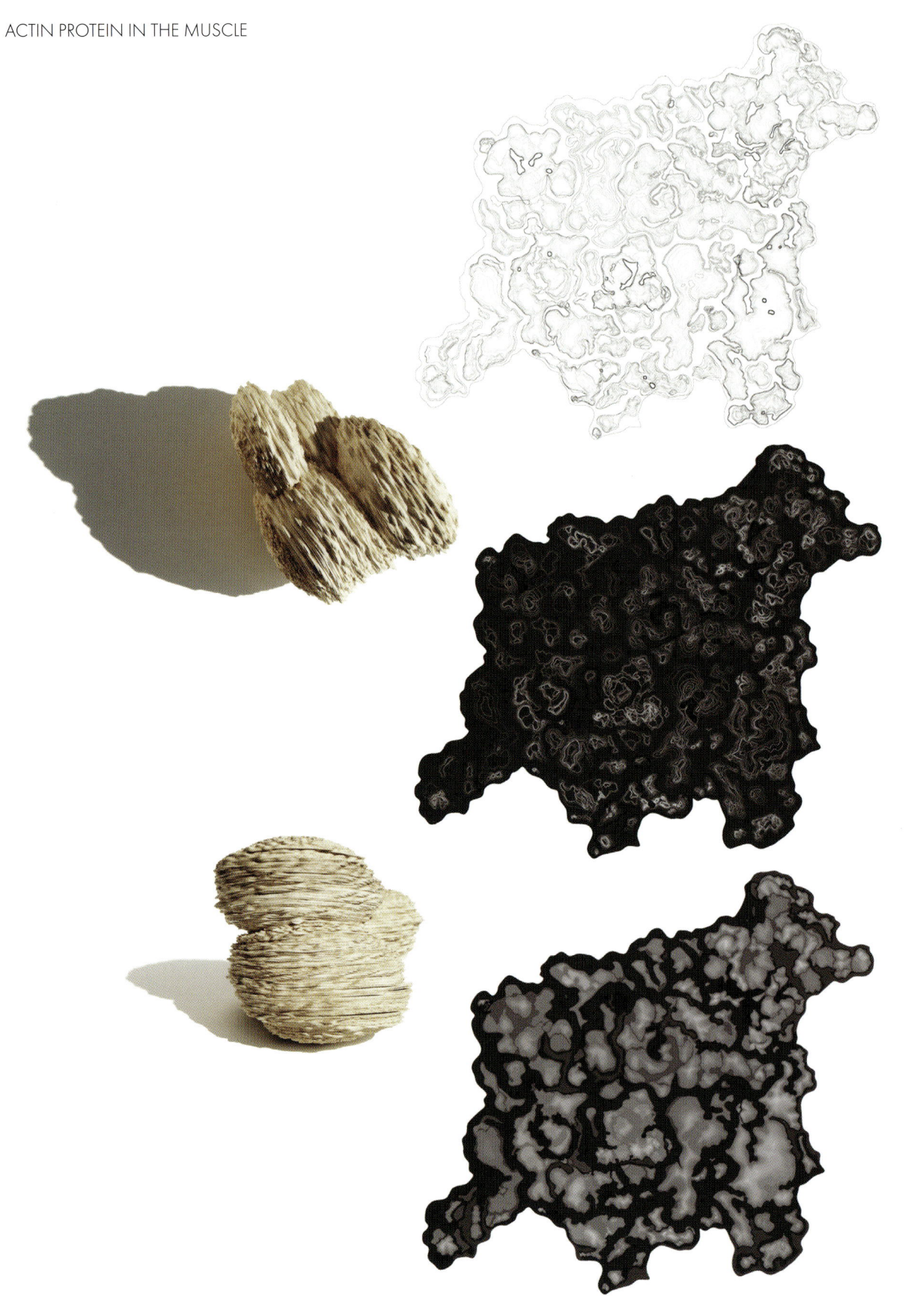

CELLULAR TRANSFORMATIONS

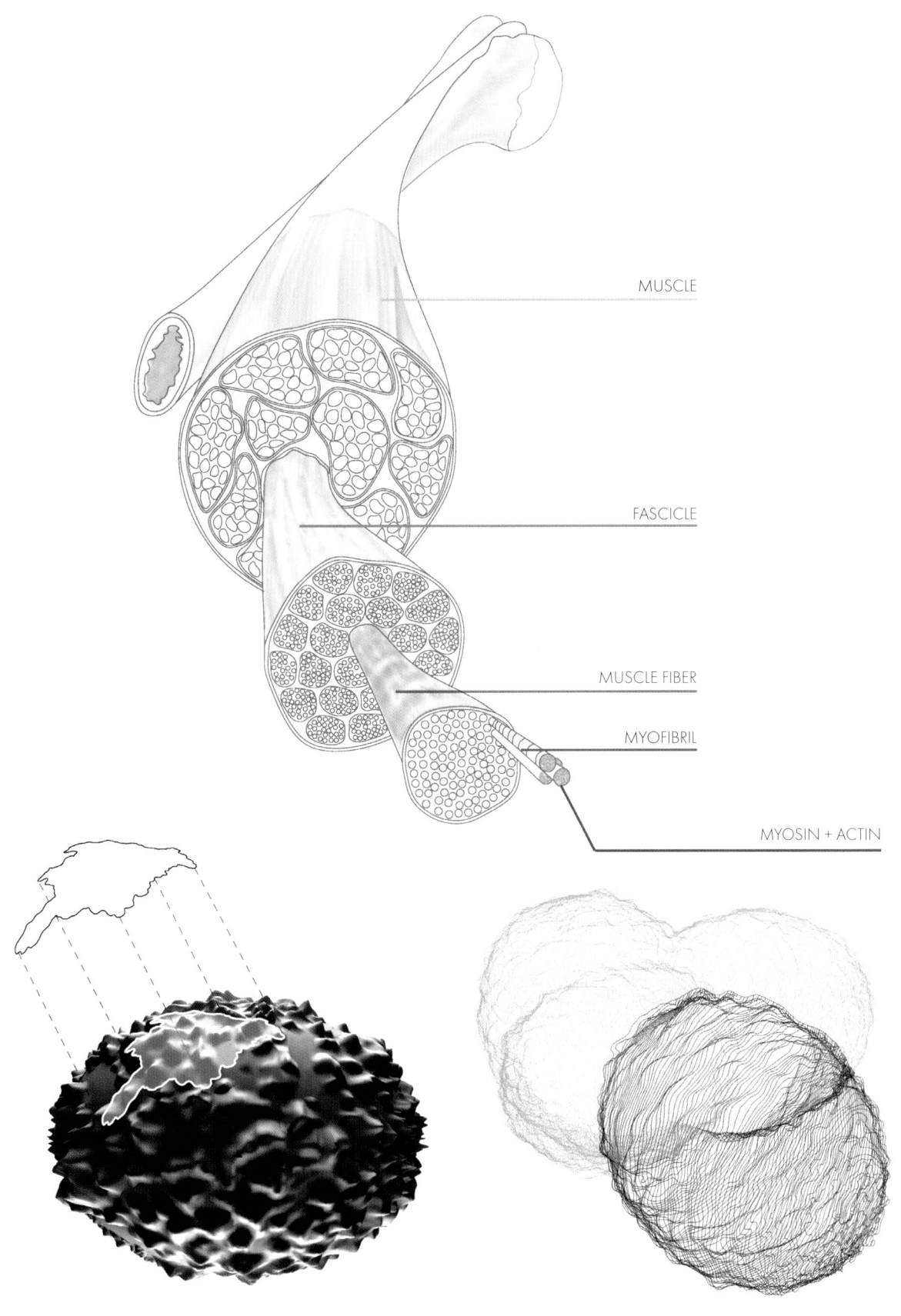

YT OH

ACTIN PROTEIN IN THE MUSCLE

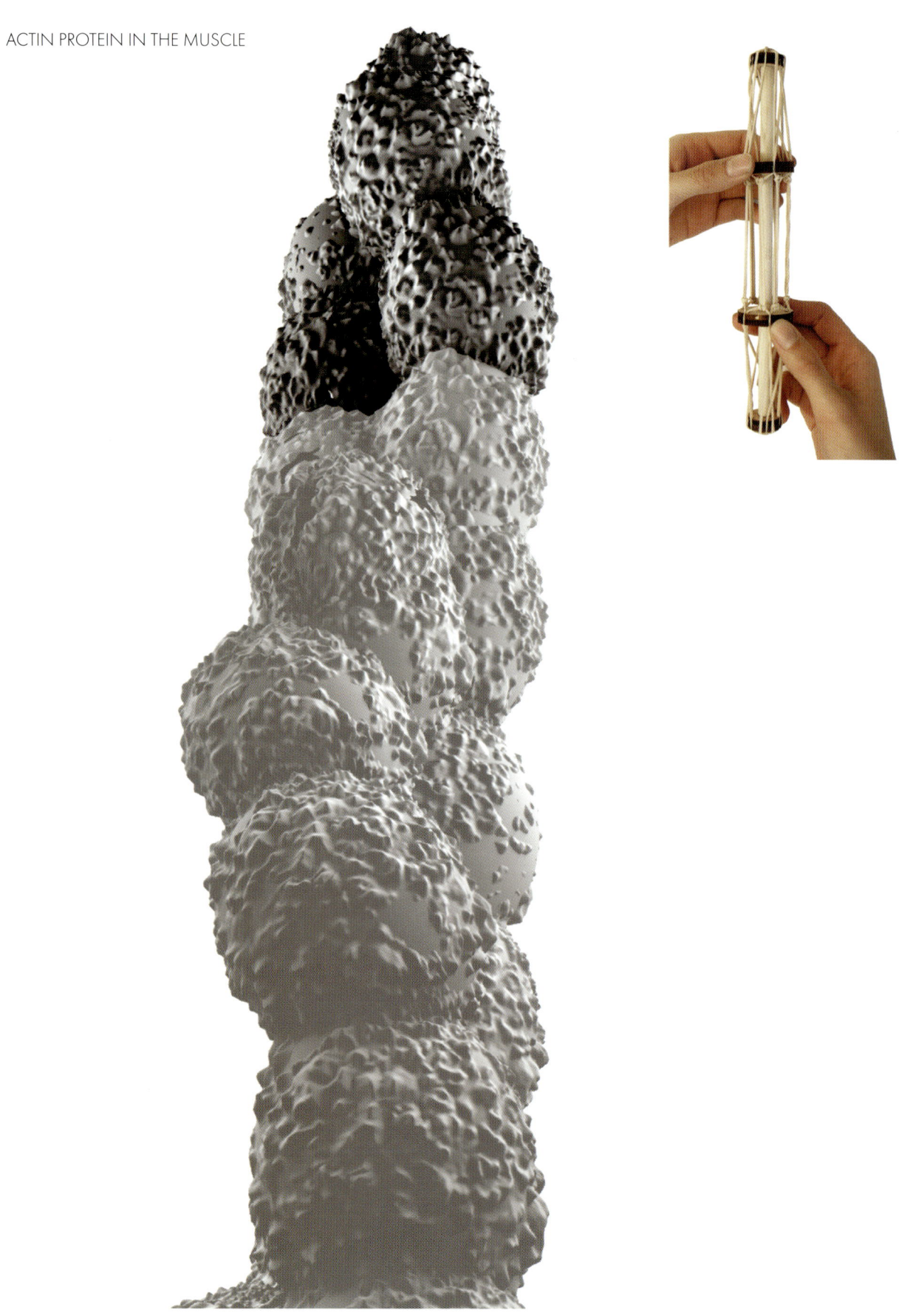

059 CELLULAR TRANSFORMATIONS

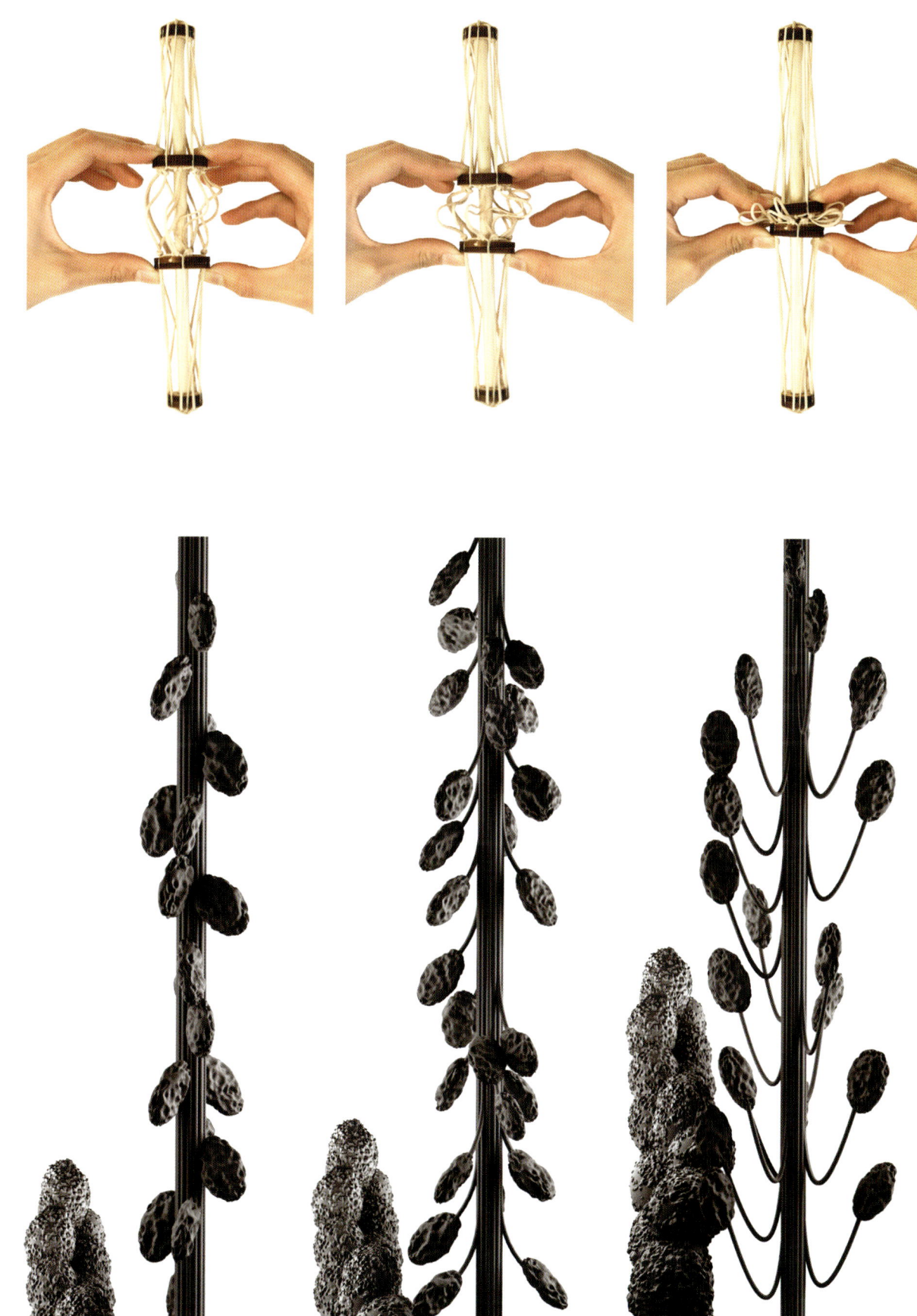

DAVID MATTHEW BOYNTON

NERVE CELLS

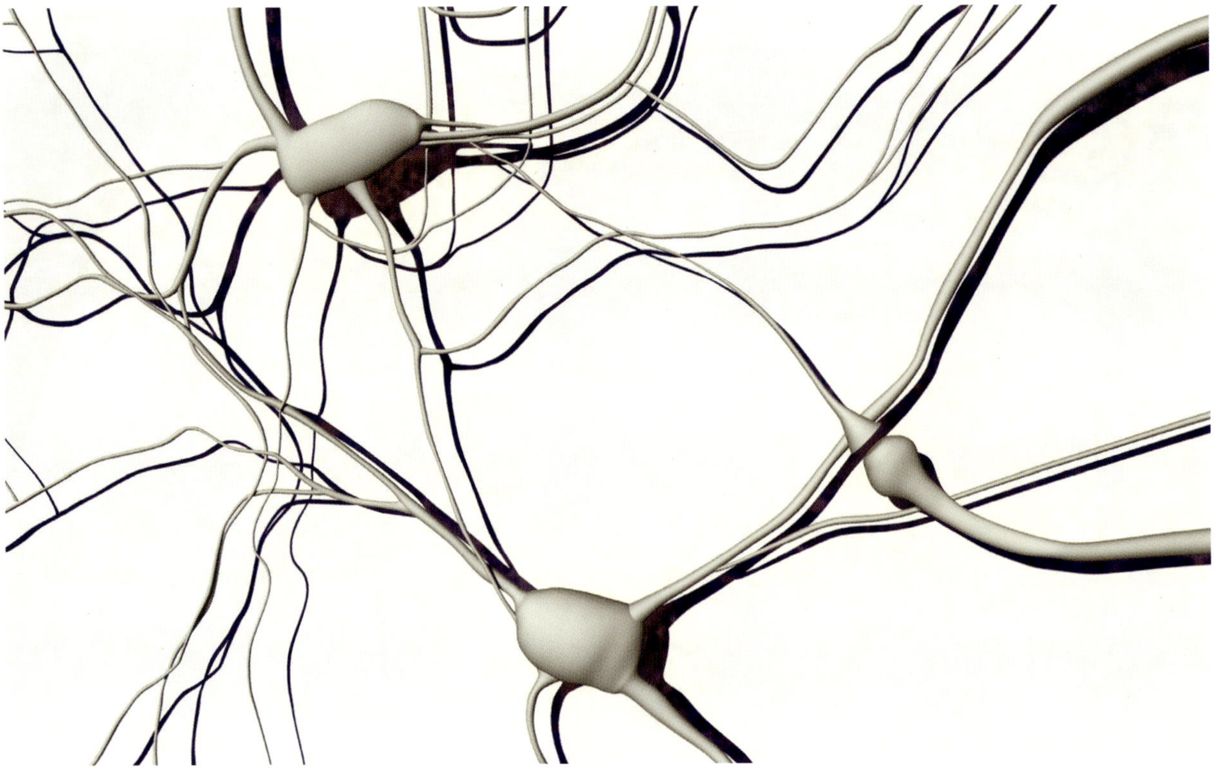

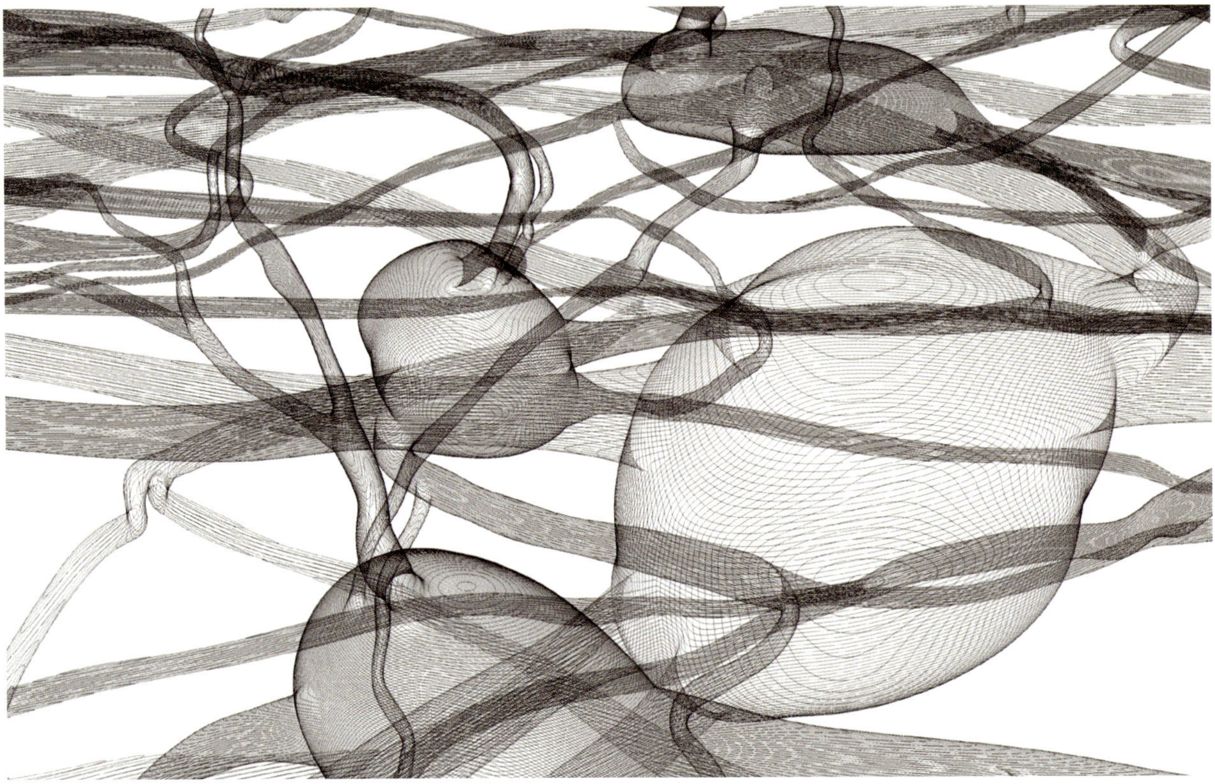

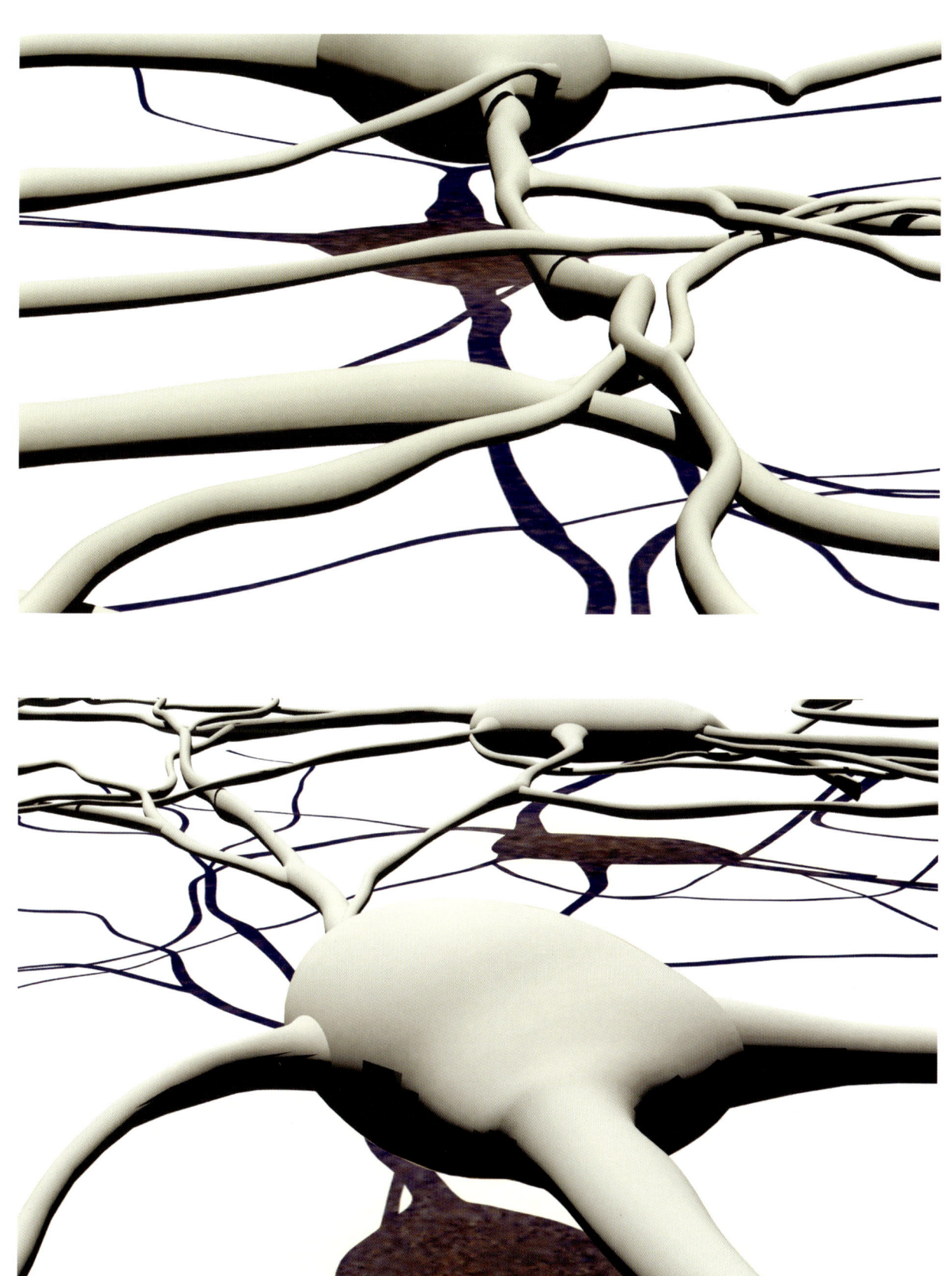

DAVID MATTHEW BOYNTON

NERVE CELLS

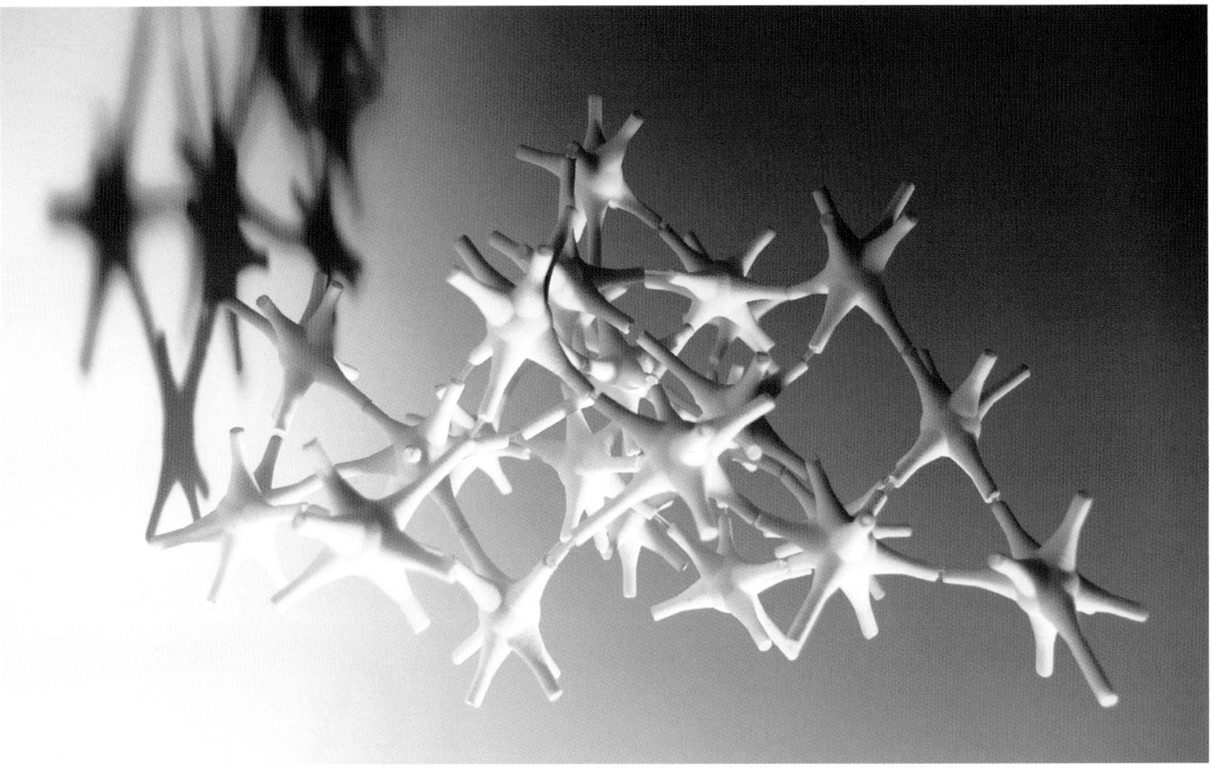

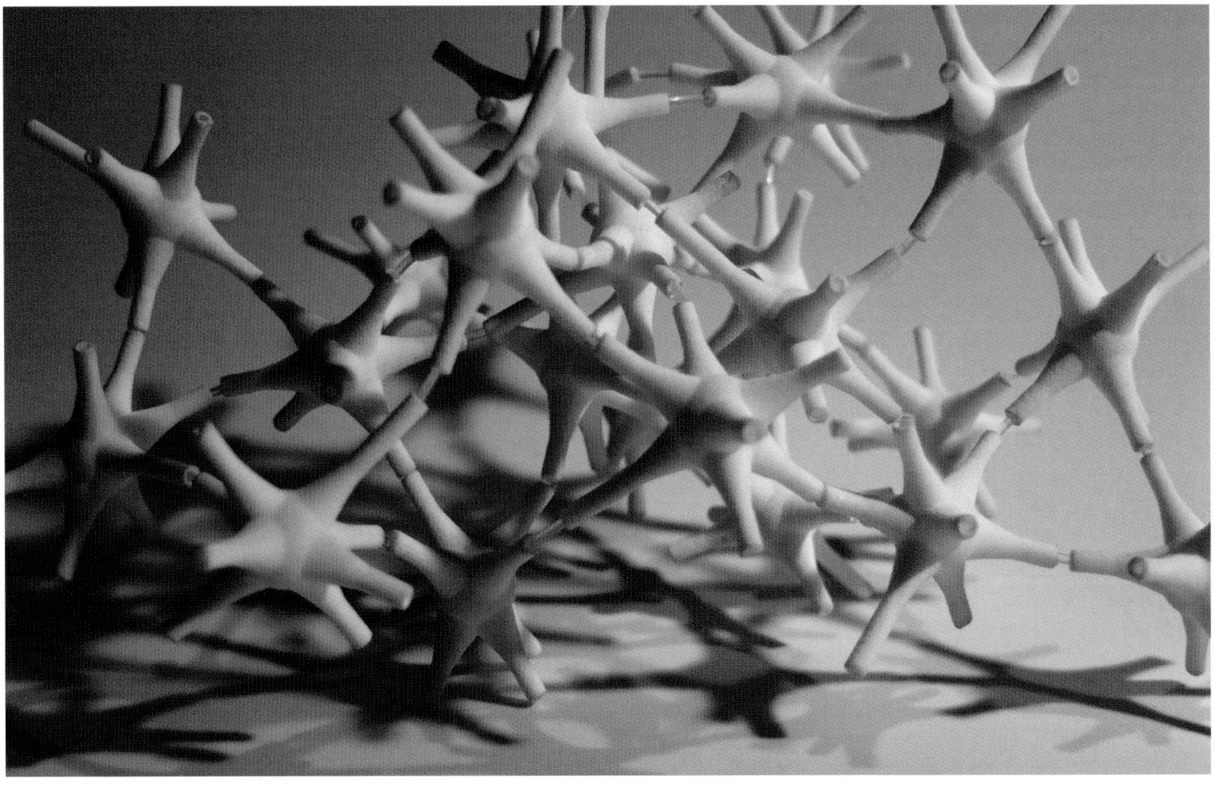

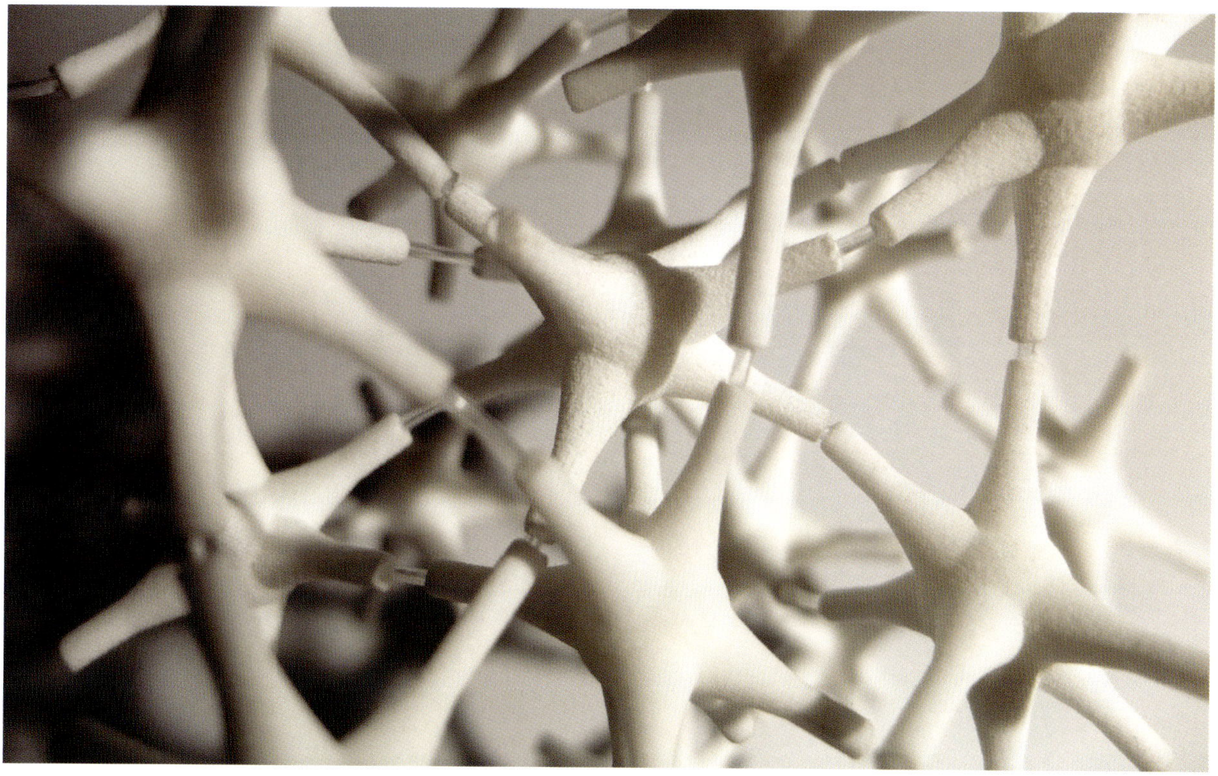

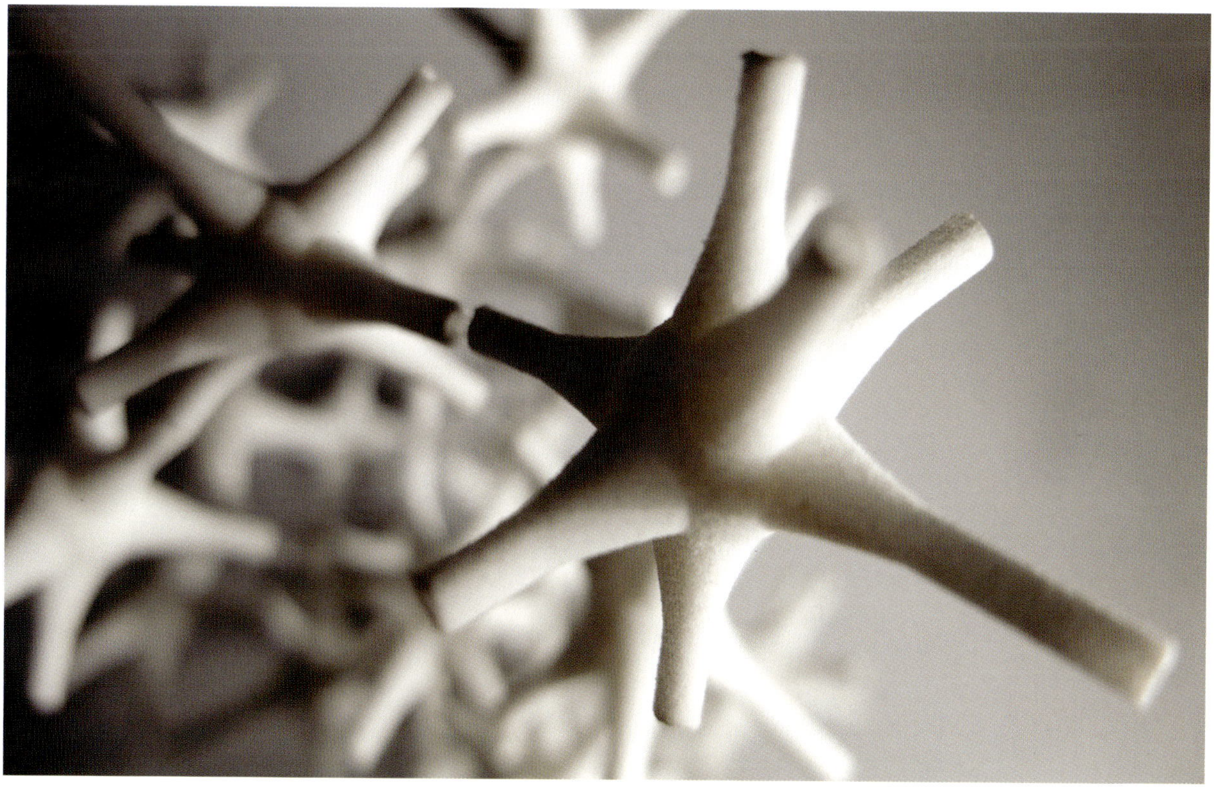

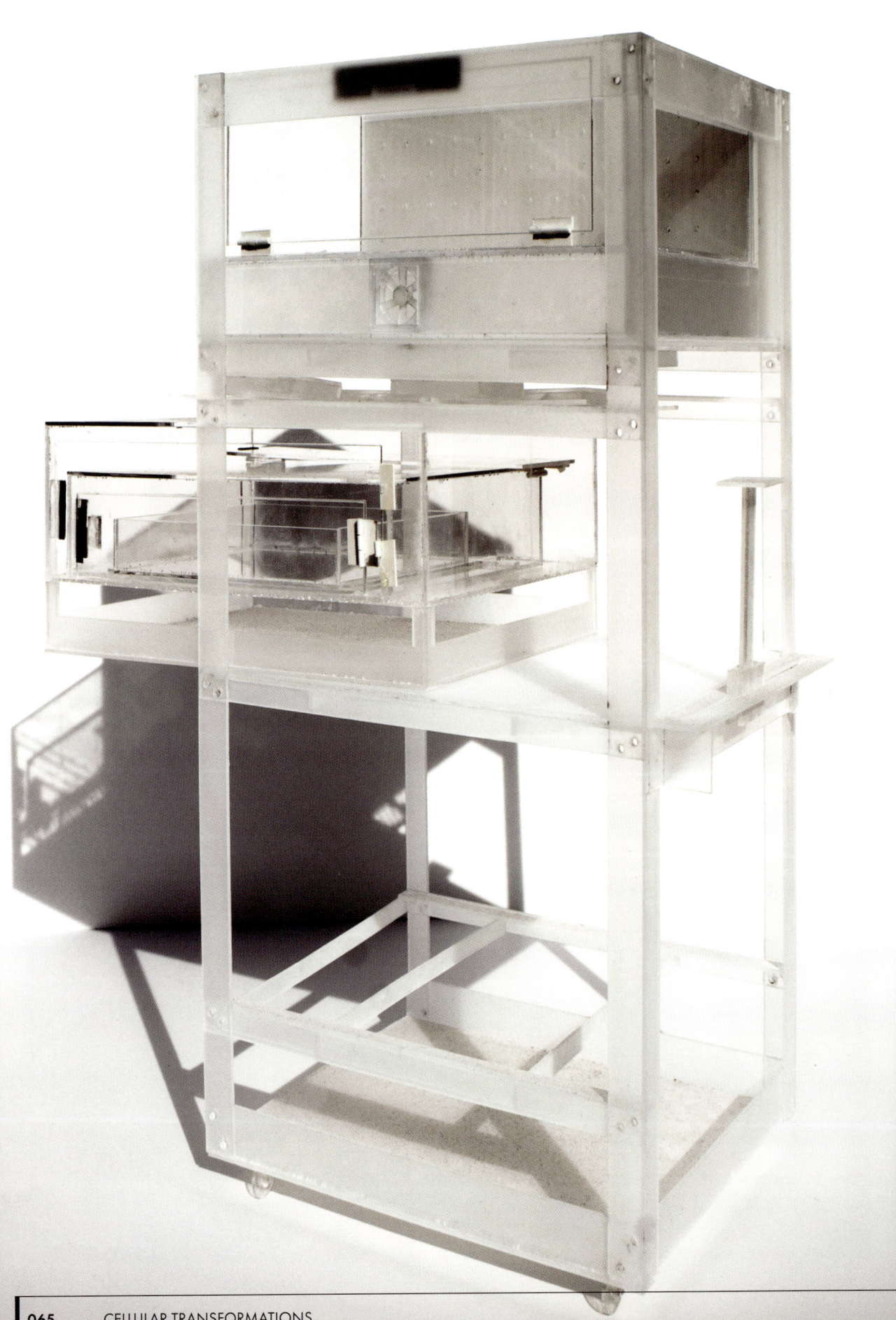

CATALYST: 2013
MOBILE CELL LAB

The Mobile Cell Lab was designed as a portable facility to grow and image plant and animal cell and tissue cultures. The intent of the mobile laboratory was for public educational and outreach programs to highlight cell biology as a discipline that can make a large impact in both the biomedical and design worlds. The Mobile Cell Lab comprised of plexi-glass enclosures assembled with aluminum structures and equipped with HEPA filters, fans, lighting, heating and various water and liquid infrastructural systems to culture cells and tissues under controlled conditions. It also houses a digital camera for monitoring and documenting the patterns of cellular growth. The design and development of this laboratory became a catalyst to bring together biology and architecture for practical applications.

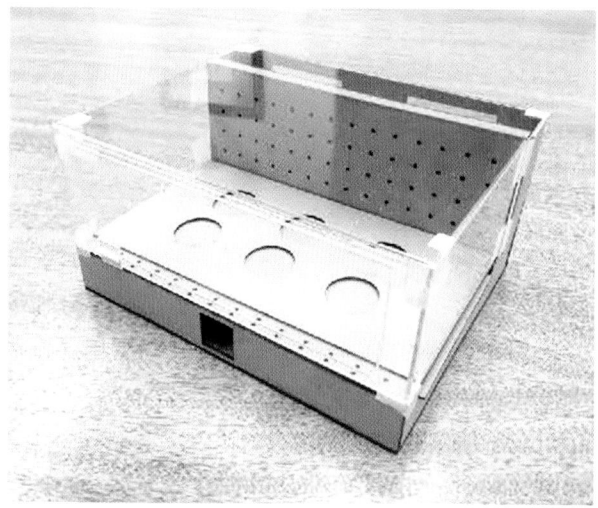
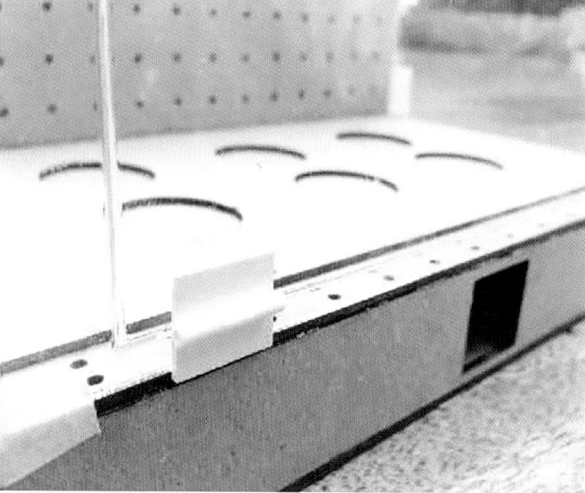

BRIAN CHO | MIN-GU JANG | XIAOMENG LI | NIKI MURATA

CELL LABS: ASSEMBLED AXON

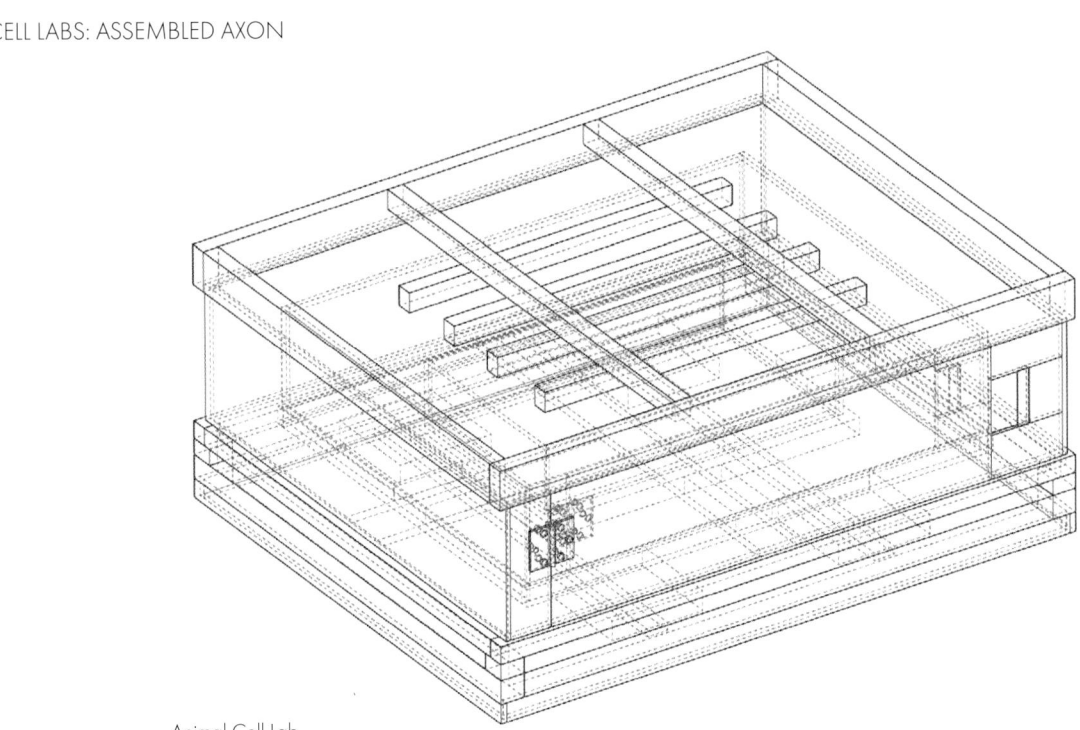

Animal Cell Lab

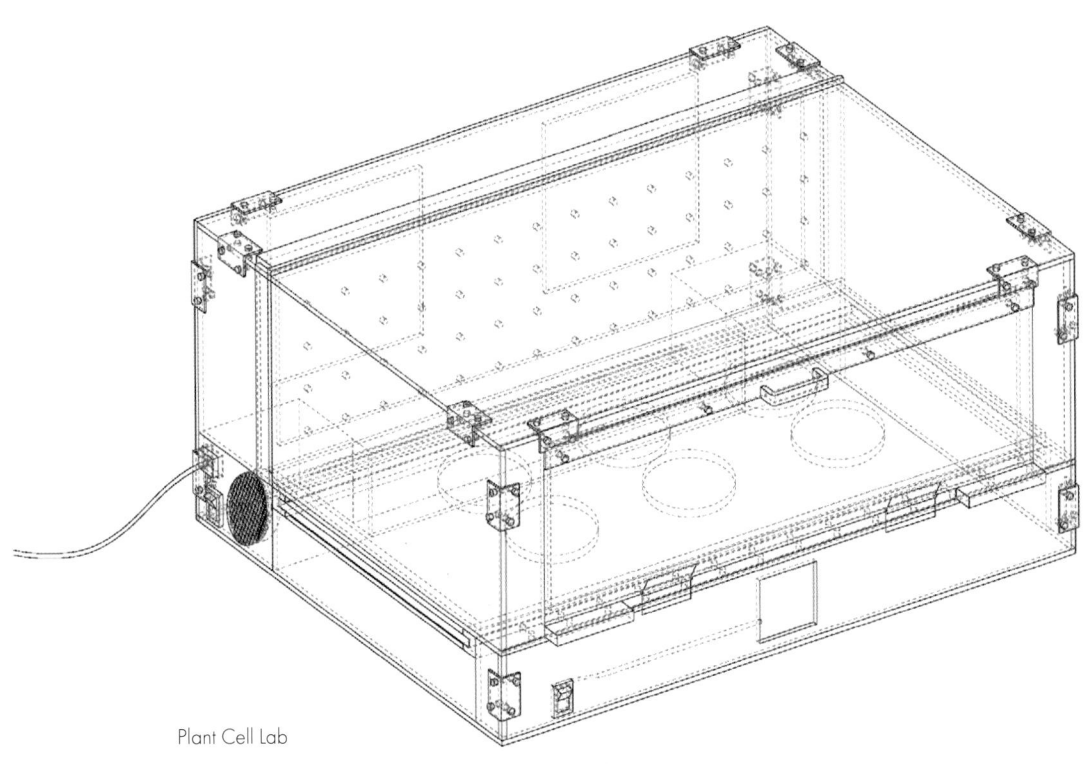

Plant Cell Lab

CELL LABS WITHIN THE FRAME: ASSEMBLED AXON

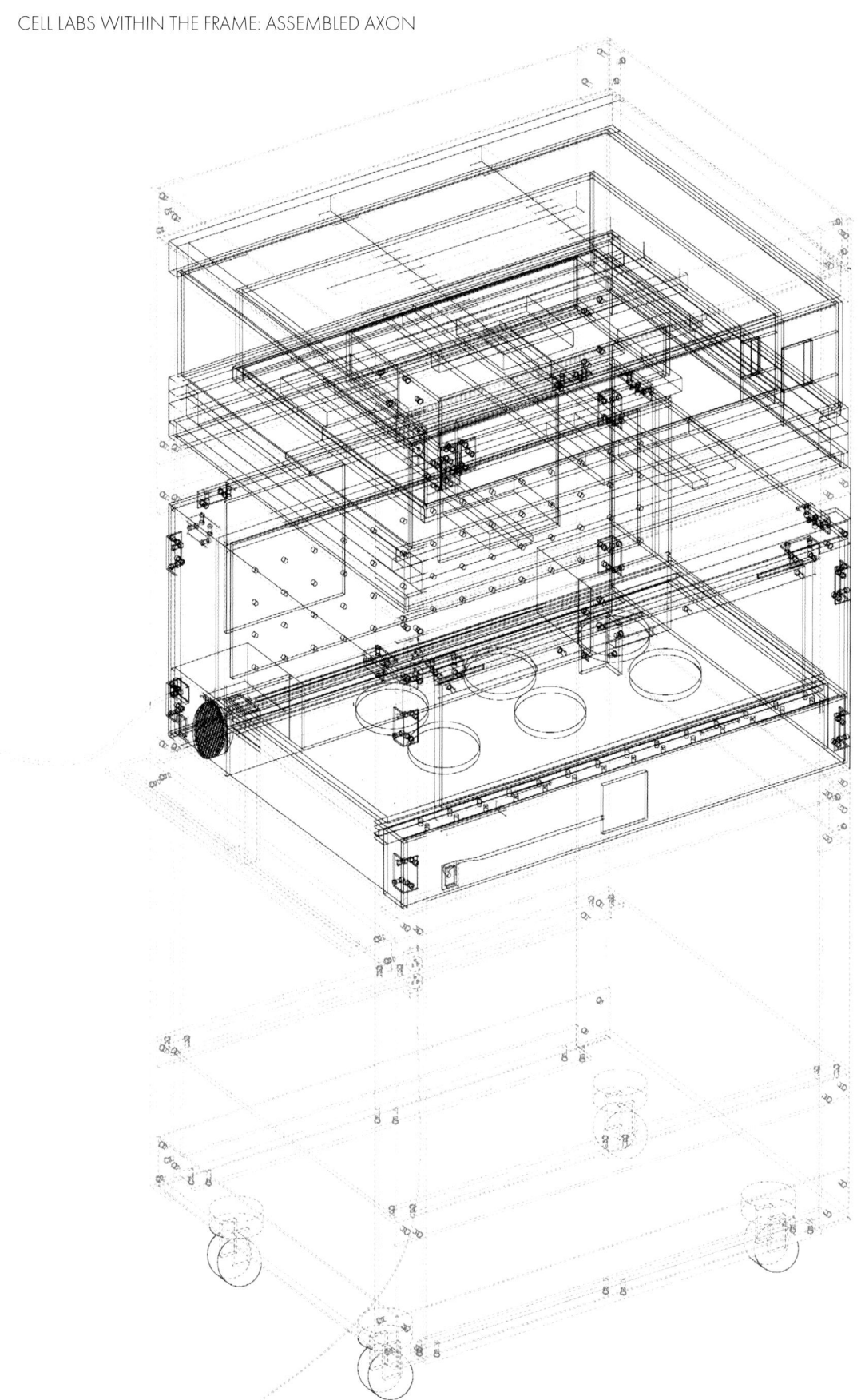

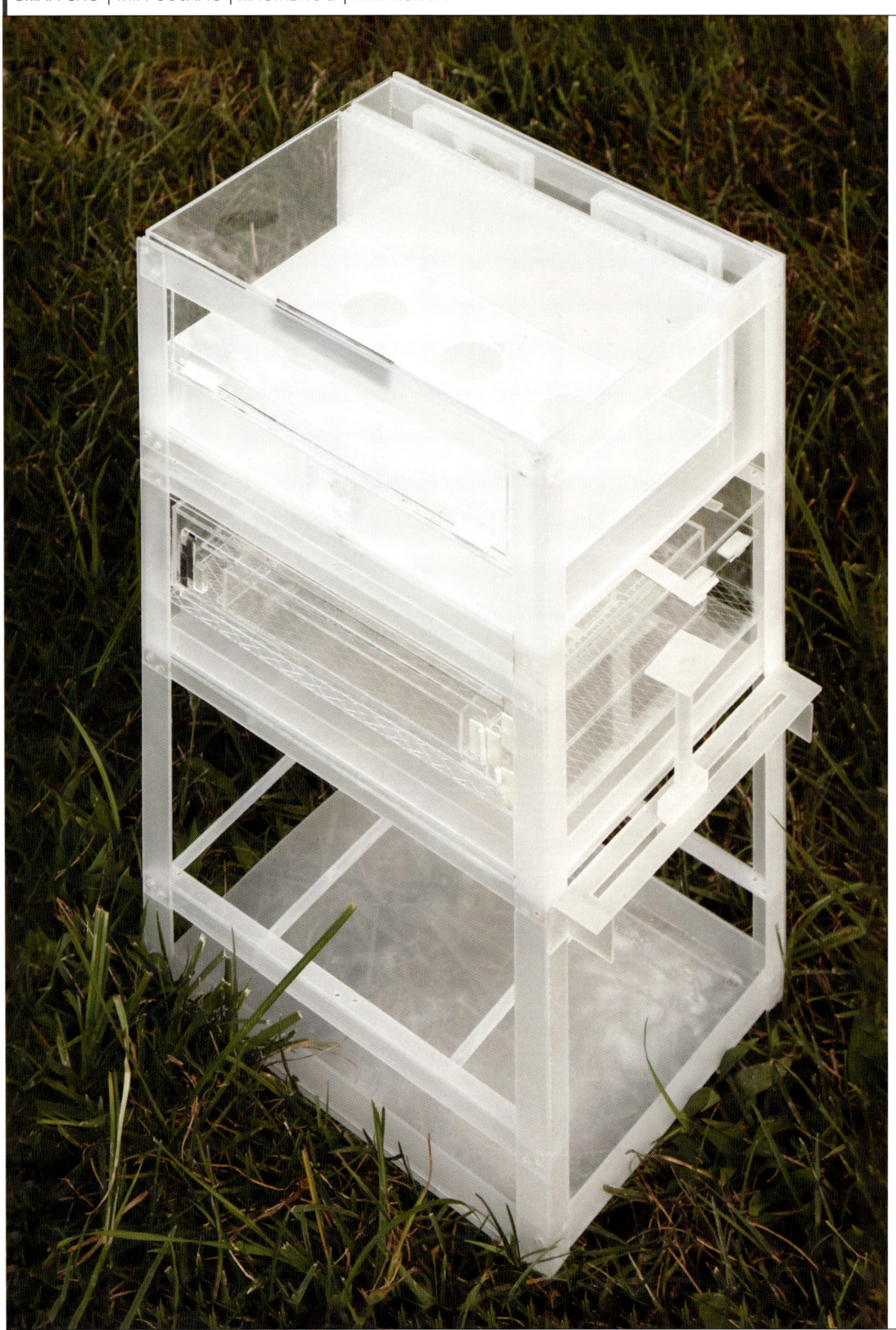

CELL LABS WITHIN THE FRAME: SECTIONS AND ELEVATIONS

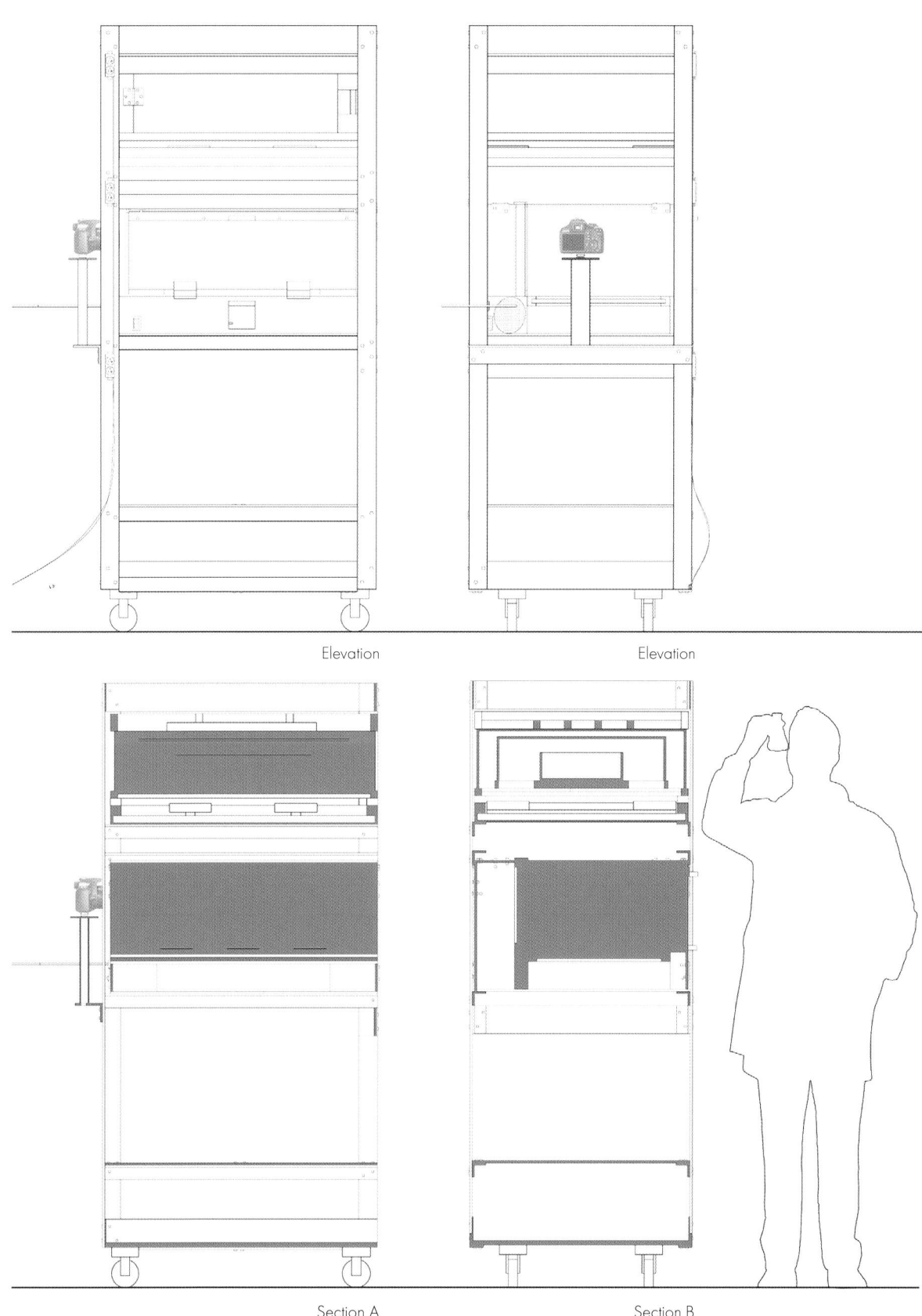

Elevation | Elevation

Section A | Section B

ELLEN NOLL | GLENN PARK | JINGWEN SHI | FEI XIE

FRAME: EXPLODED AXON

A. ALUMINUM STRUCTURAL FRAME (TOP)
B. MAIN ALUMINUM STRUCTURAL COLUMNS
C. L-BEAMS (ANIMAL CELL LAB)
D. RIVETS
E. L-BEAMS (PLANT CELL LAB)
F. CAMERA HOLDER (ADJUSTABLE)
G. L-BEAMS (CAMERA)
H. ALUMINUM STRUCTURAL FRAME (BOTTOM)
I. WHEELS

BRIAN CHO | MIN-GU JANG | XIAOMENG LI | NIKI MURATA

FRAME: ASSEMBLED AXON

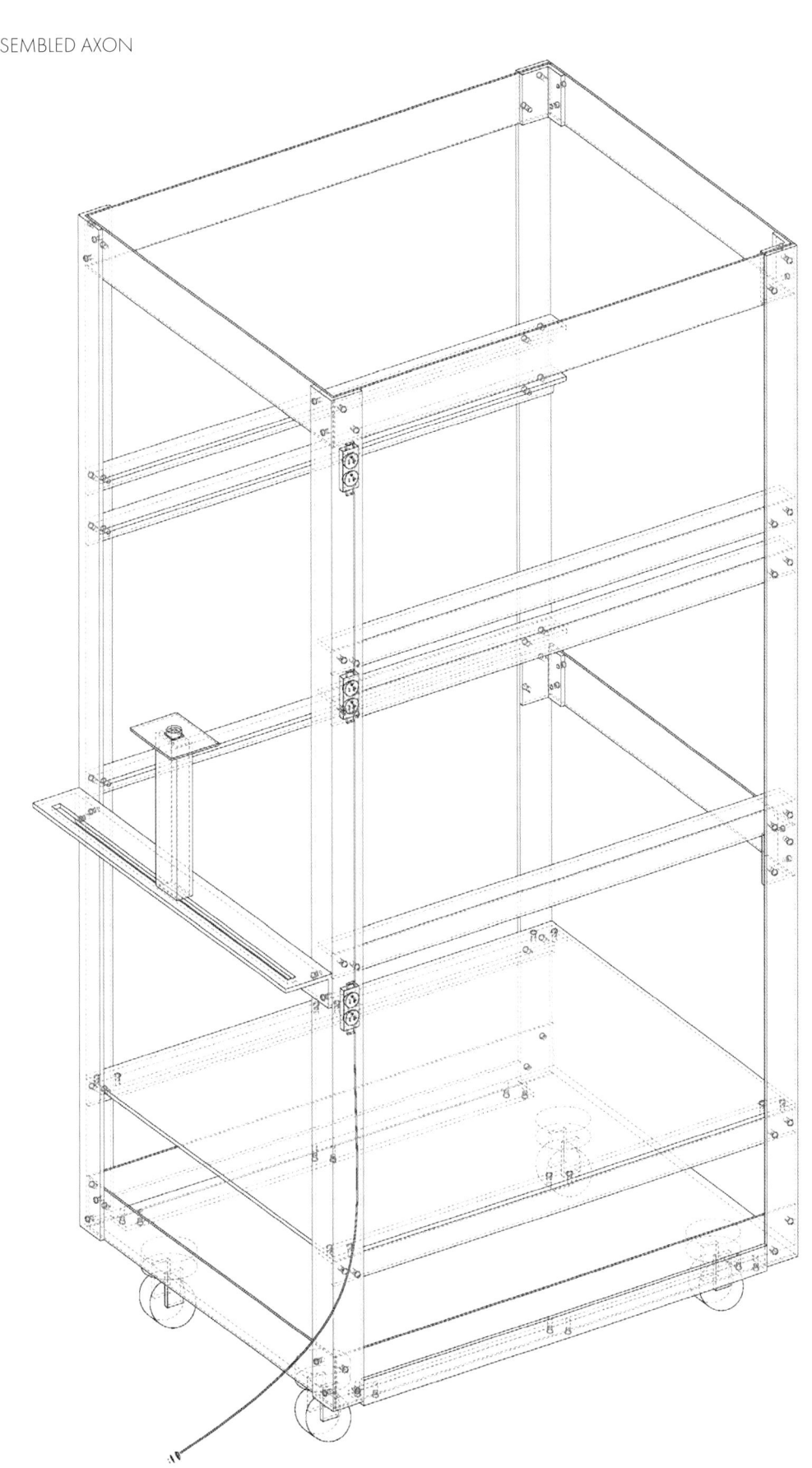

PLANT CELL LAB: EXPLODED AXON

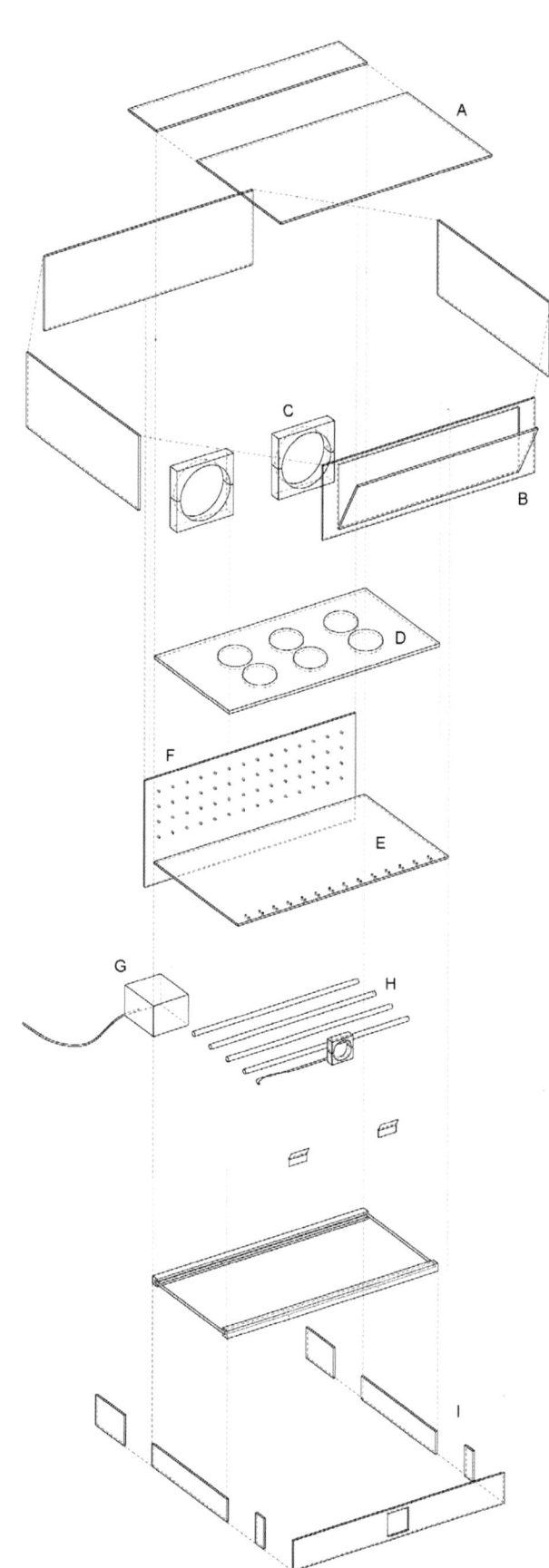

A. COVER (PLEXIGLASS)
B. DOOR (PLEXIGLASS)
C. 8" COMPUTER FAN
D. PETRI DISH TRAY
E. FILTER CASE
F. PERFORATED STEEL CASING
G. POWER SUPPLY
H. FLOURESCENT LIGHTS
I. LIGHTING/ HEATING BOX

BRIAN CHO | MIN-GU JANG | XIAOMENG LI | NIKI MURATA

ANIMAL CELL LAB: EXPLODED AXON

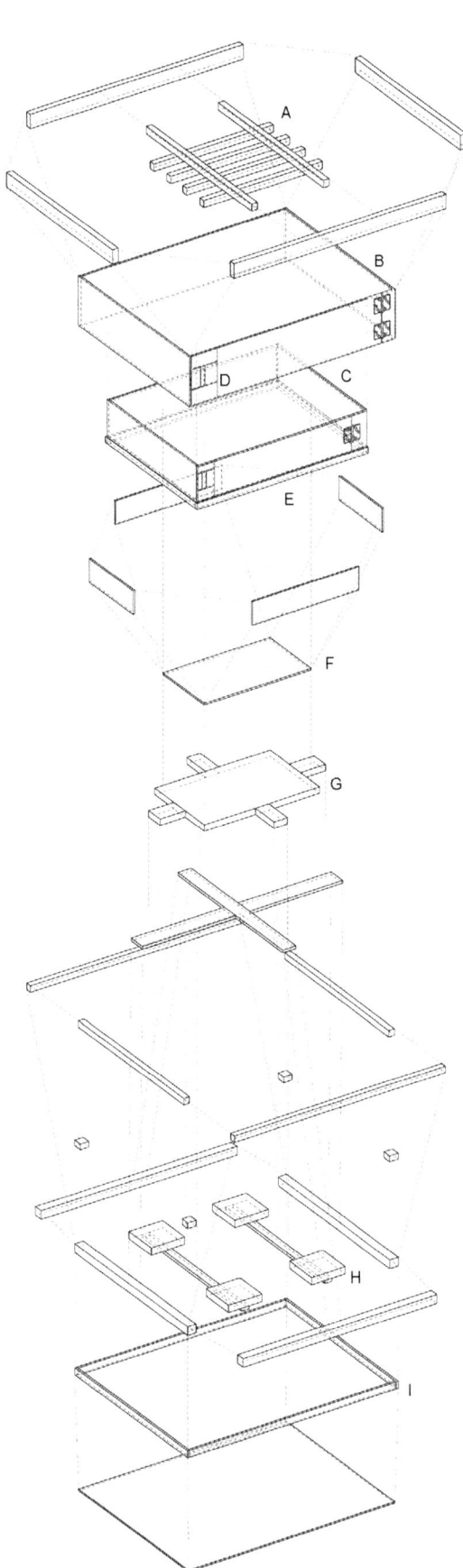

A. LIGHTS
B. COVER (PLEXIGLASS)
C. NEXINE COVER (PLEXIGLASS)
D. HINGE
E. DOOR (PLEXIGLASS)
F. CULTURE DISH (PLEXIGLASS)
G. FILTER
H. FANS
I. WATERTANK

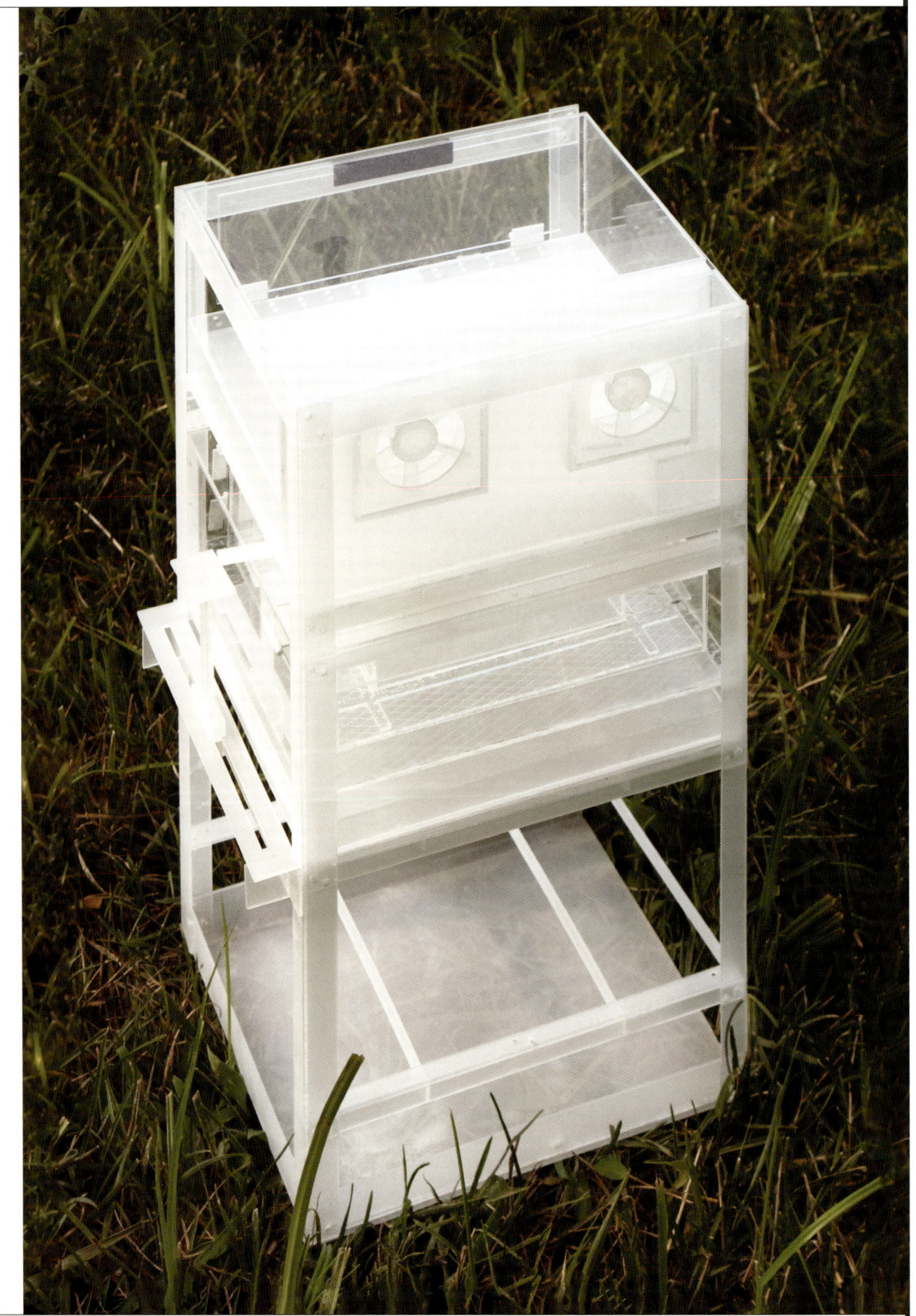

CELL LABS WITHIN THE FRAME: PLANS

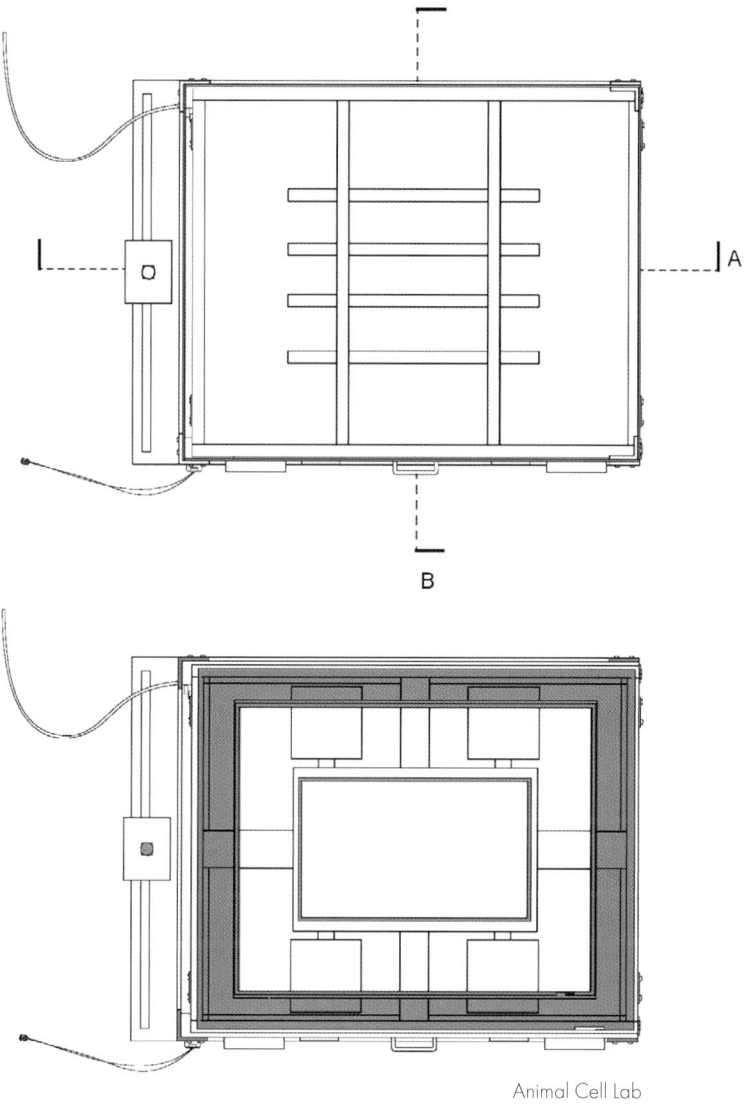

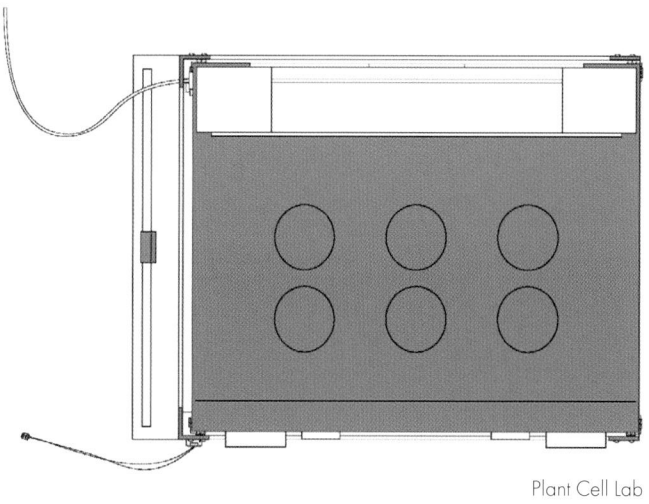

Animal Cell Lab

Plant Cell Lab

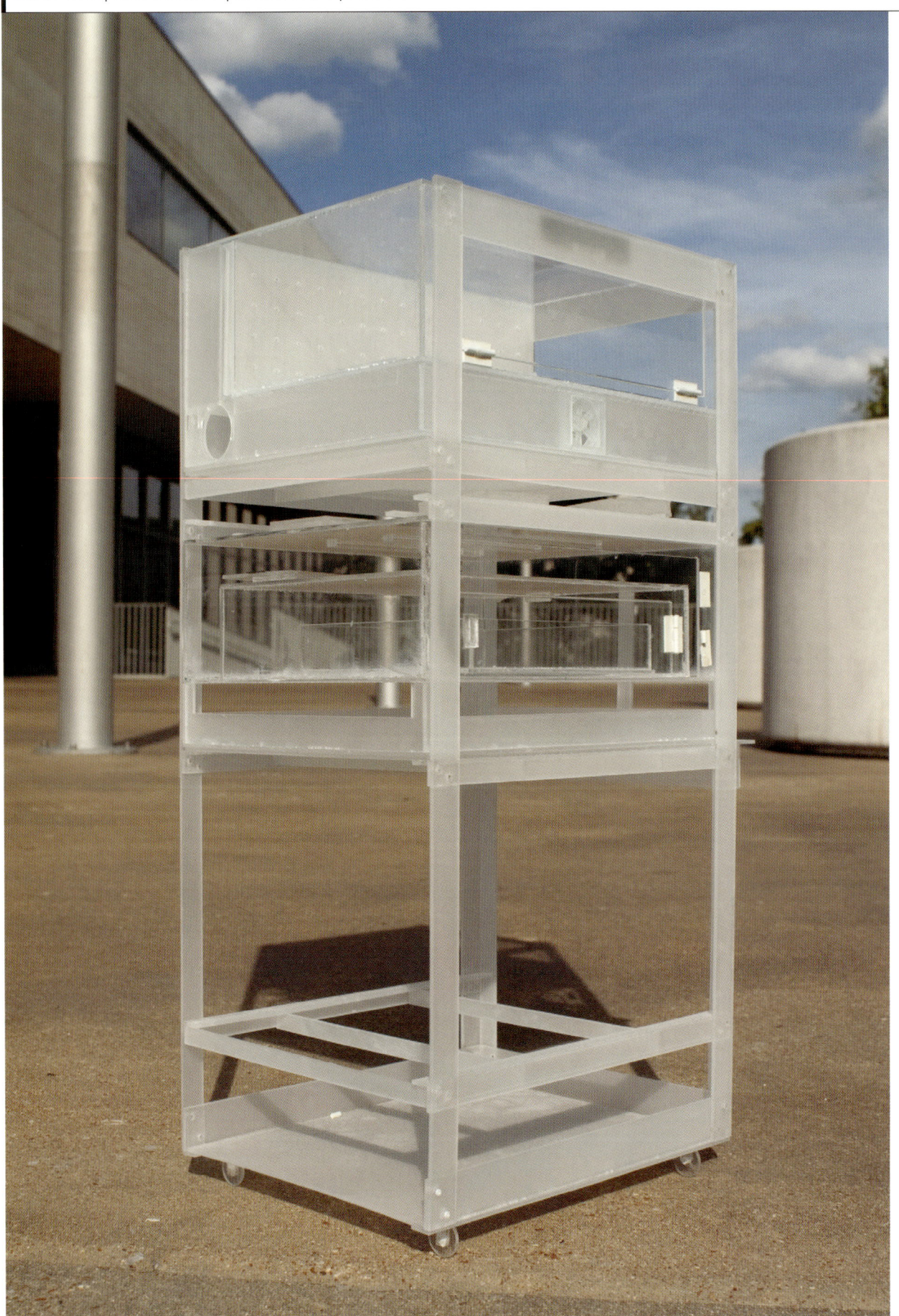

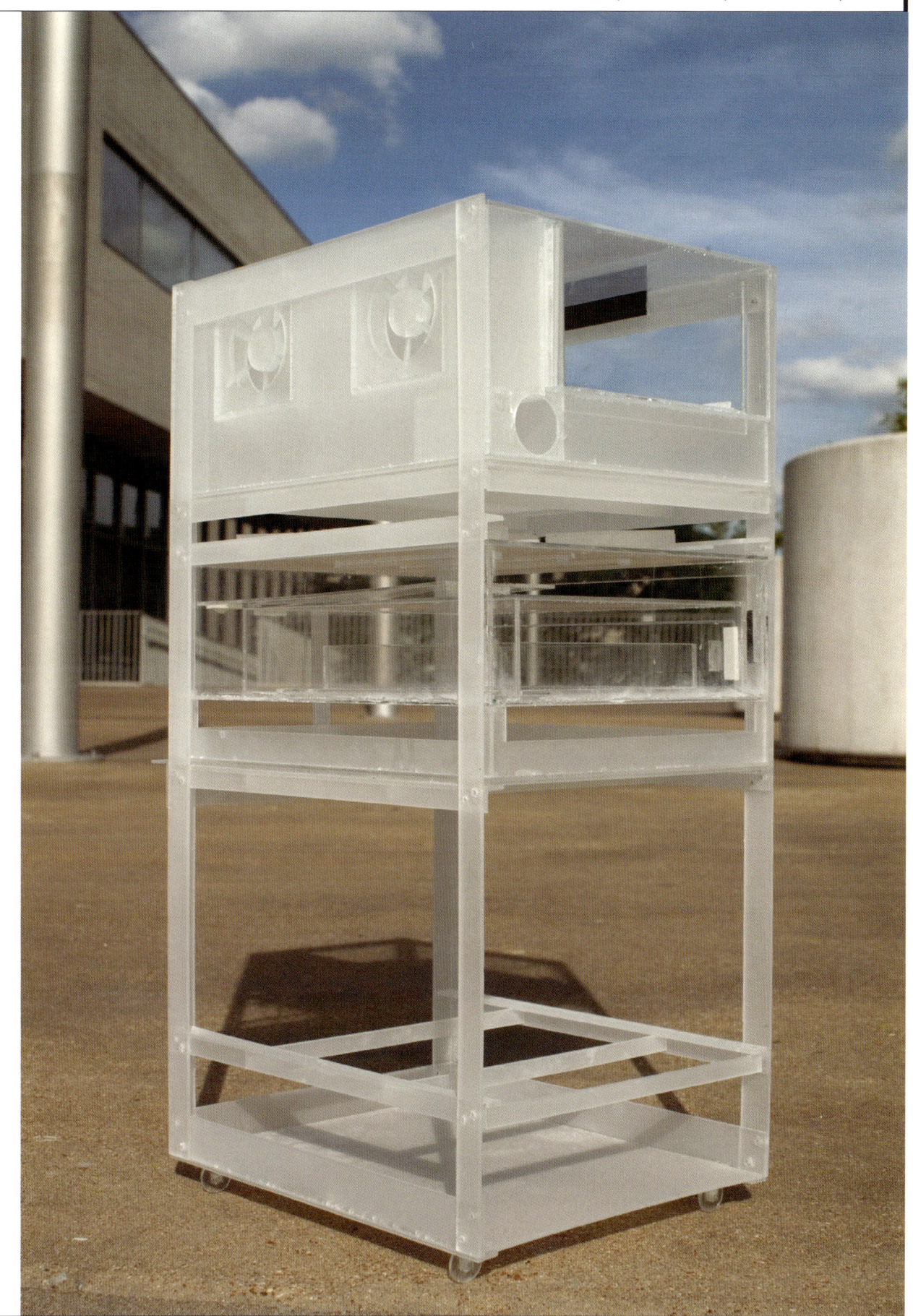

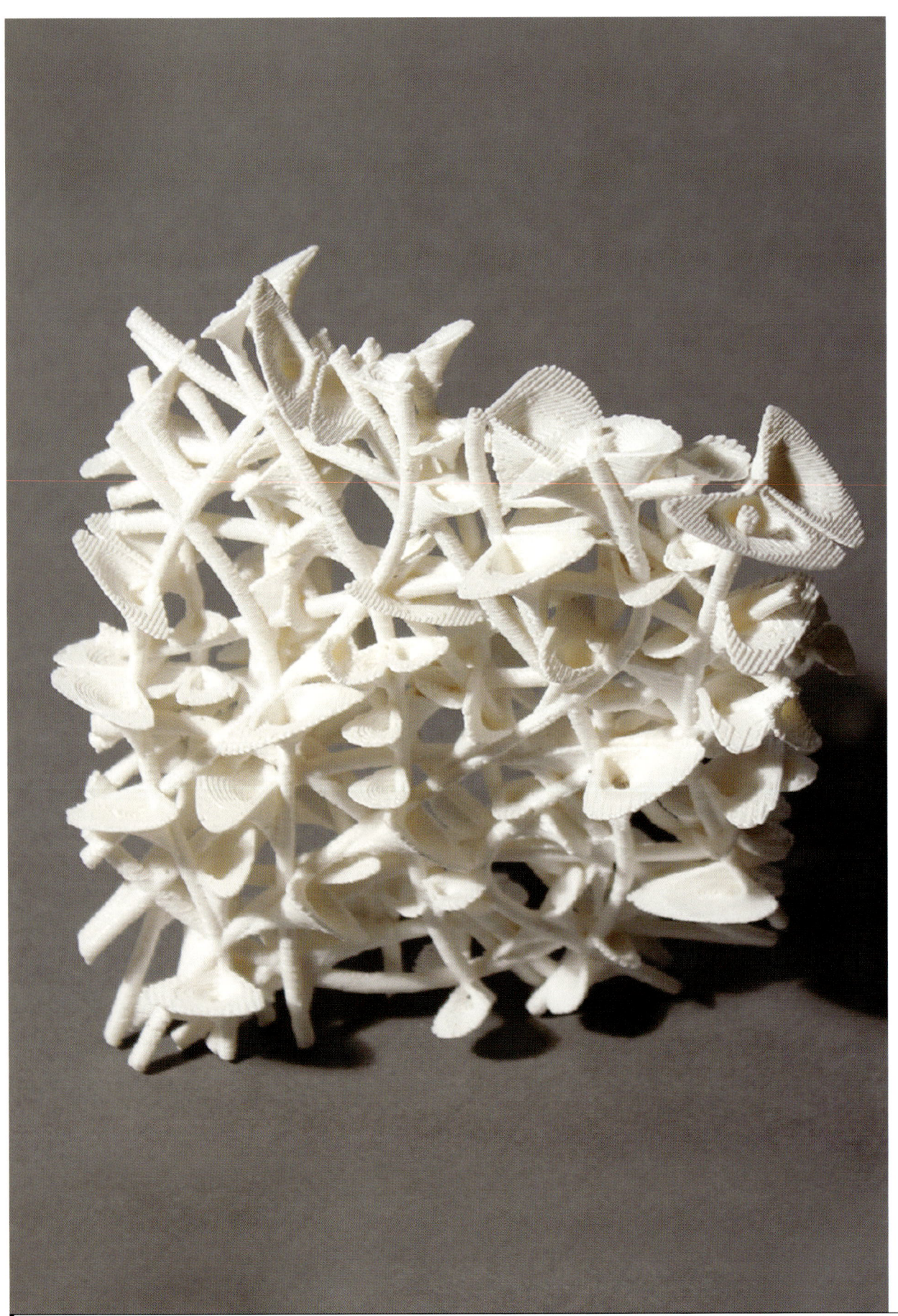

EMERGING: 2013
SCAFFOLDING RESEARCH

Scaffolding Research was a design development project to fabricate physical frameworks to grow moss, a nonvascular plant that typically grows as a colony on various surfaces. The project used Physcomitrella patens, a moss species used as a model organism in plant biology, to grow from its filamentous protonemata stage to a mature organism containing leafy gametophores that enable sexual reproduction. The research explored properties of scaffolds that enabled robust moss growth by optimizing light, water and mineral availability. Students used sterile culture techniques to prevent contamination of moss during long-term growth and observation. Scaffolding Research was an important aspect of the Cellular Transformations course because it enabled the design and development of hybrid structures.

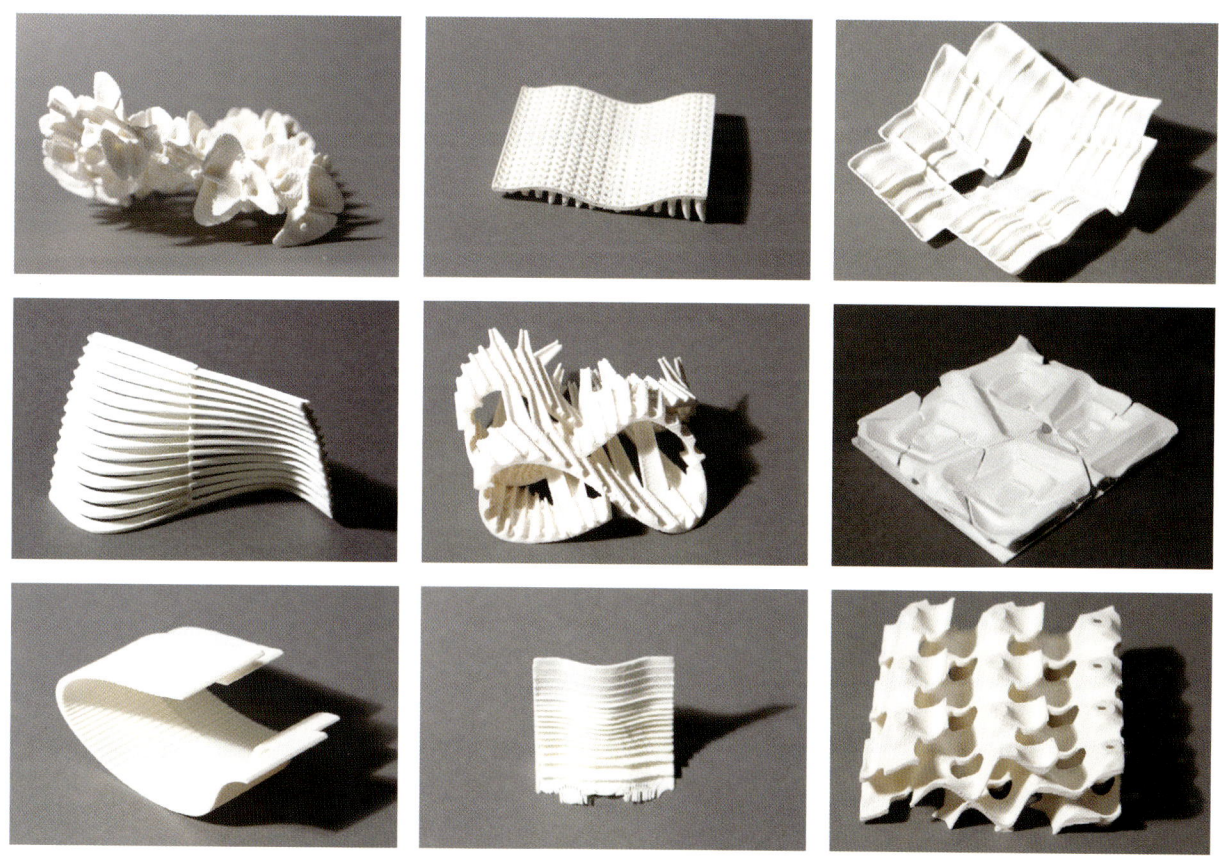

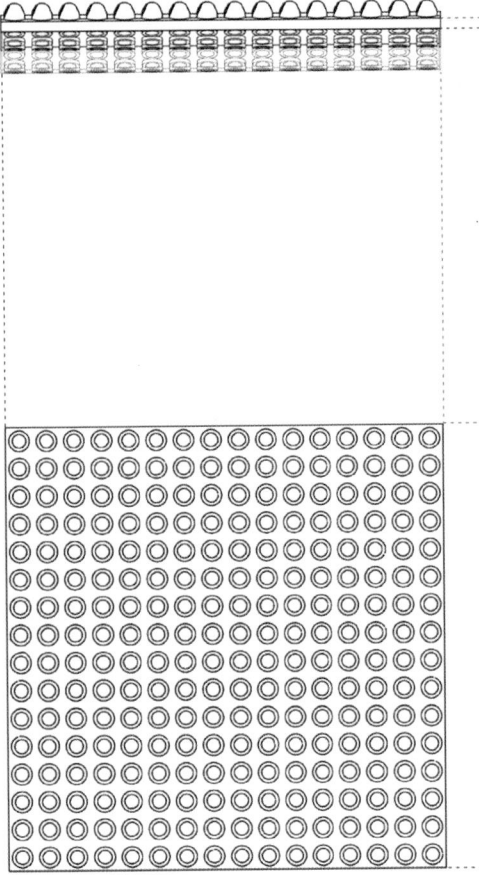
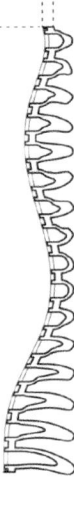
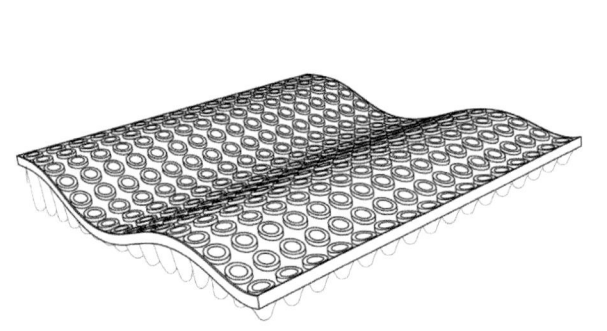
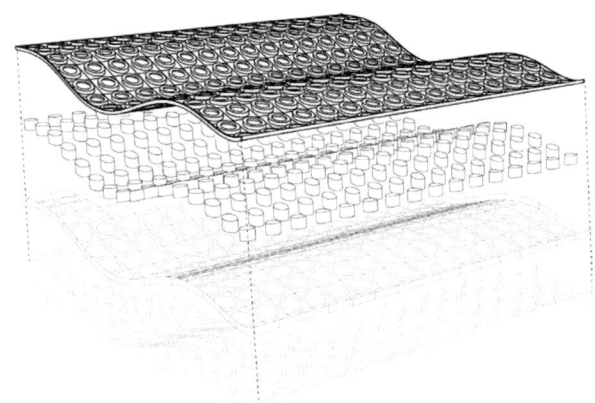

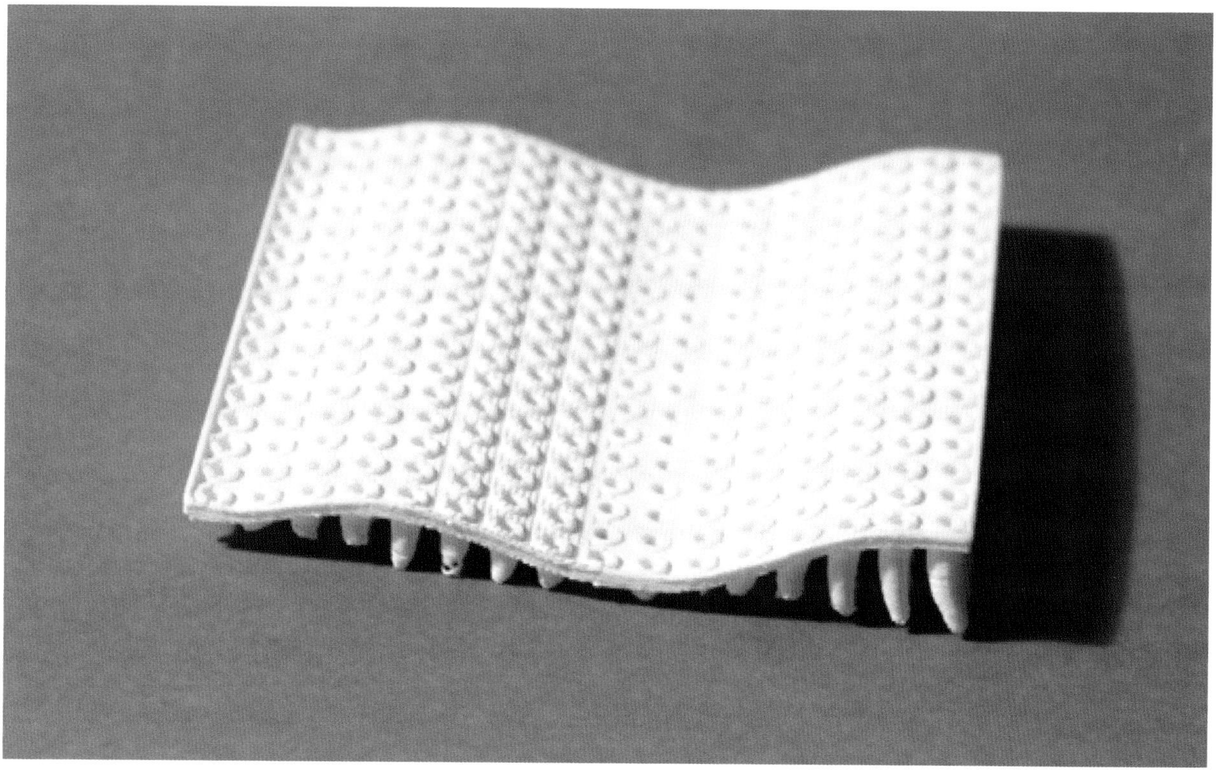

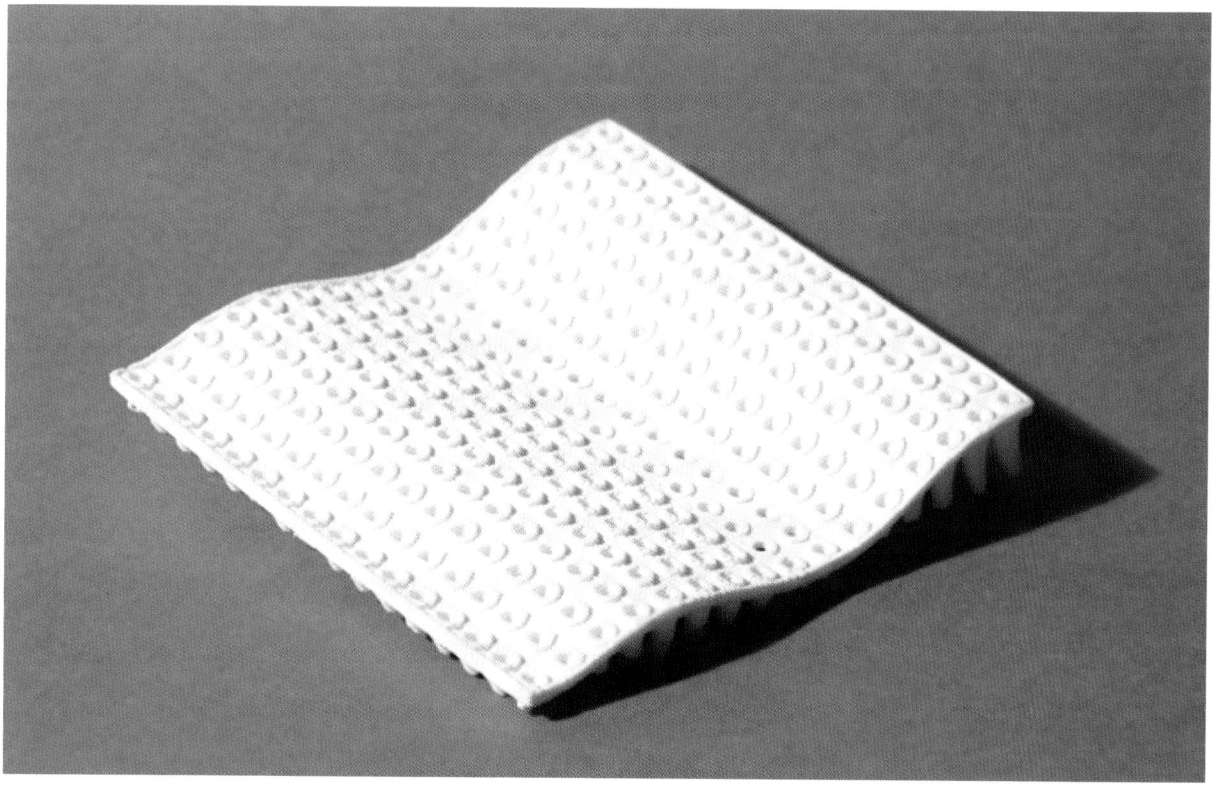

AMBER IBARRA

SCAFFOLDING RESEARCH

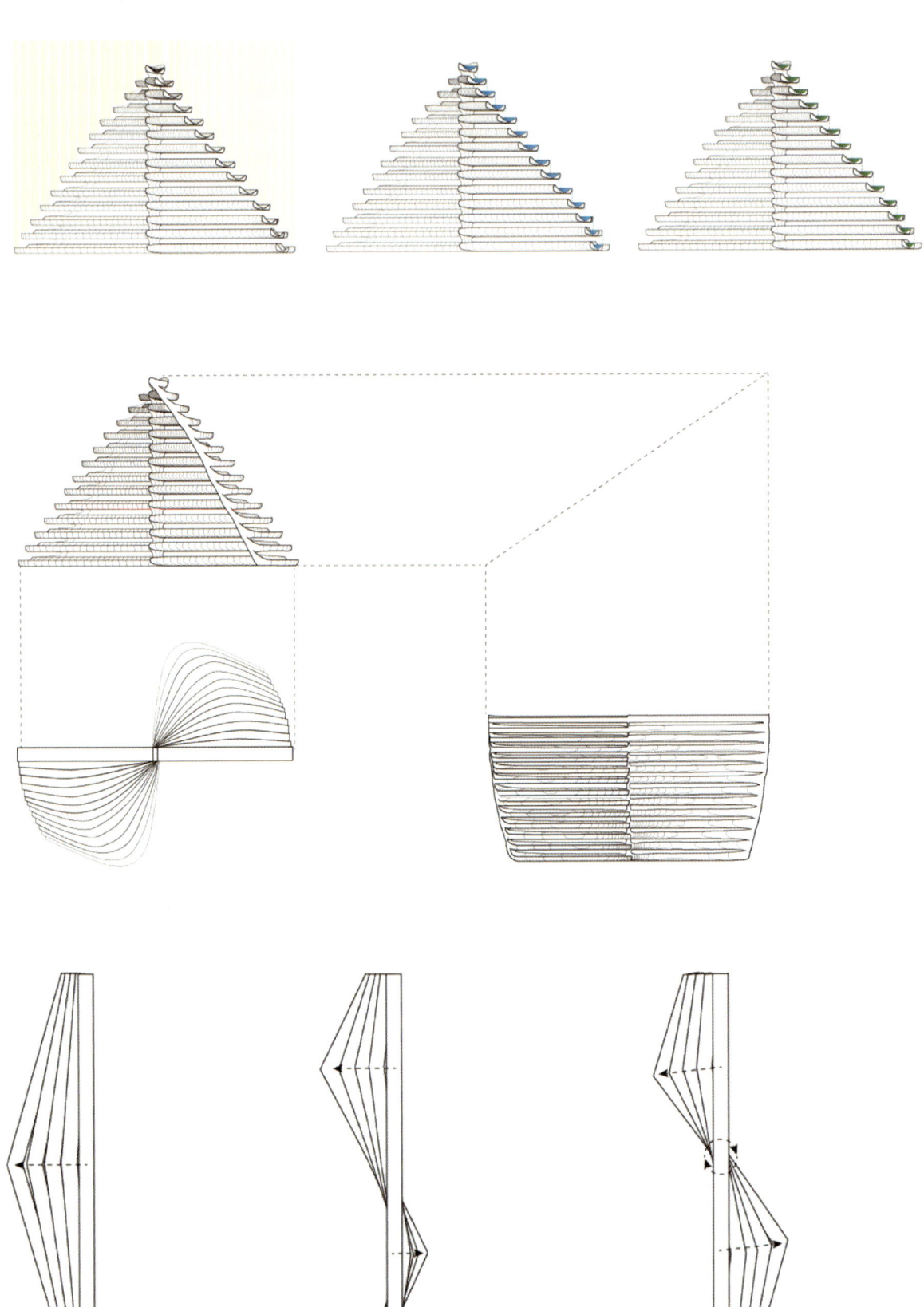

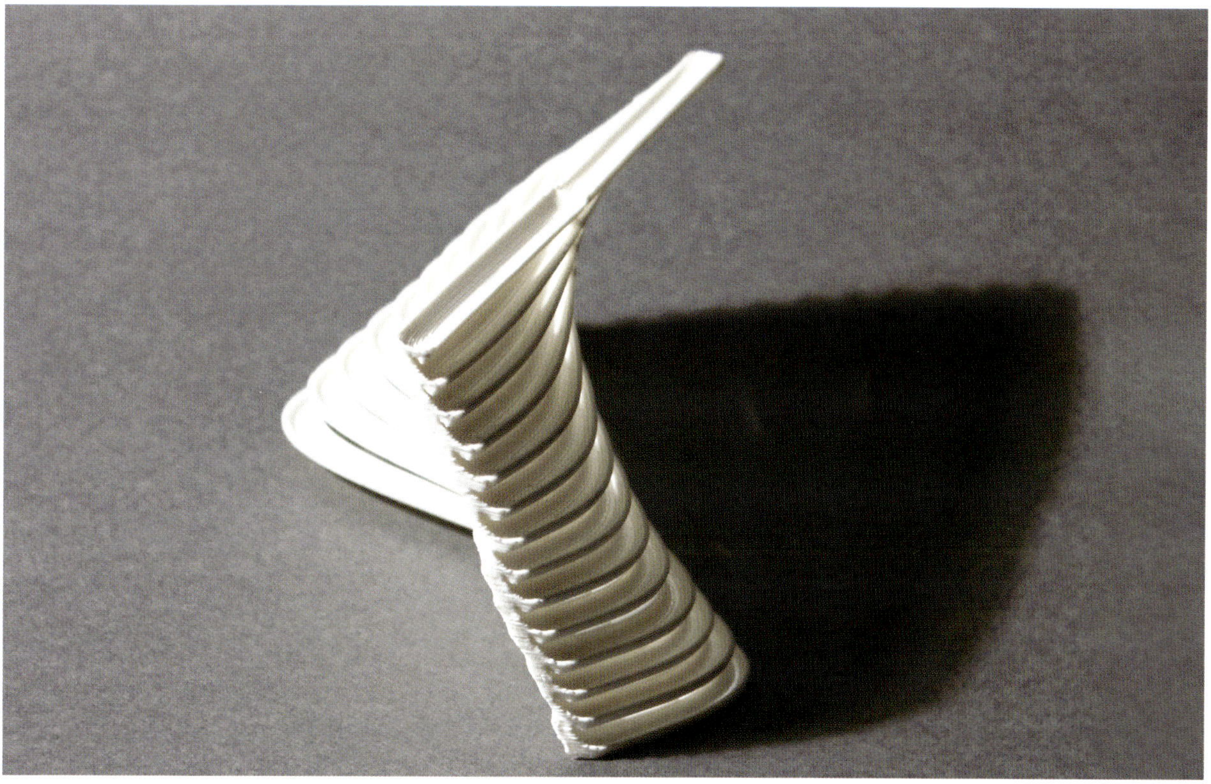

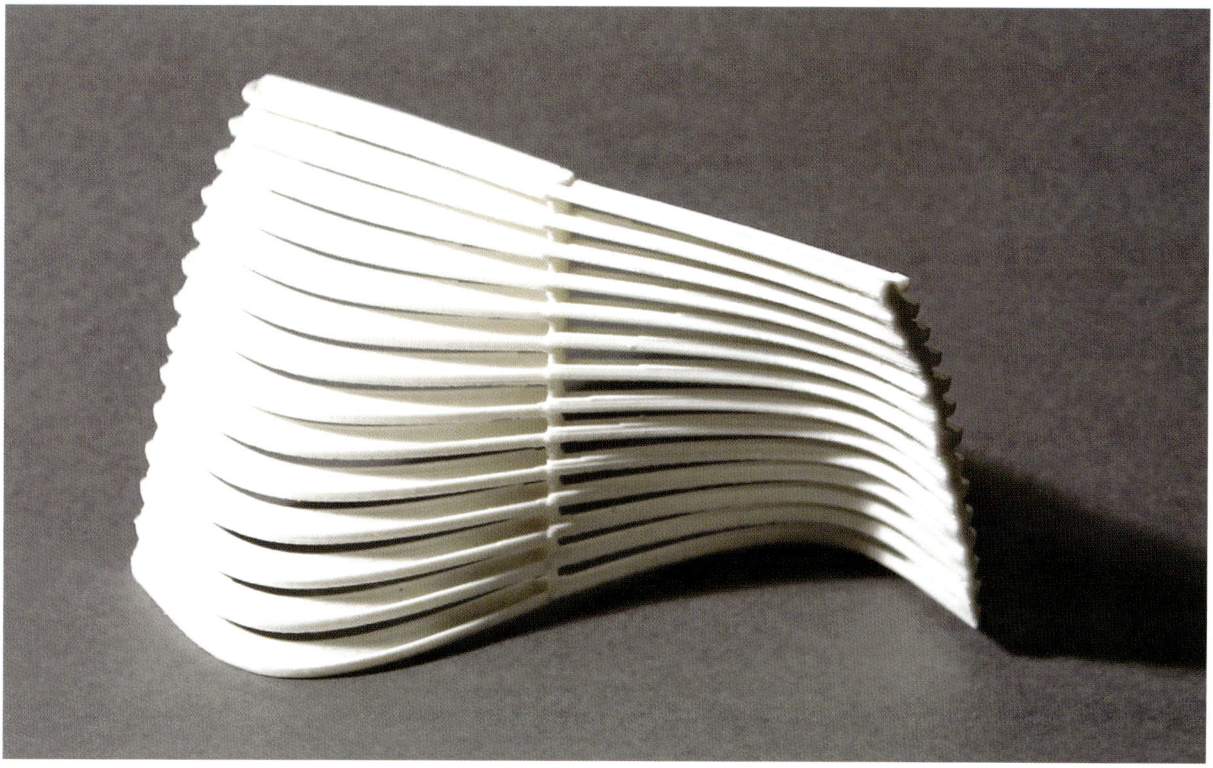

MICHAEL POLITTE

SCAFFOLDING RESEARCH

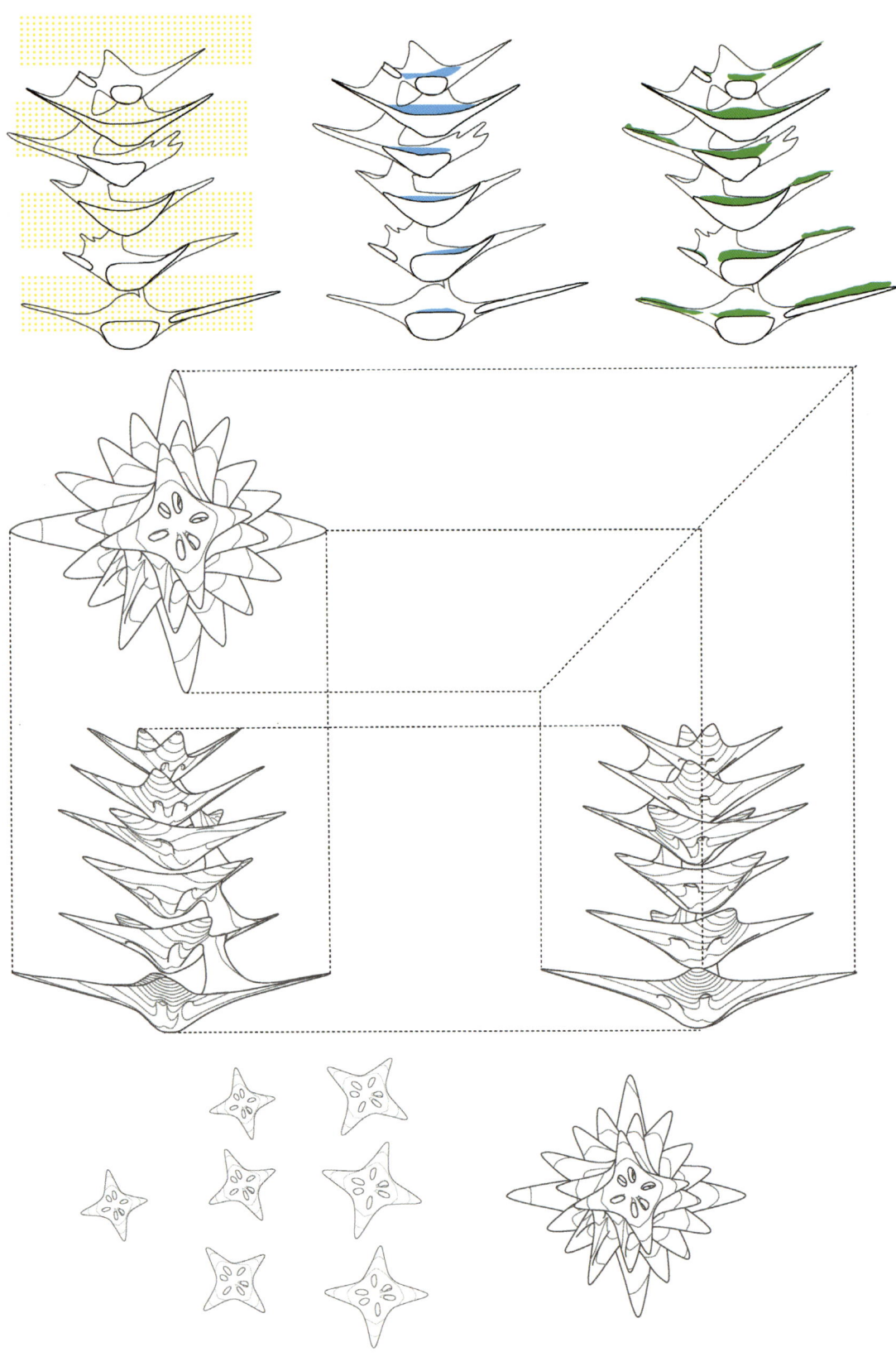

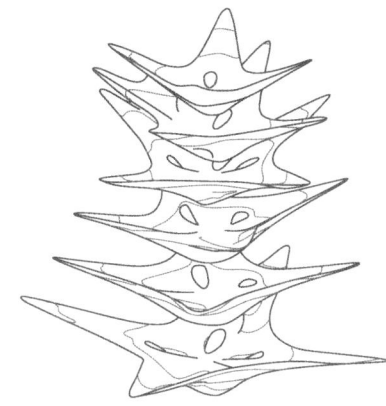
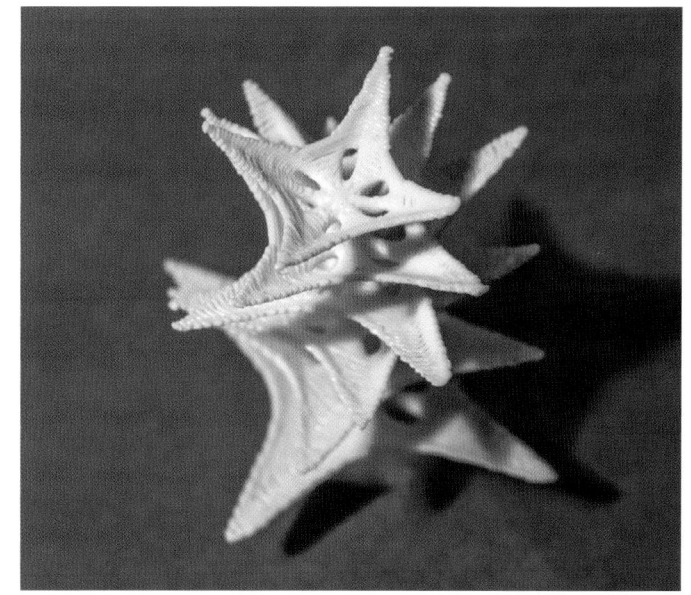
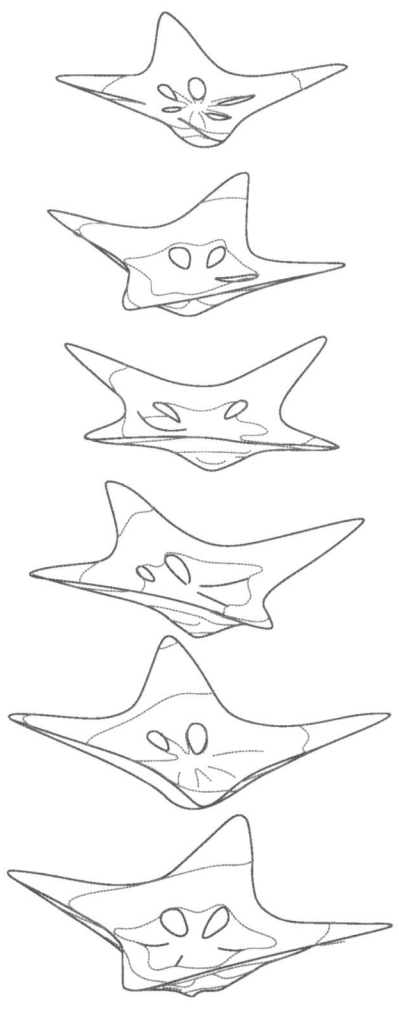
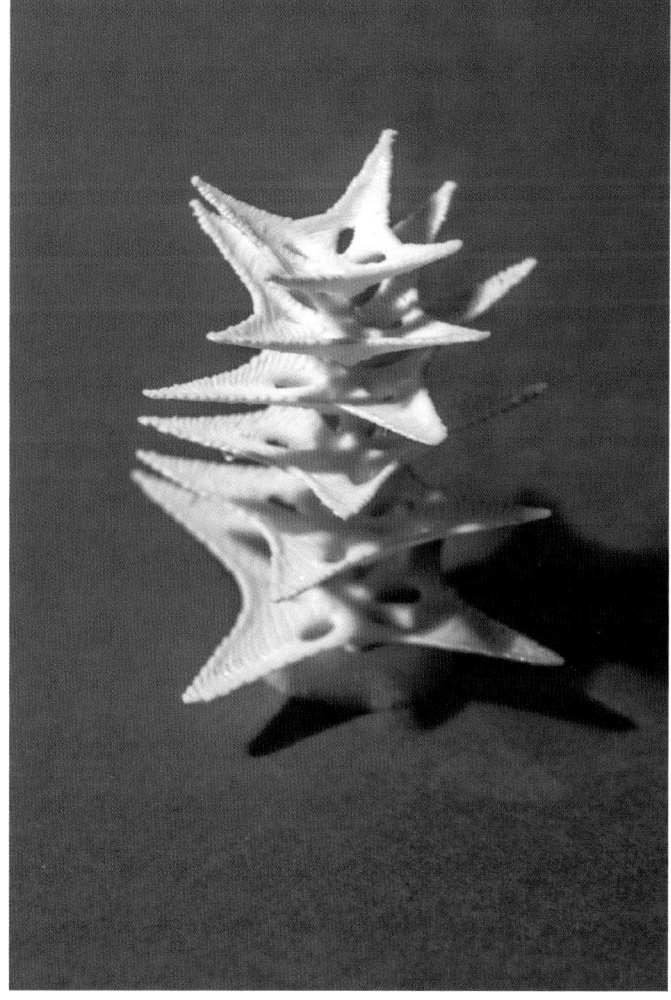

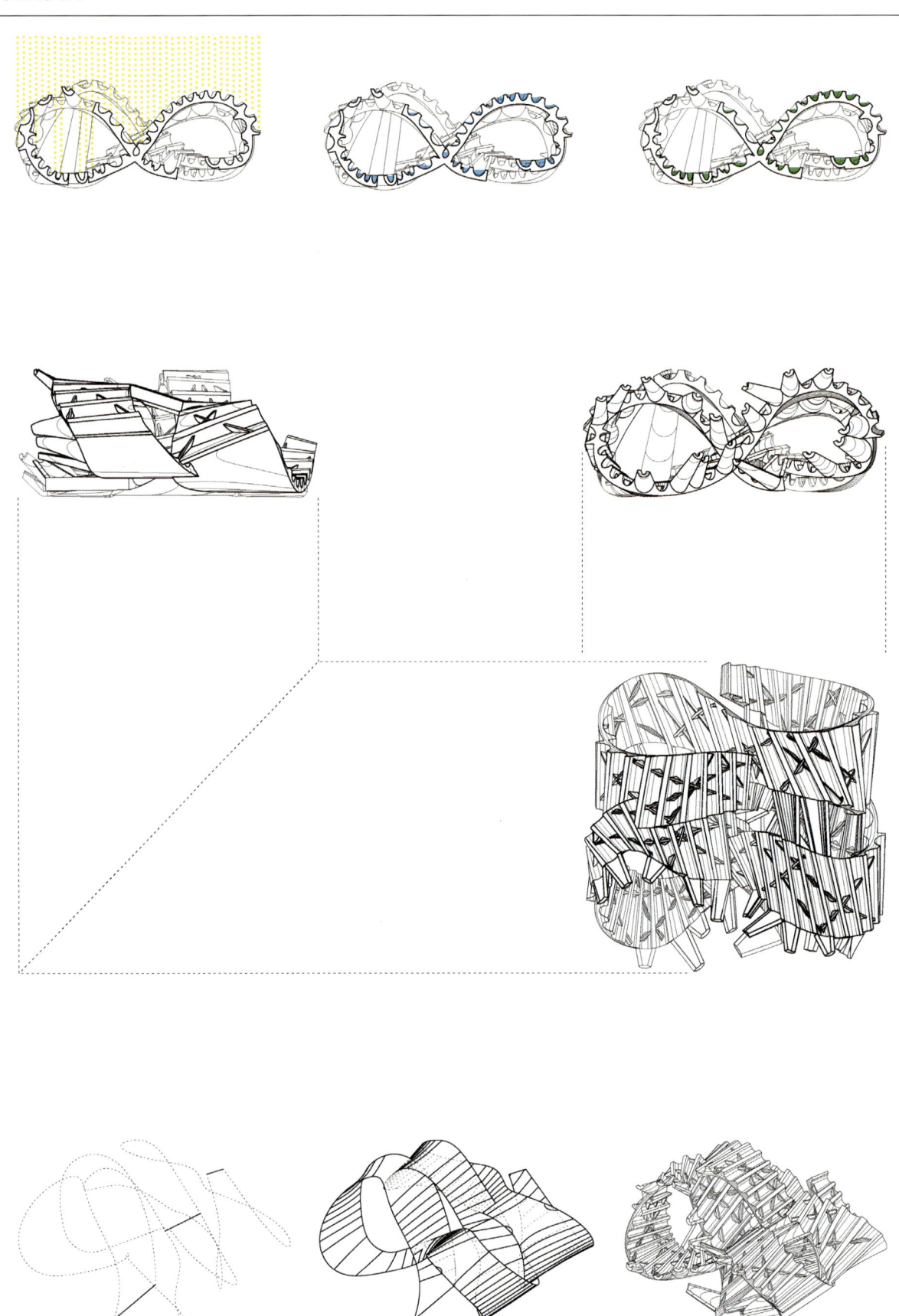

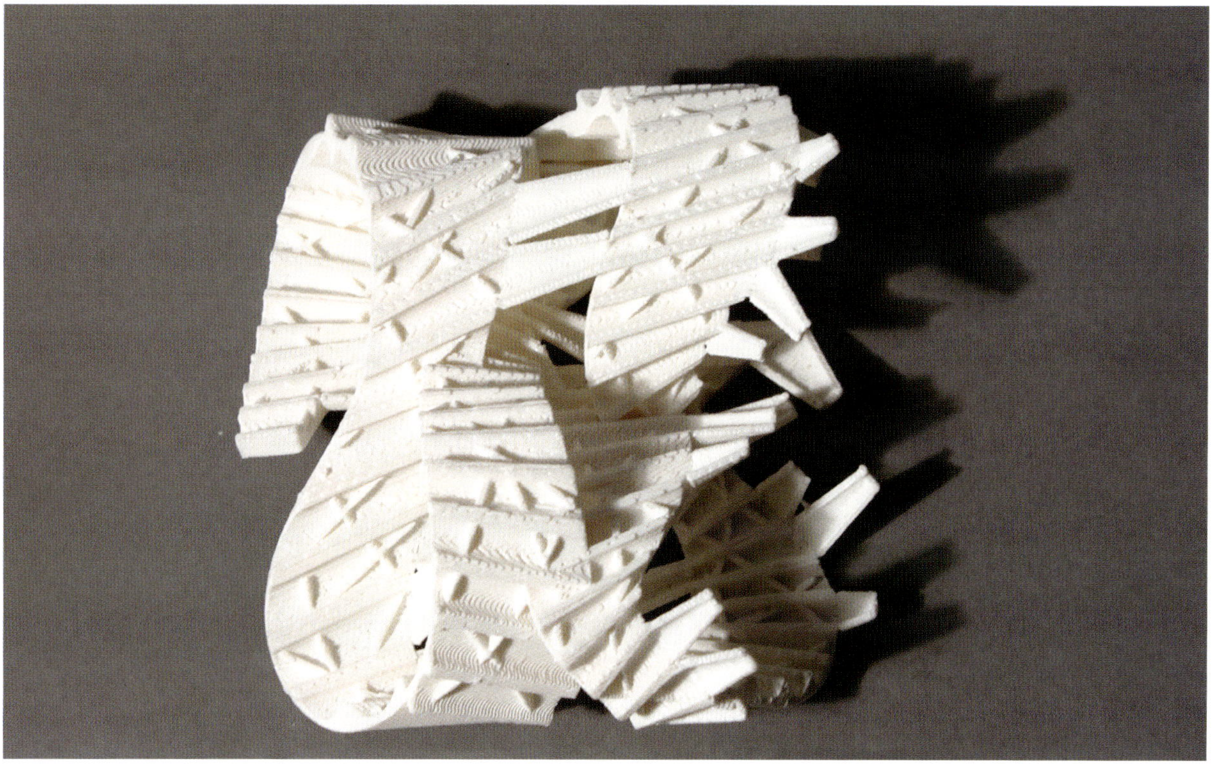

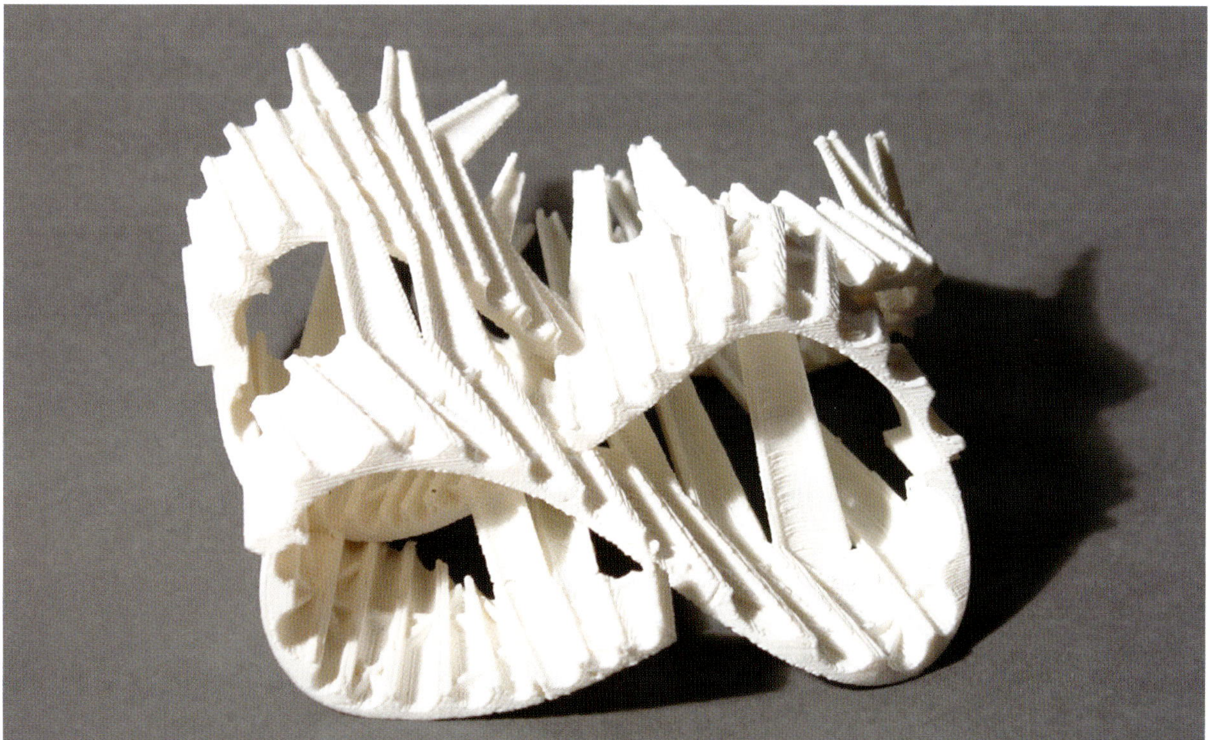

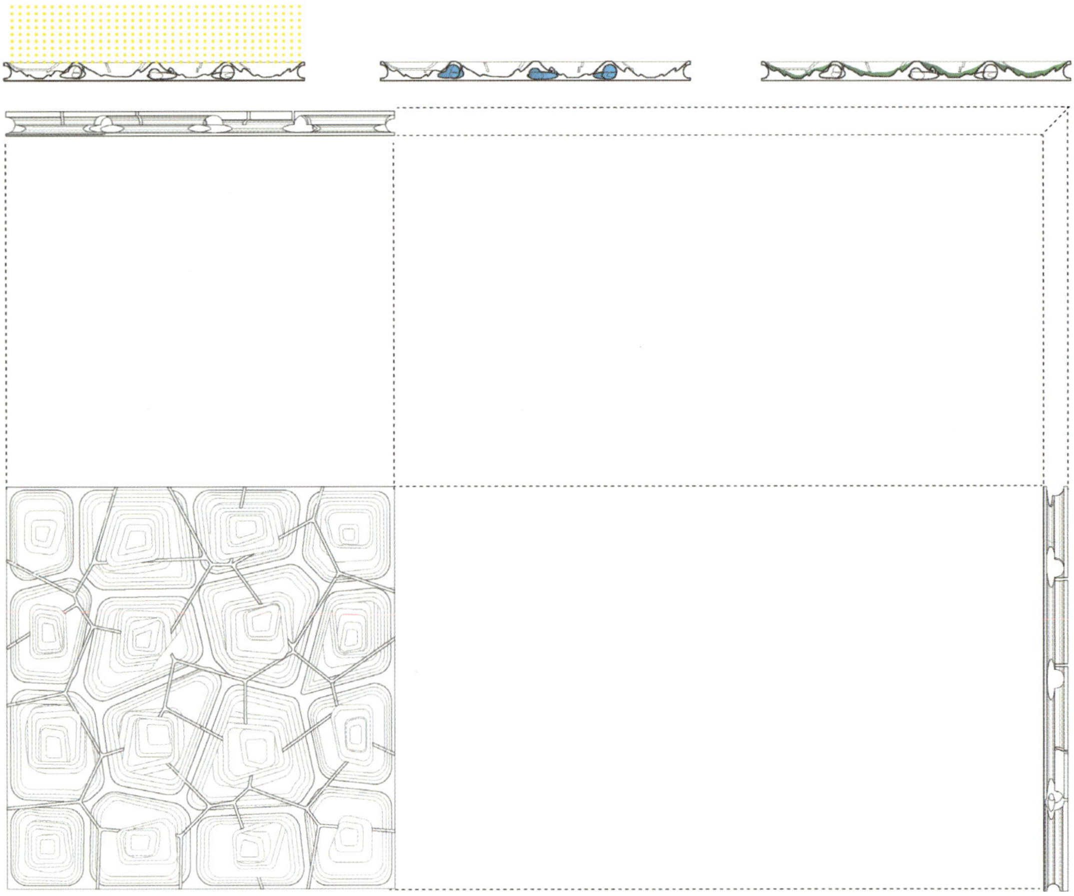

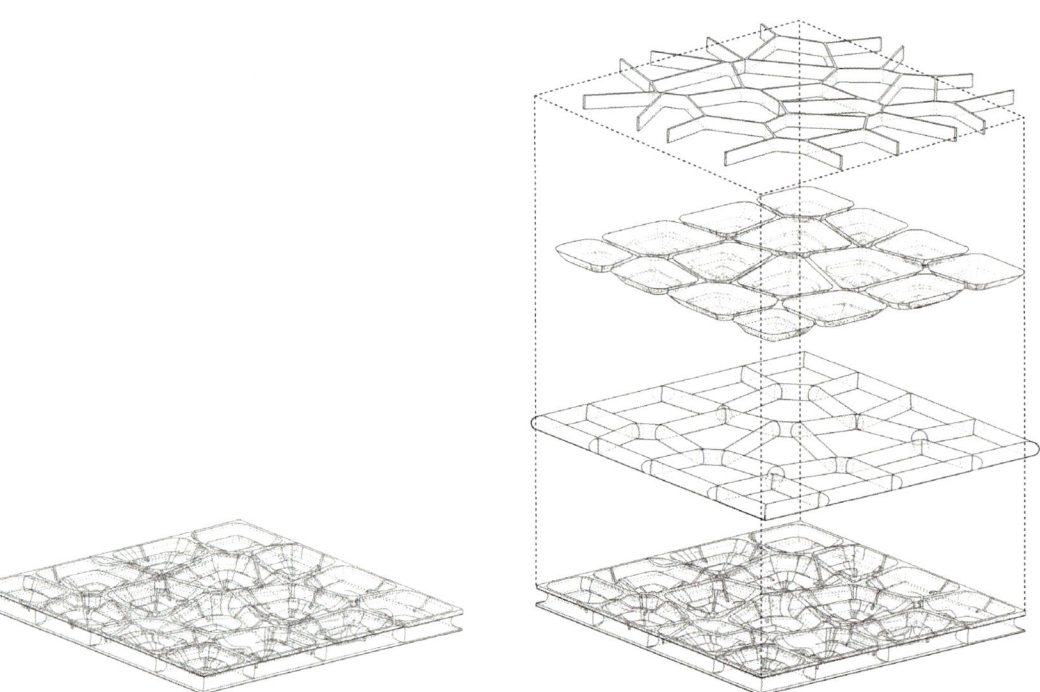

CELLULAR TRANSFORMATIONS

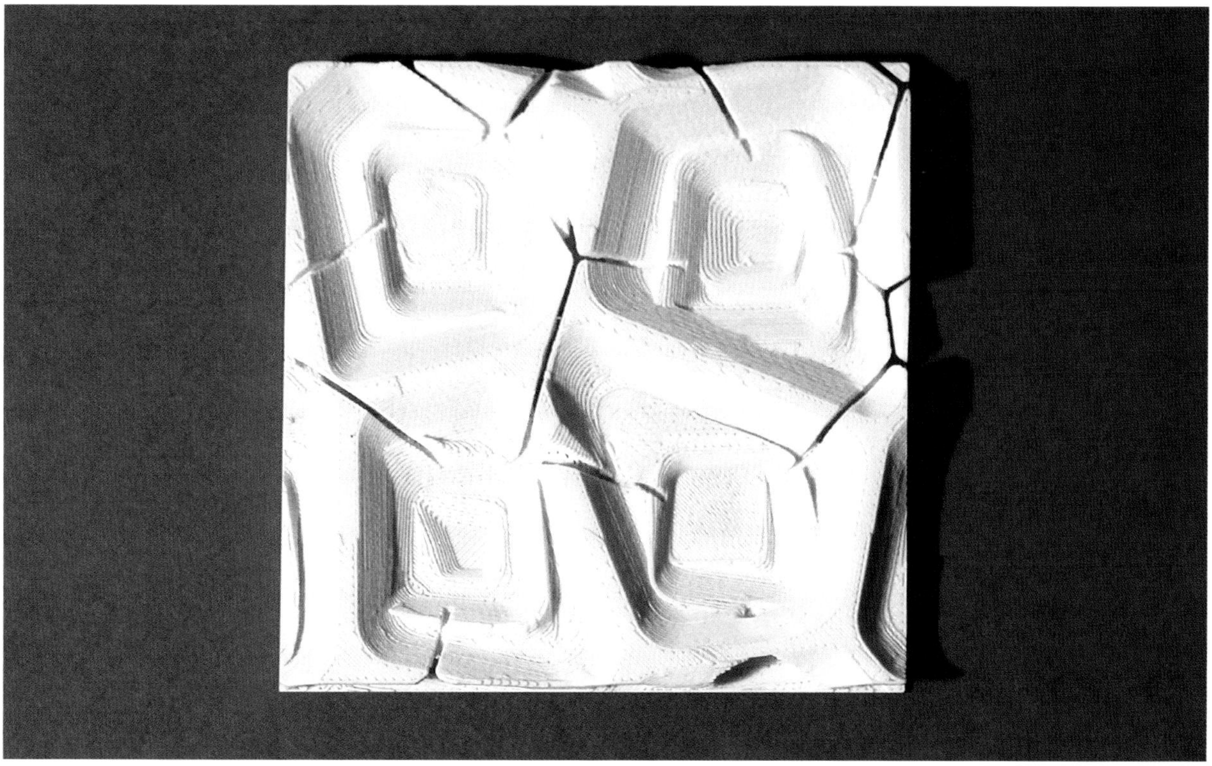

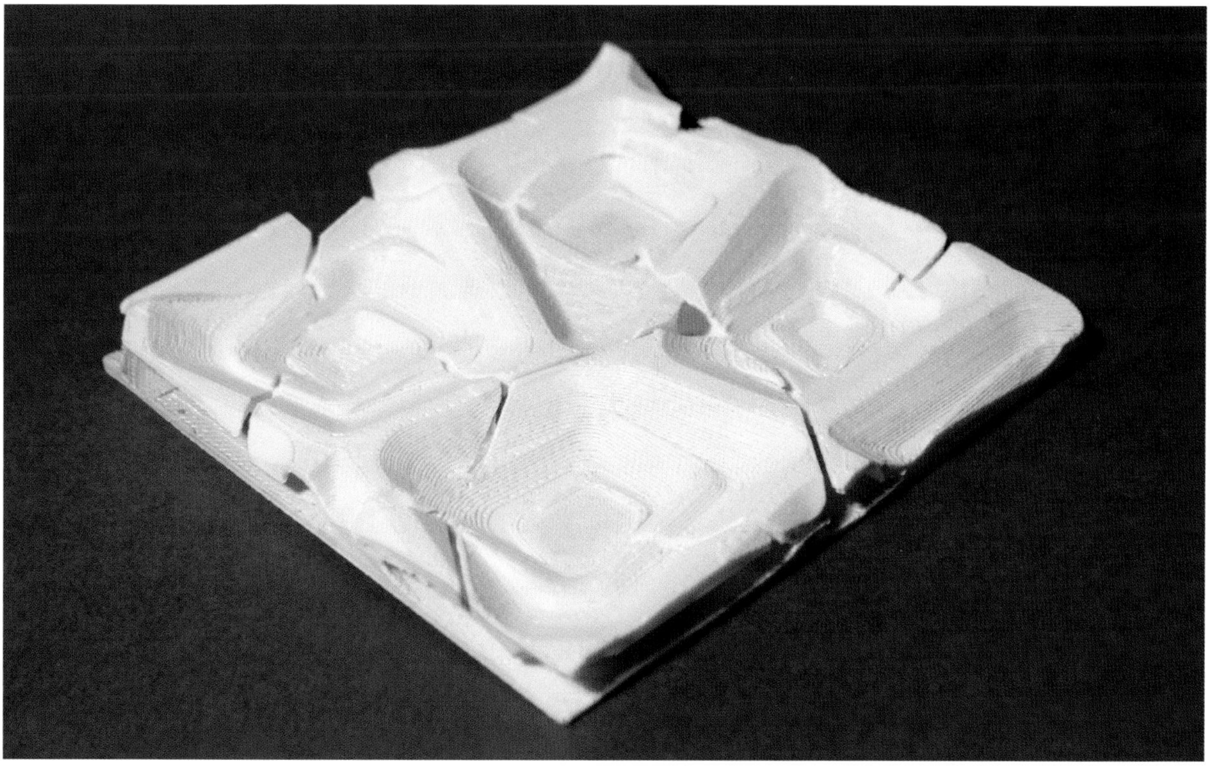

ERIN WONG

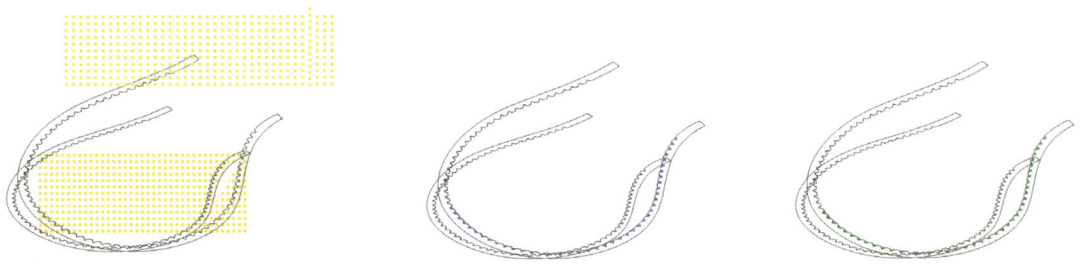

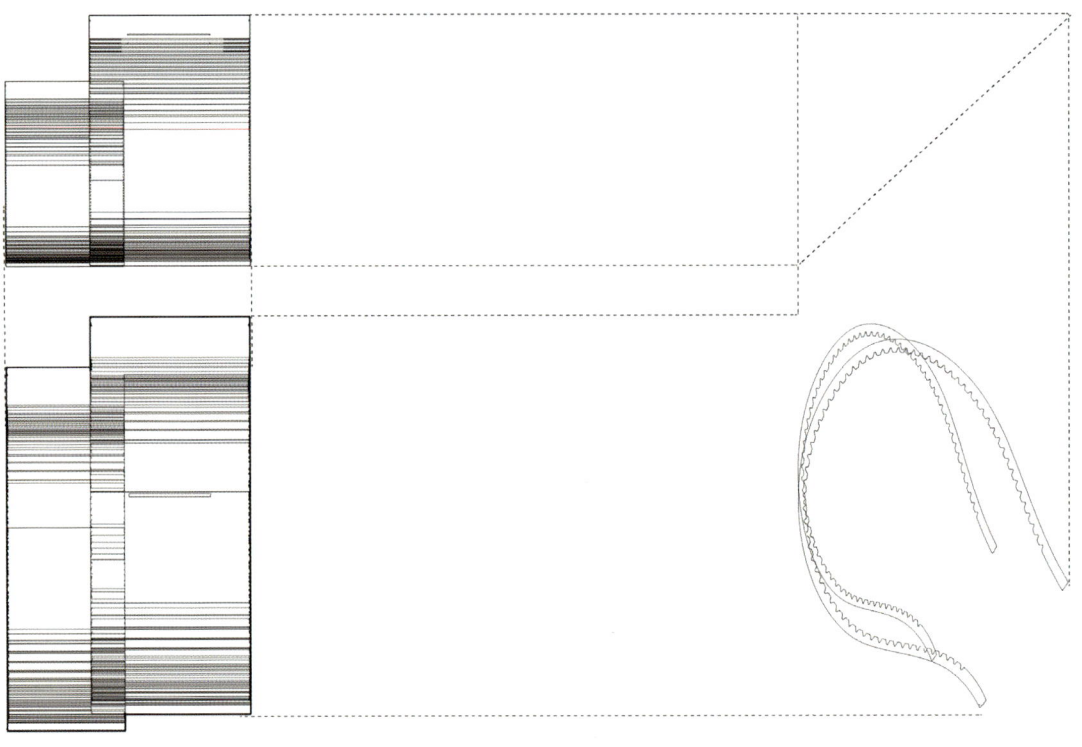

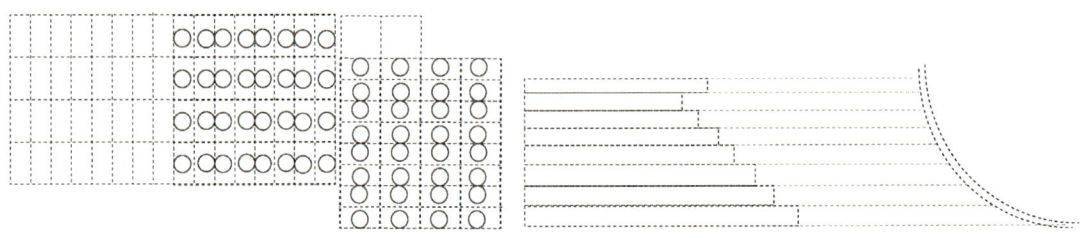

CELLULAR TRANSFORMATIONS

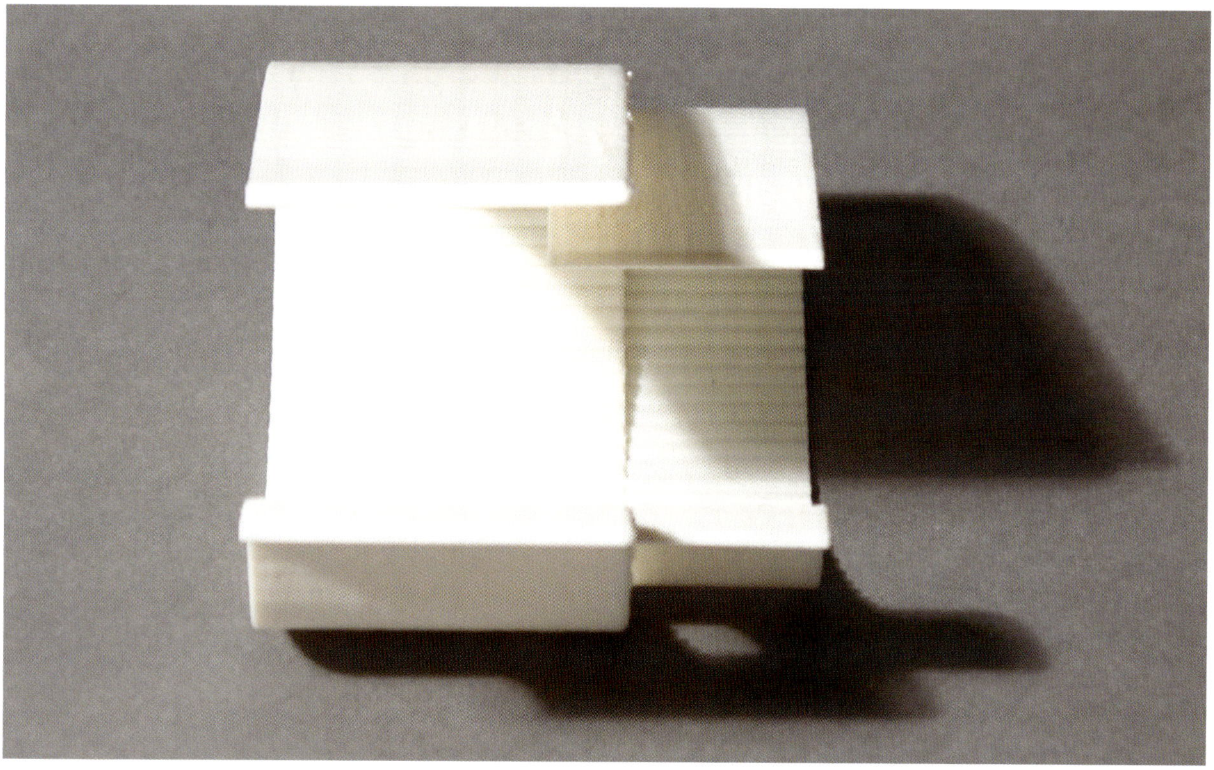

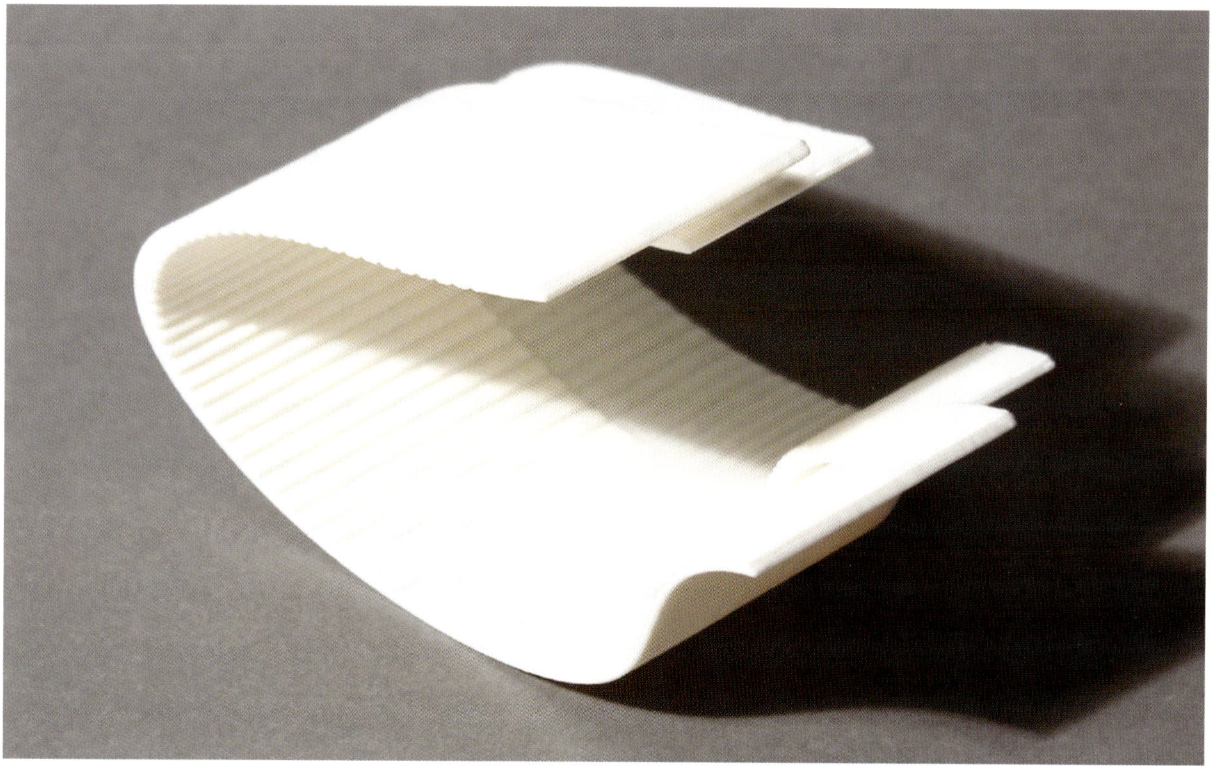

ERIN WONG

SCAFFOLDING RESEARCH

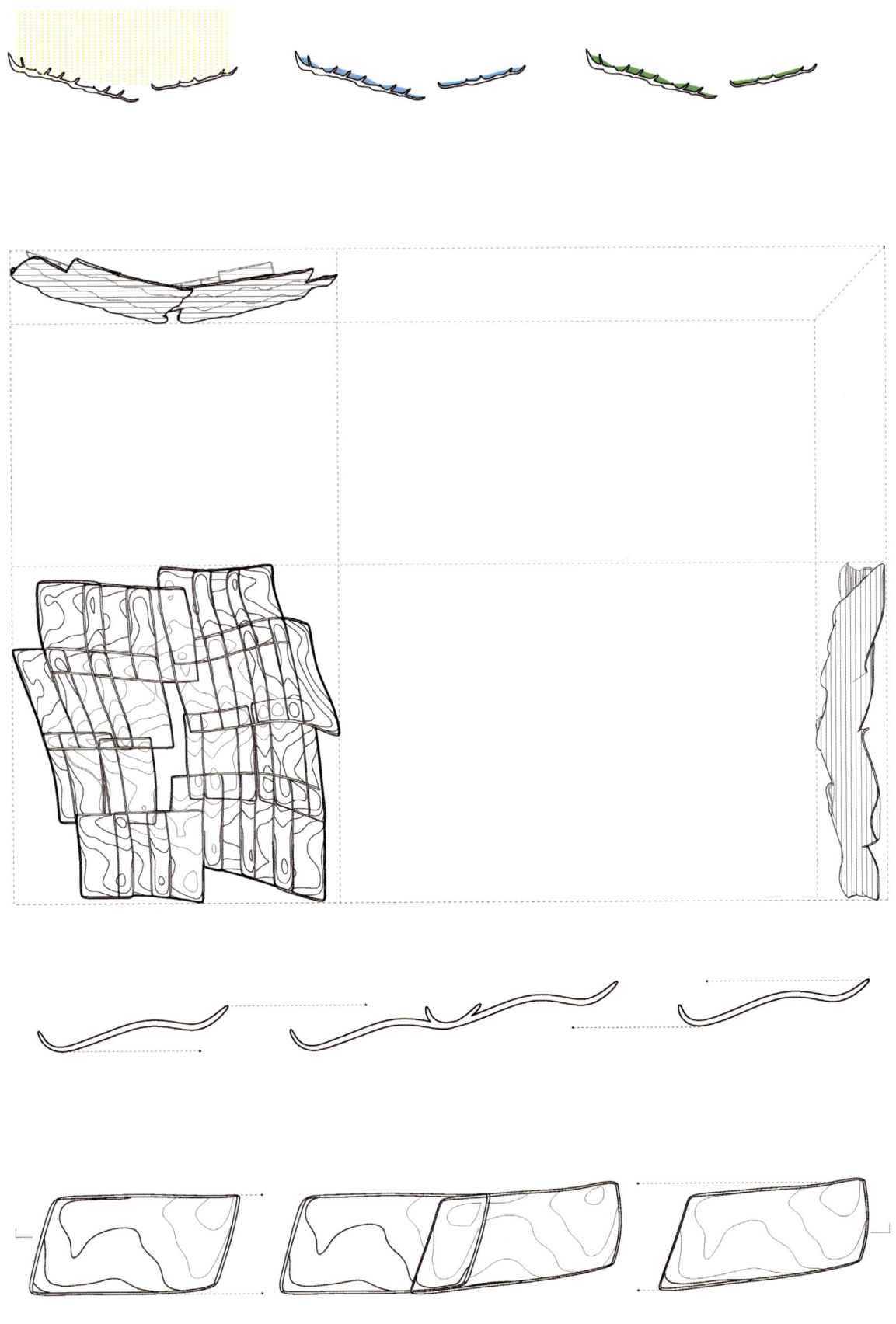

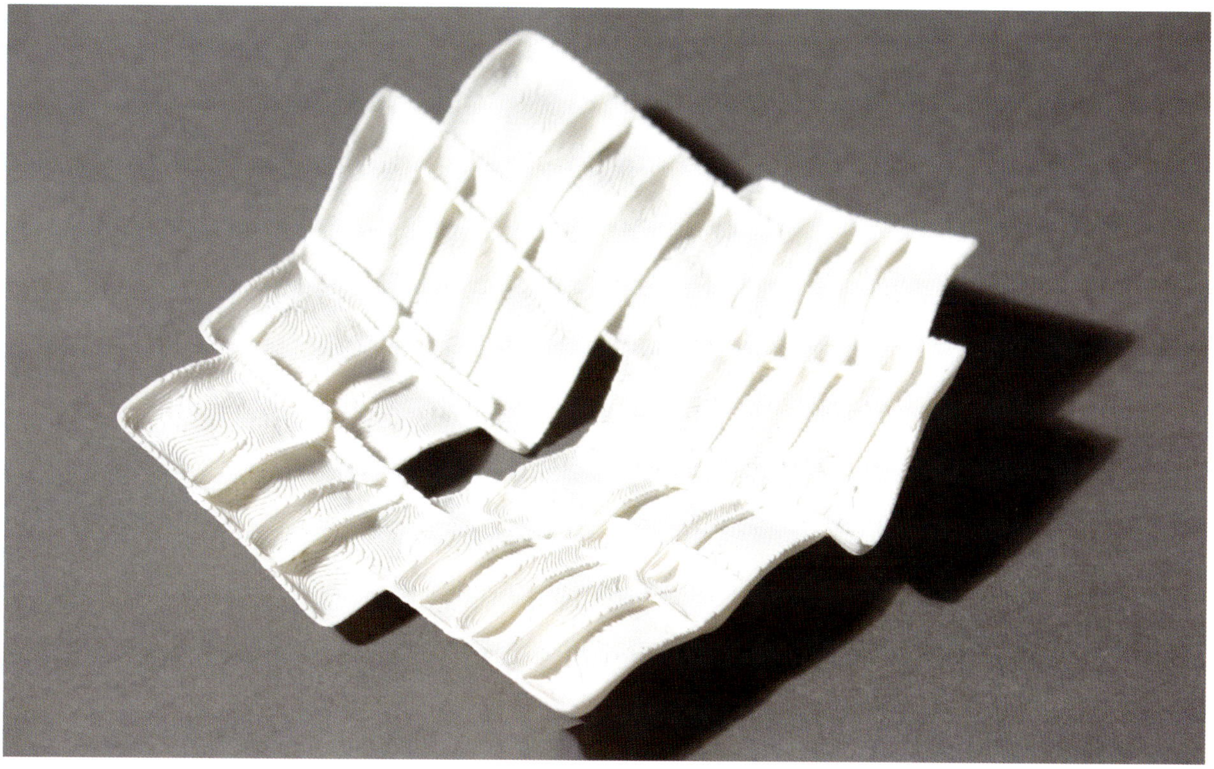

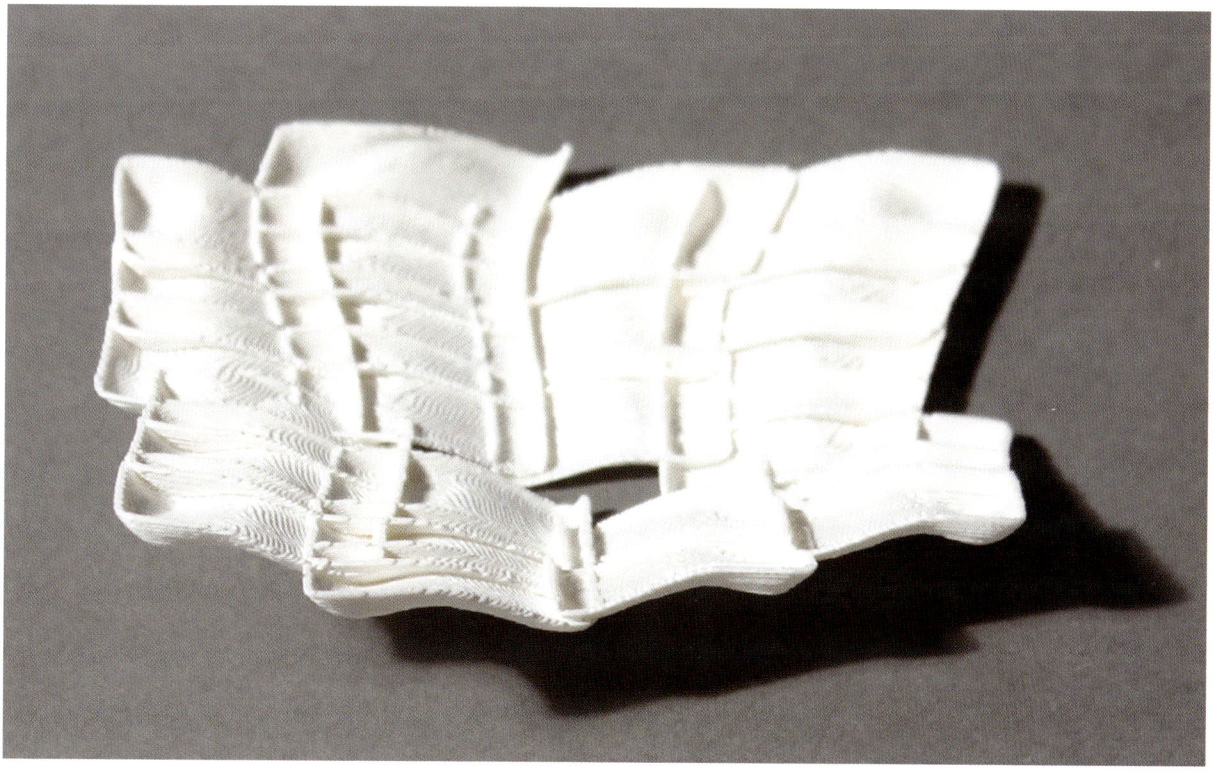

CAITLIN SANDER

SCAFFOLDING RESEARCH 094

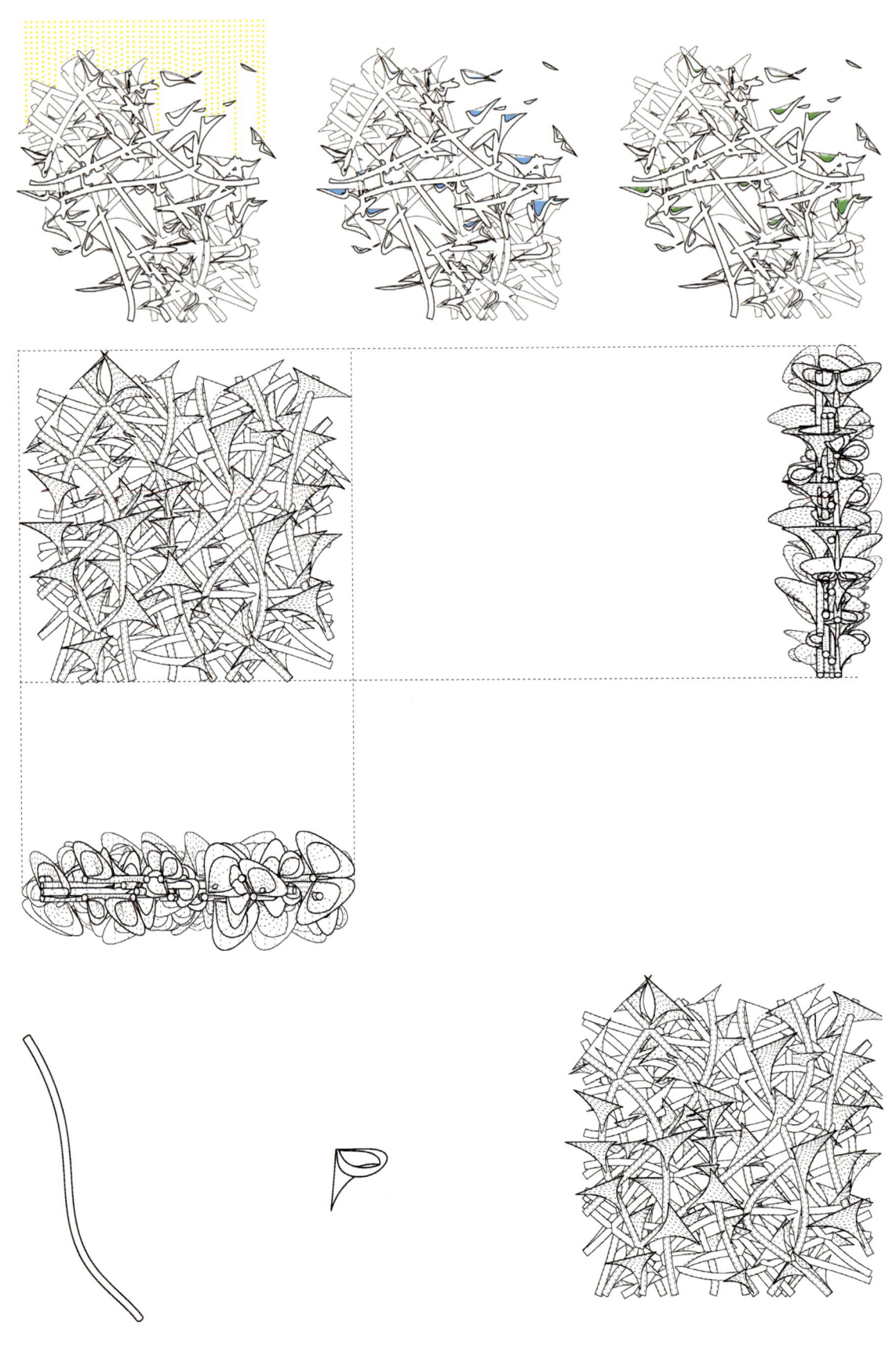

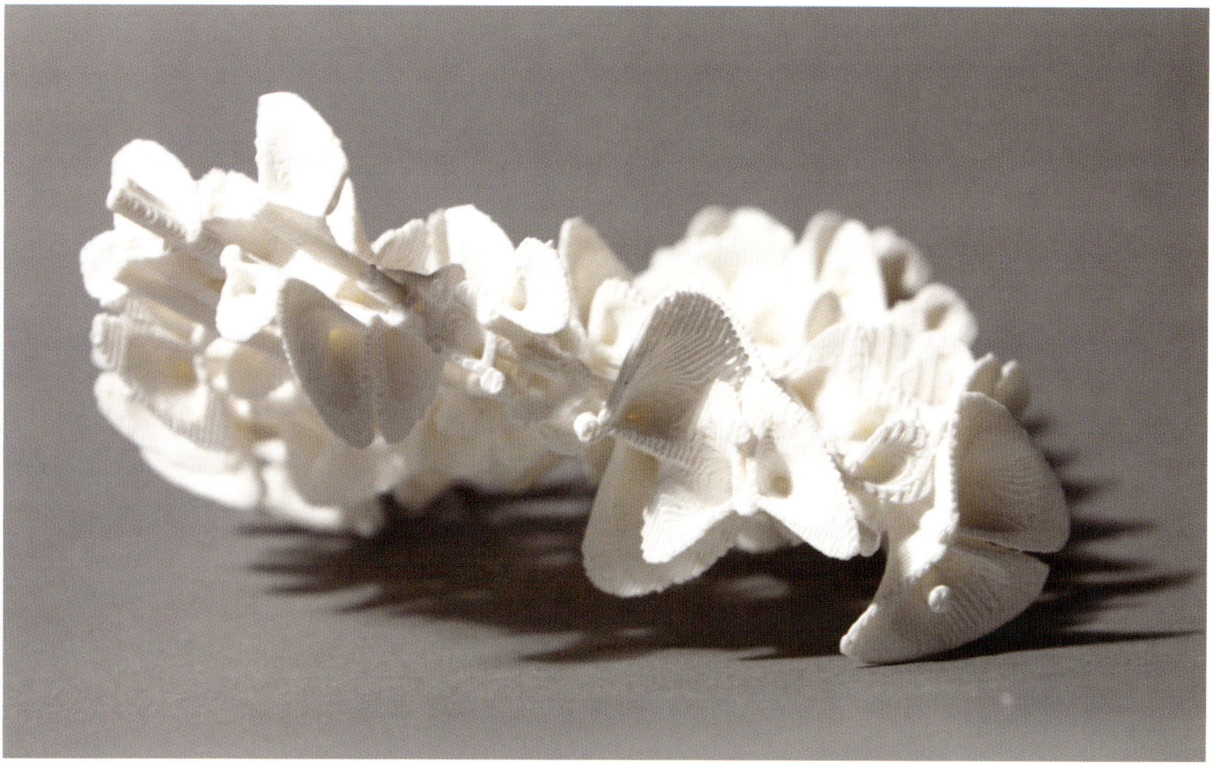

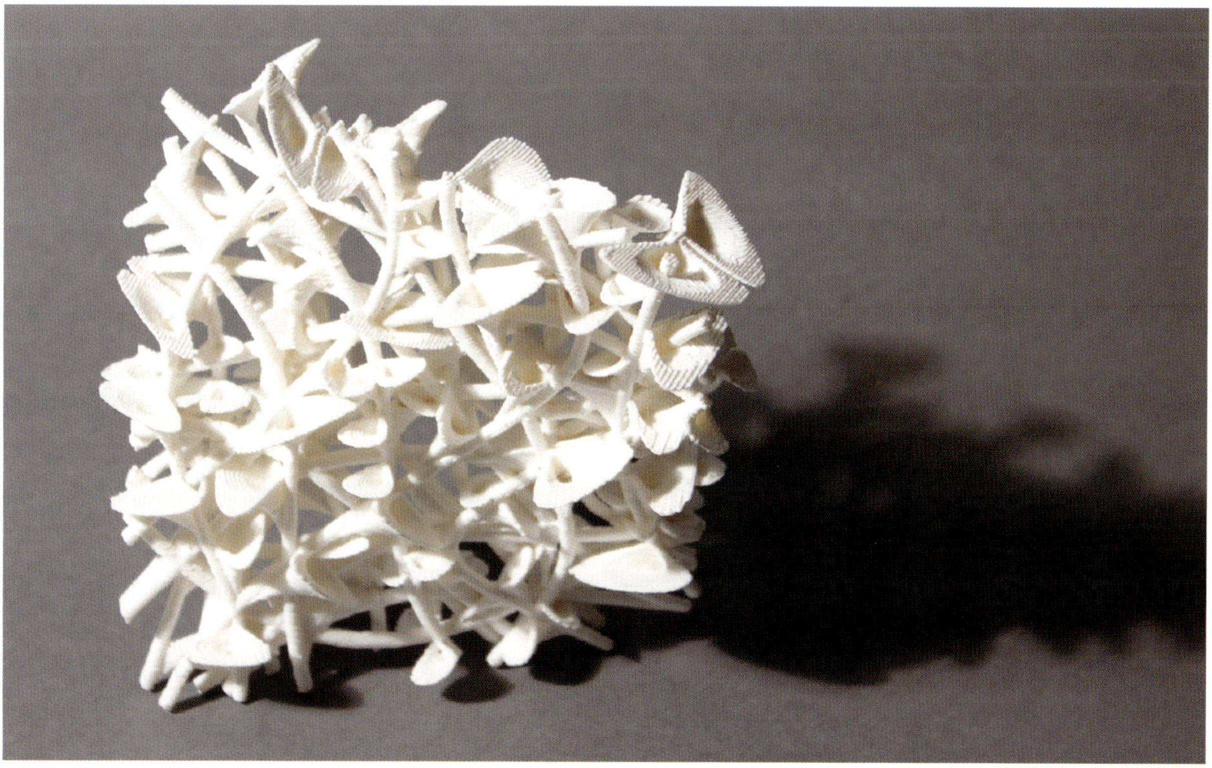

WEN YANG LIN

SCAFFOLDING RESEARCH

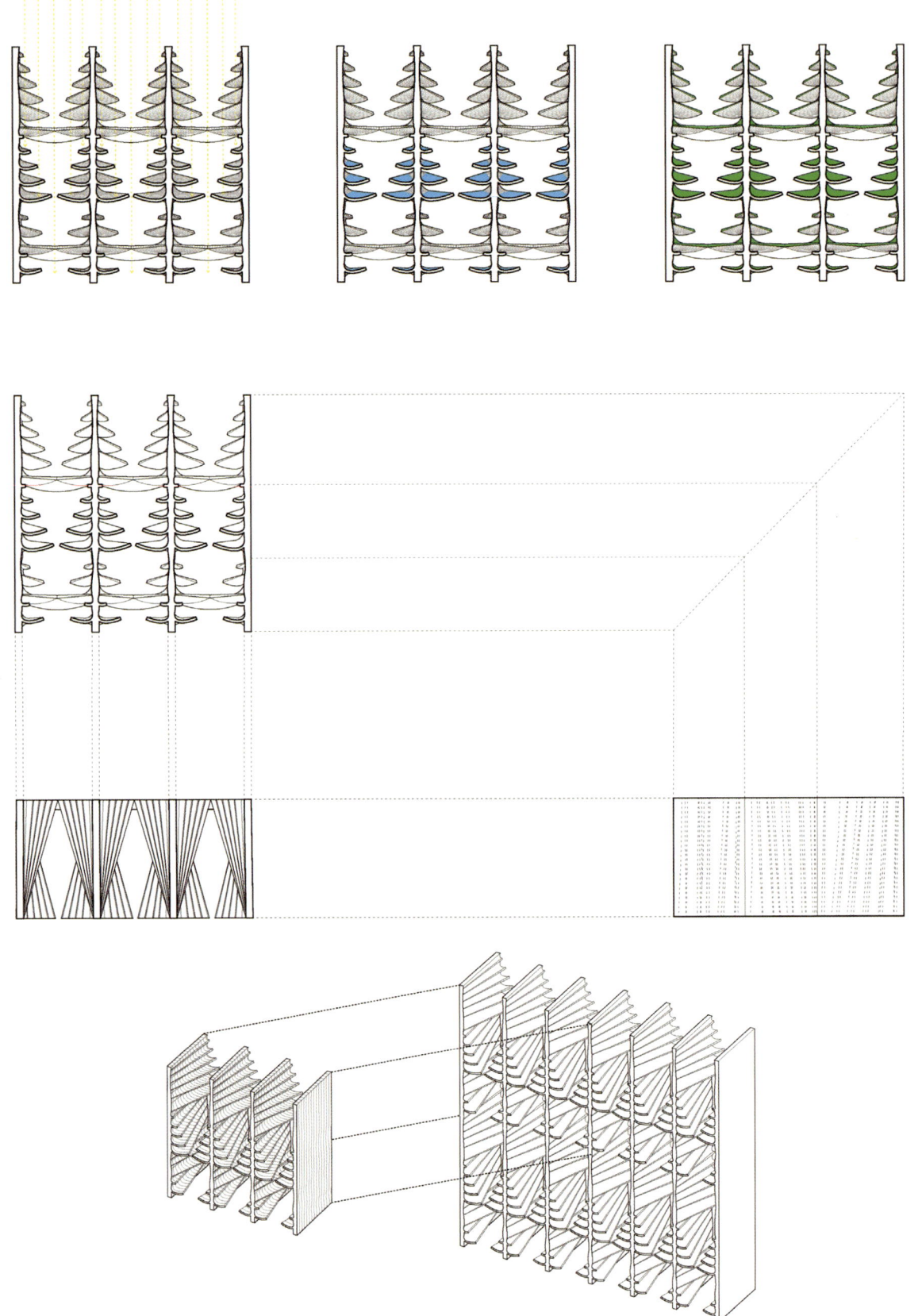

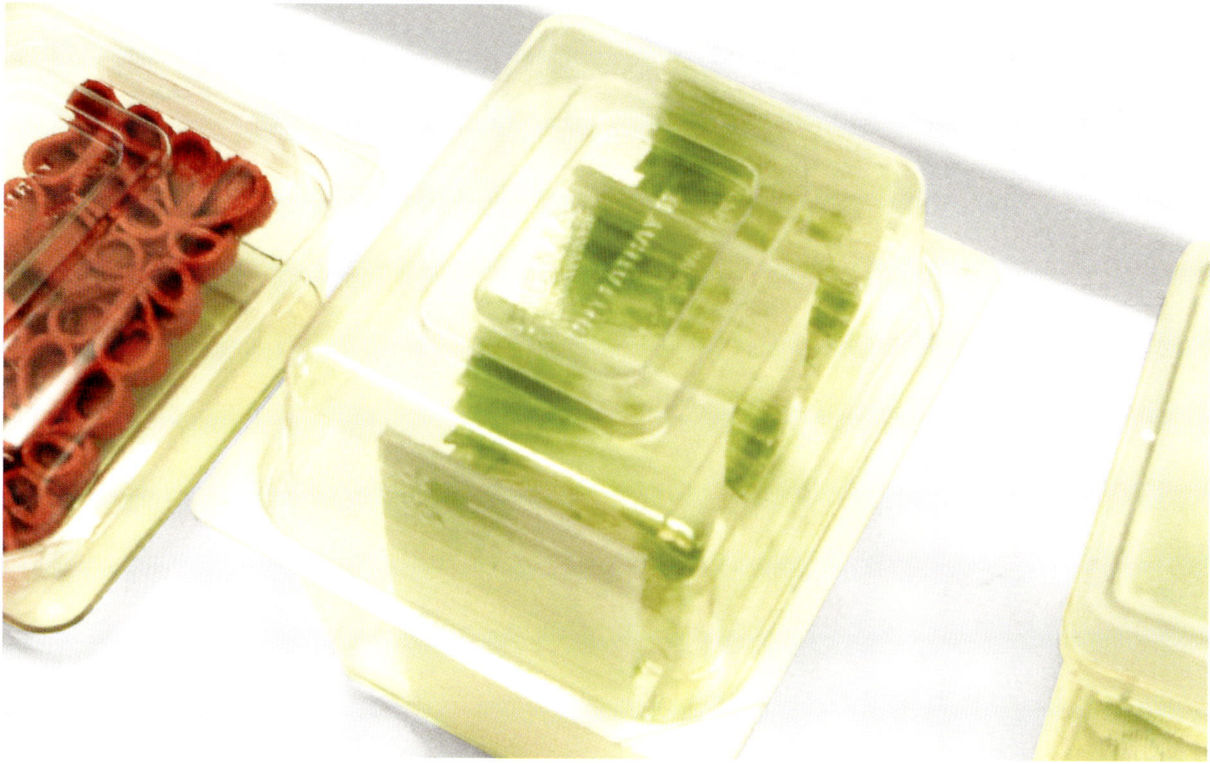

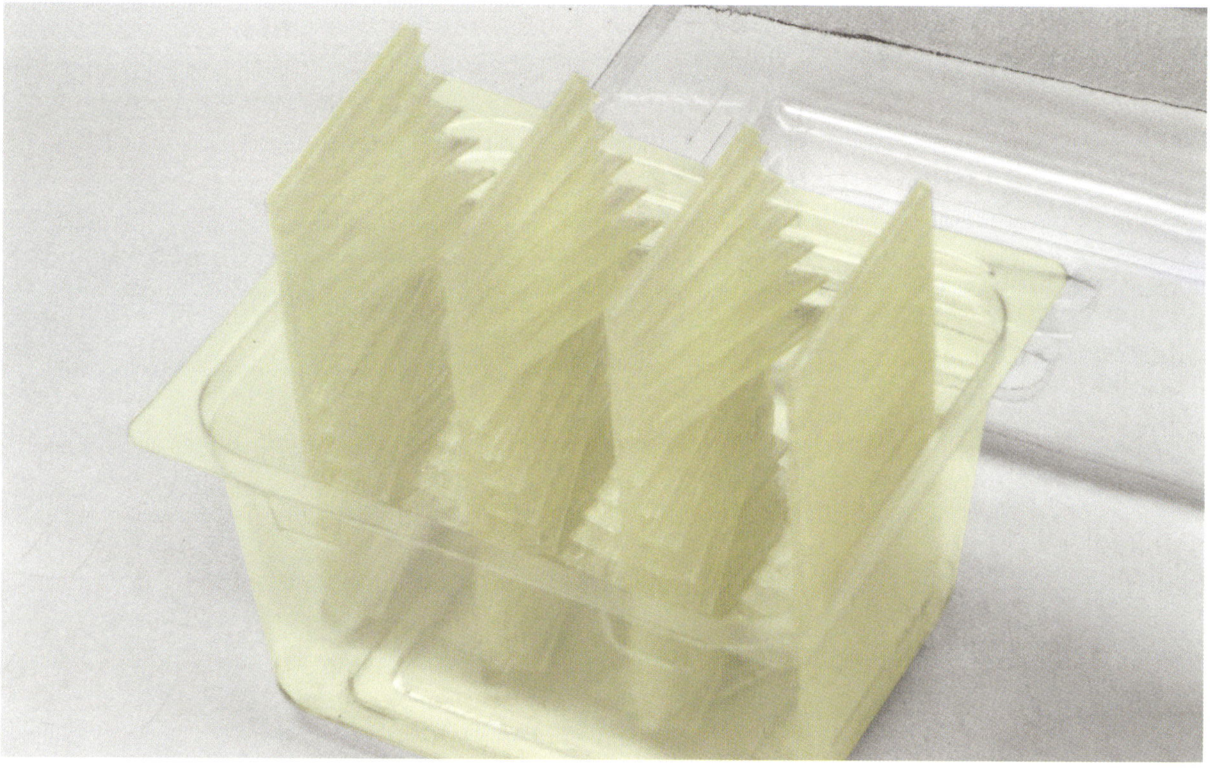

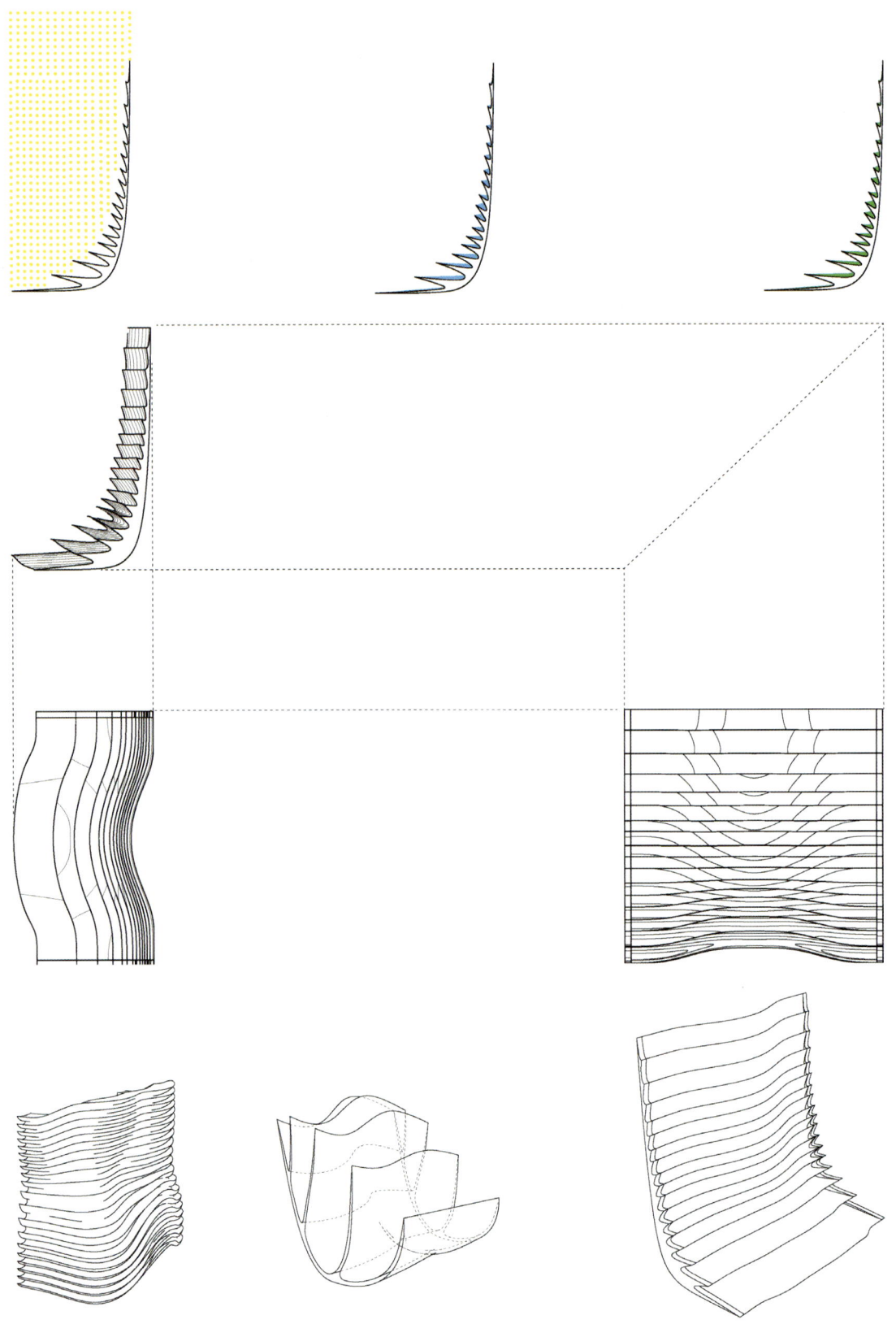

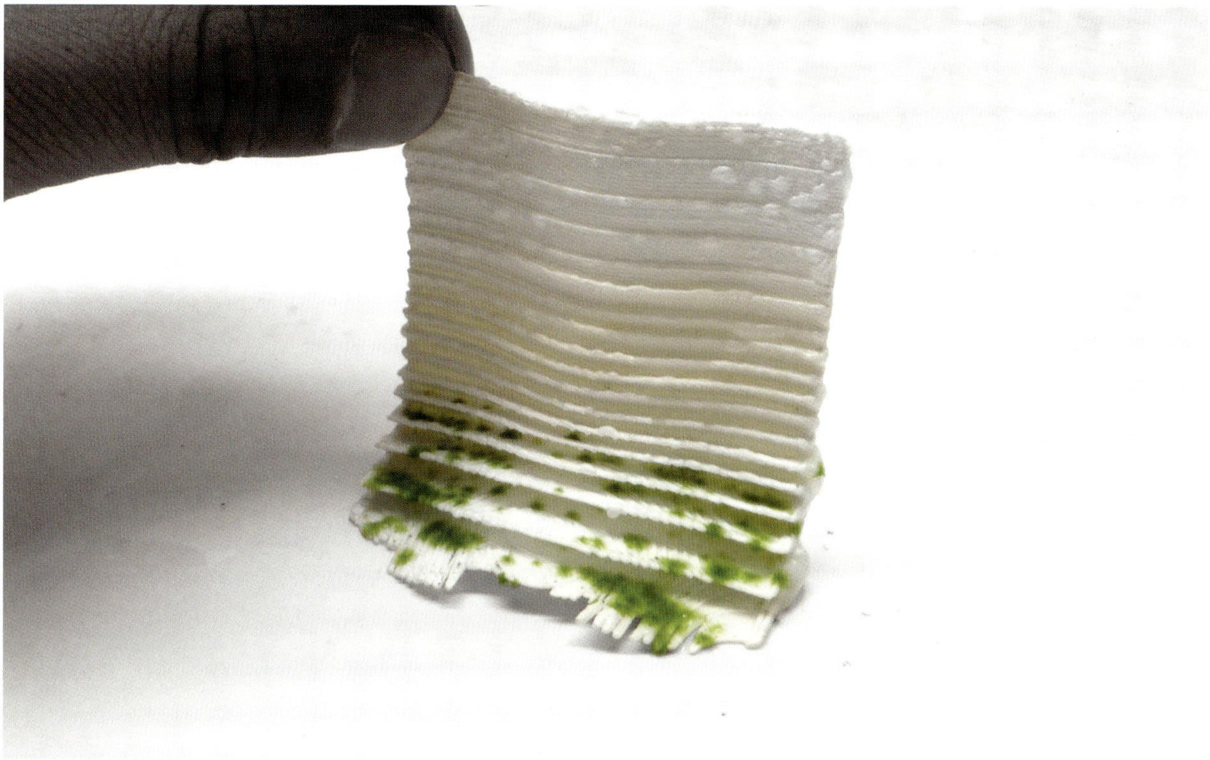

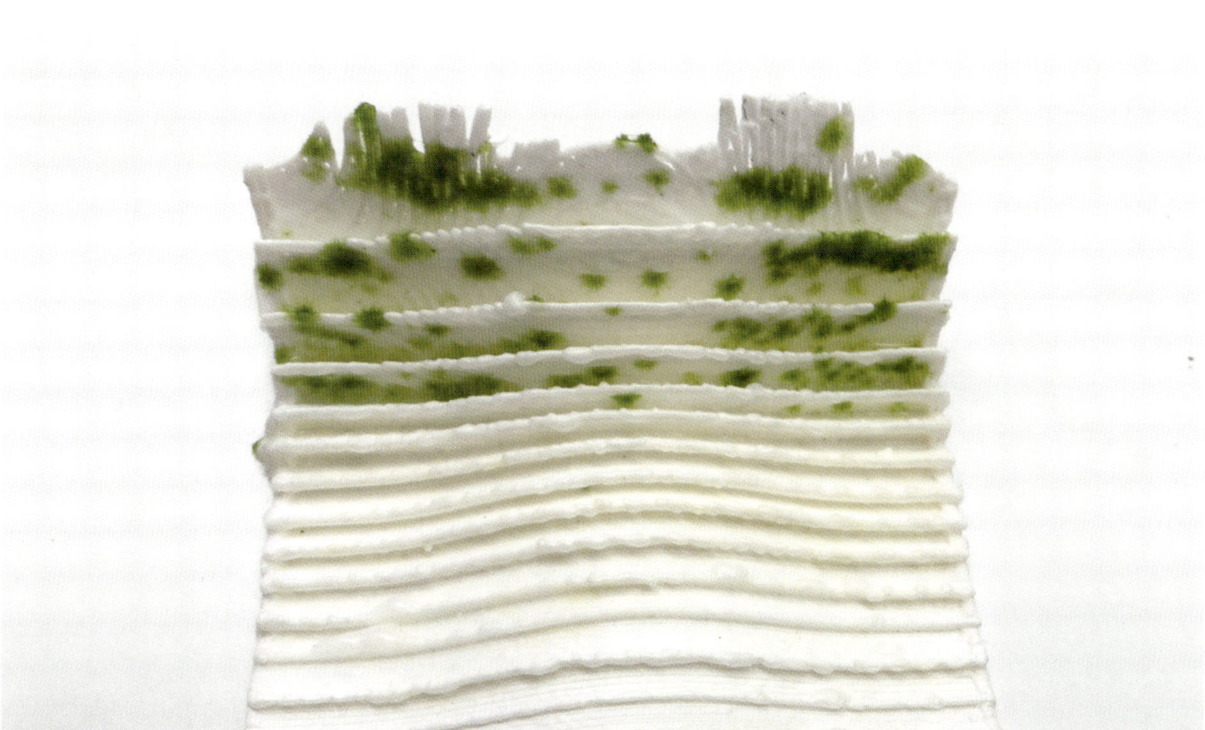

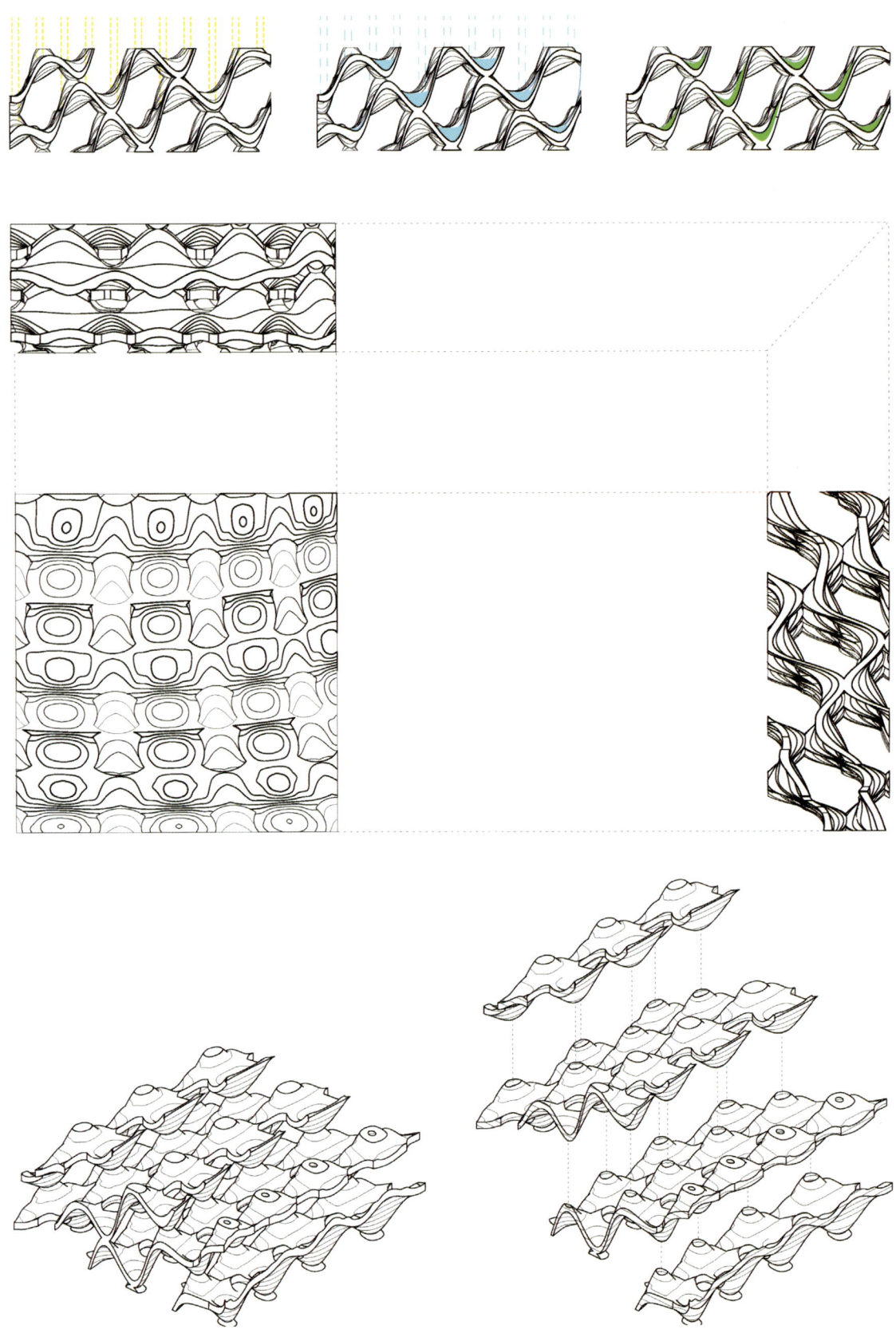

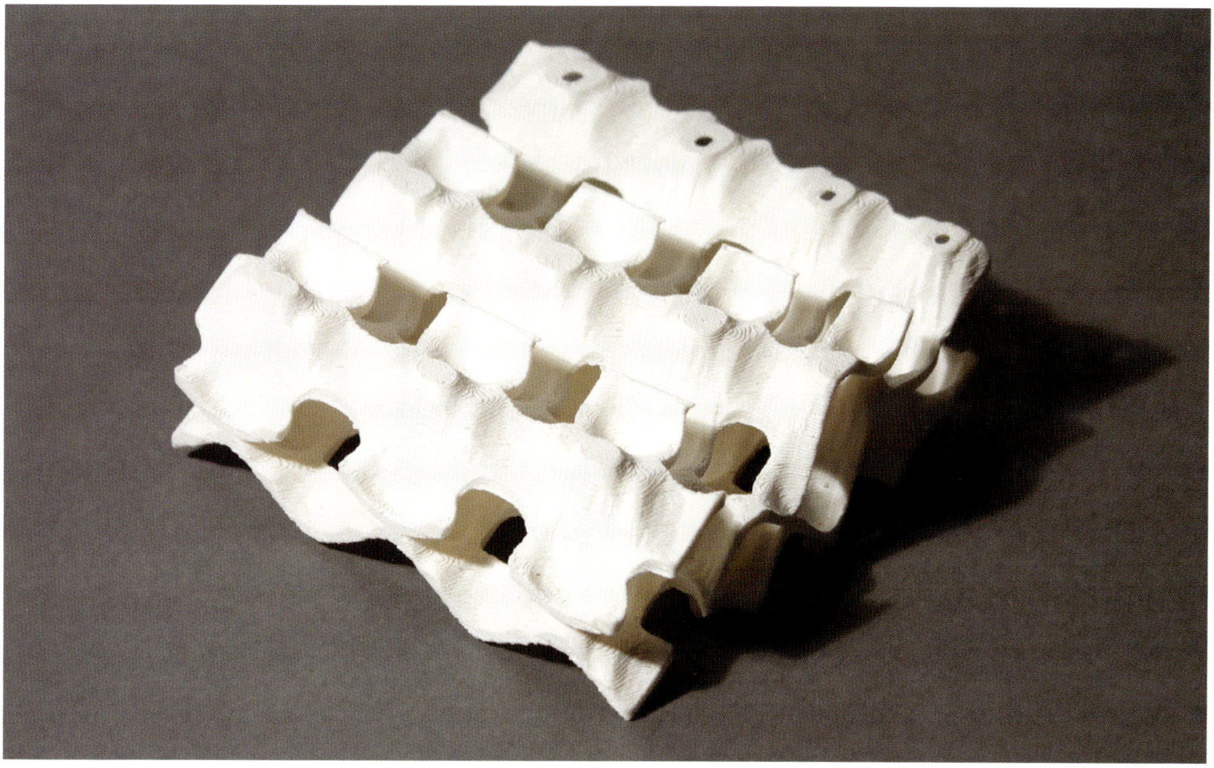

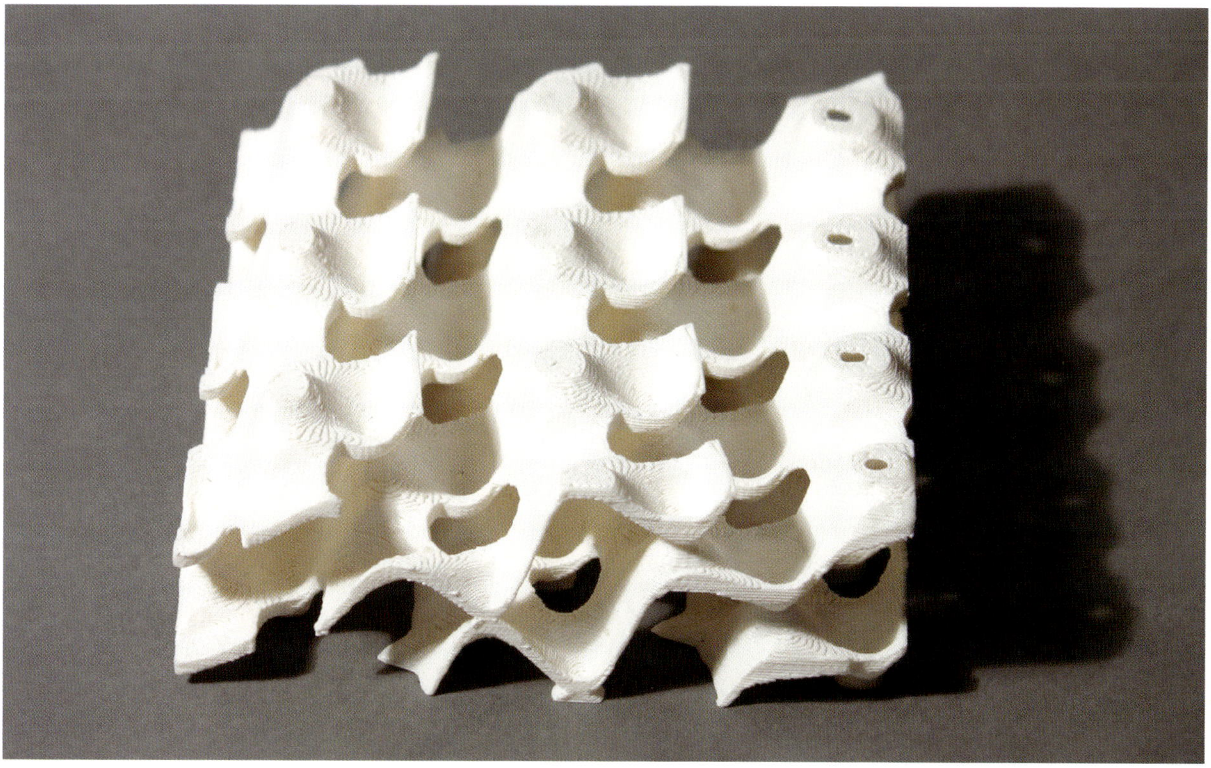

ALLISON BERNETT

SCAFFOLDING RESEARCH

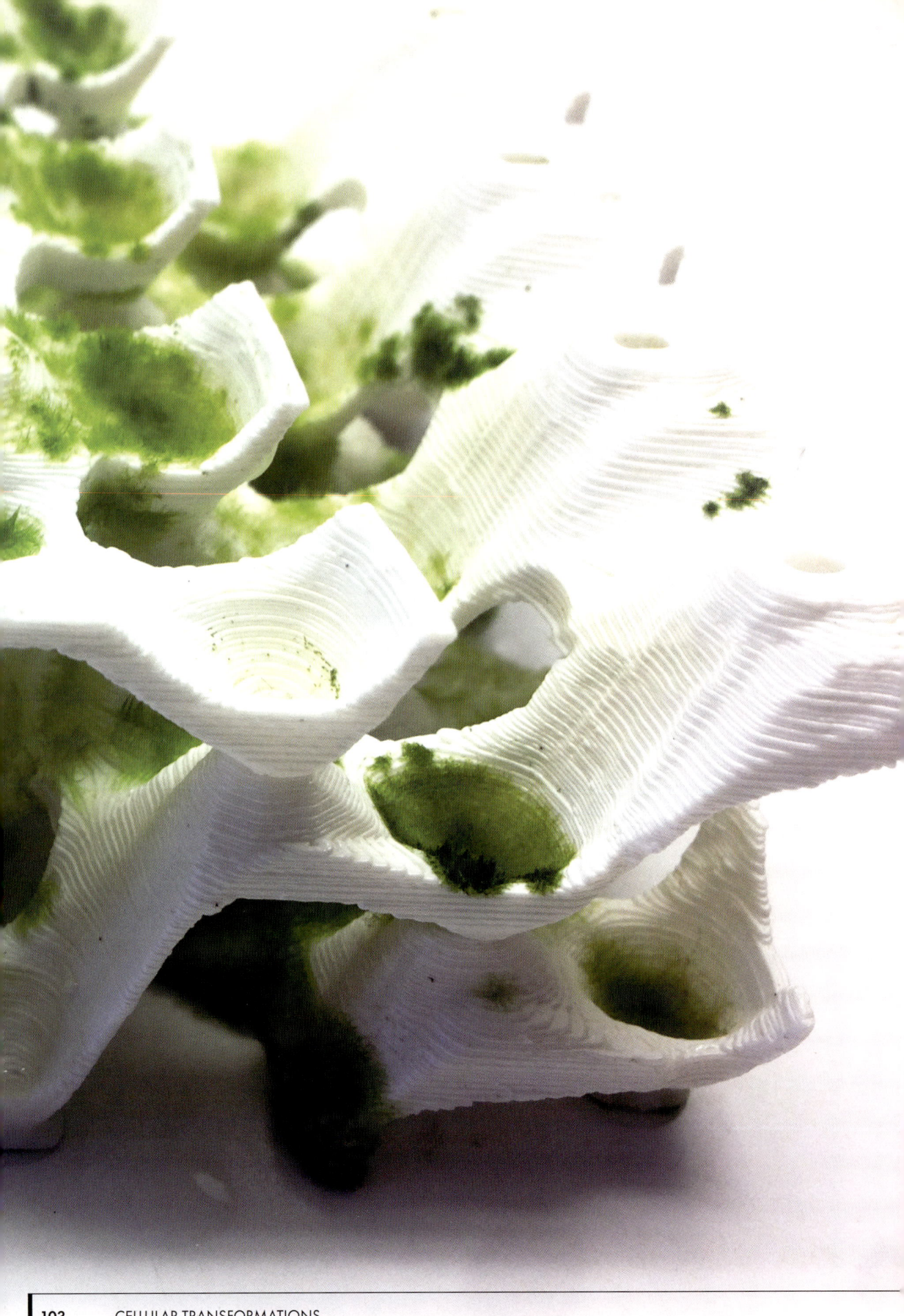

SCAFFOLDINGS: 2013
MICRO-ENVIRONMENTS

Micro-Environments was an extension of the Scaffolding Research project to improve the development of hybrid structures. Generative digital modeling was used to design and optimize artificial scaffolding. Students predicted and tested scaffold performance for nutrient delivery and light penetration as assessed from overall moss growth and surface colonization. This process included multiple design iterations and alterations of the successful designs. The scaffolding was produced using 3D printing technology and the resolutions of the scaffolding printouts created texture elements that enabled water and nutrient channeling to varying degrees based on the design. Thus, the artificial scaffolds served as a form of bioprinting to control cell growth and this project explored the implementation of organic matter into design solutions with potential real-world applications.

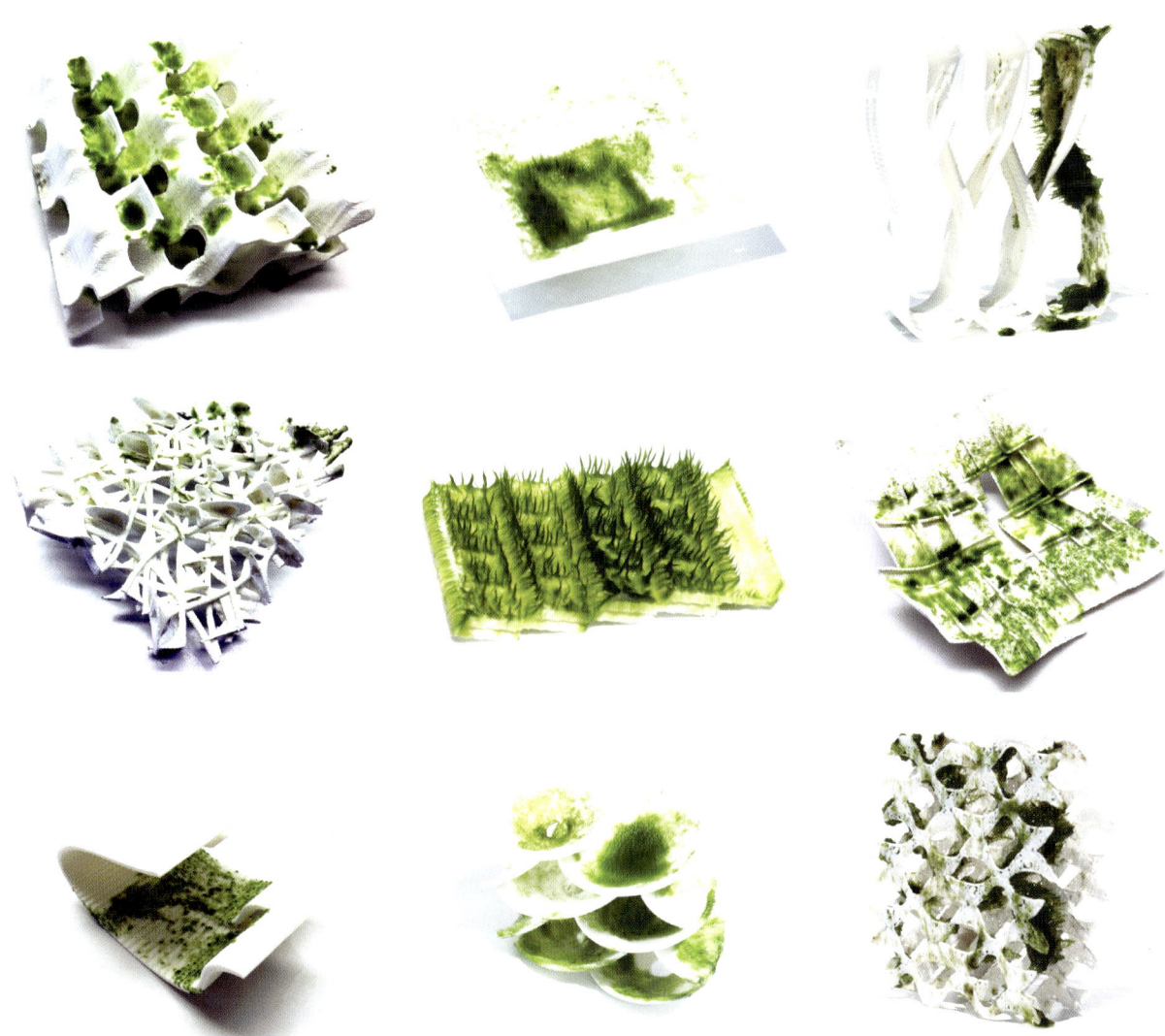

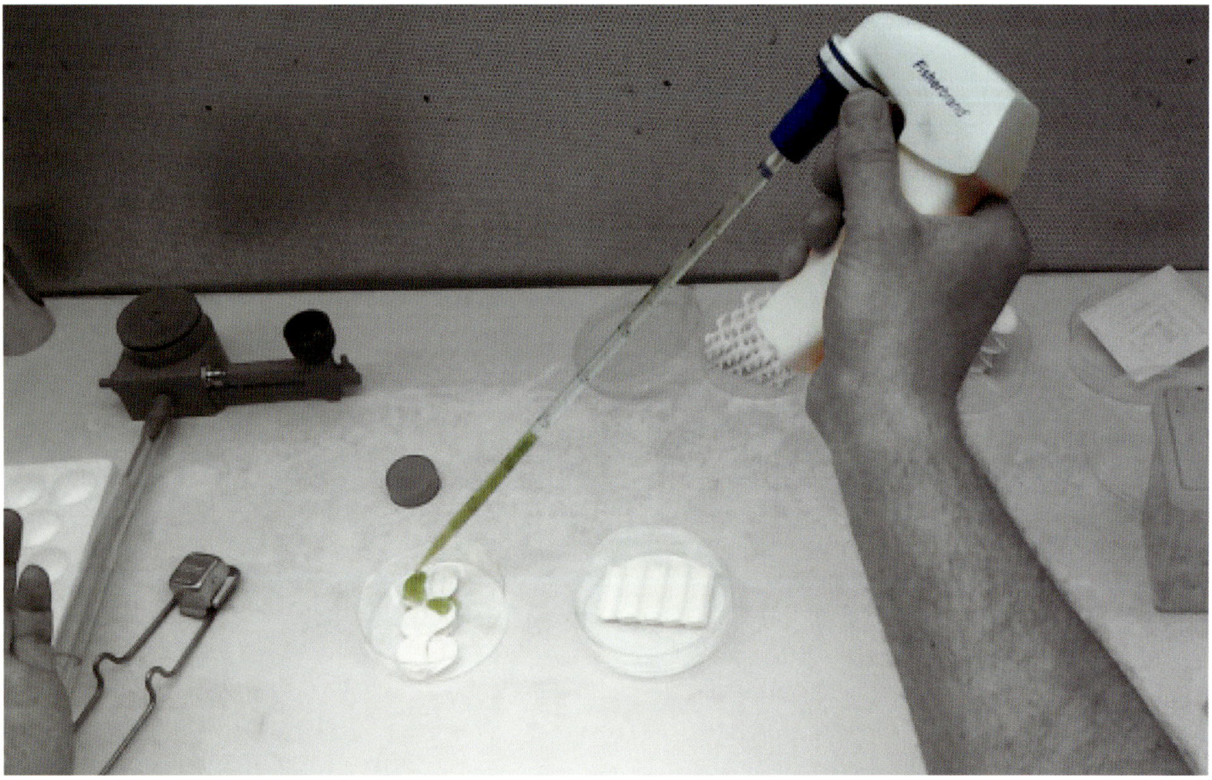

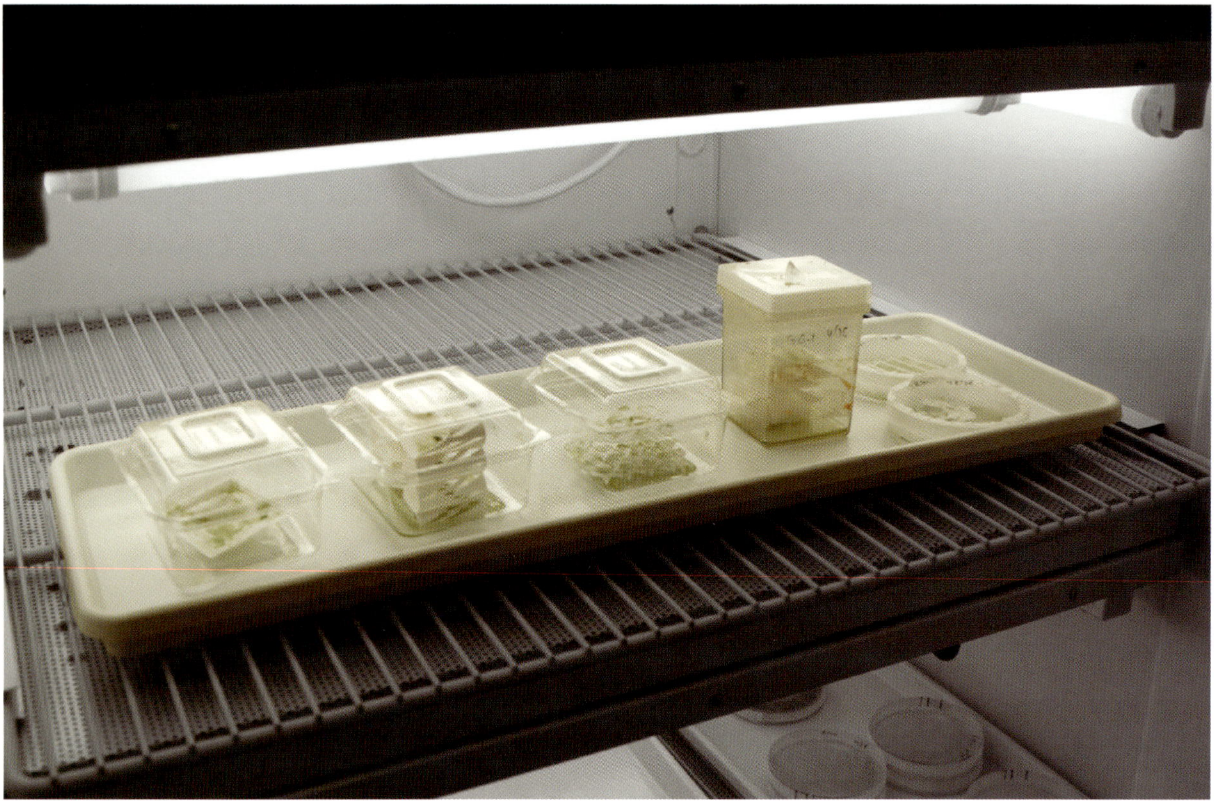

MENGYING BAI | ALLISON BERNETT | AMBER IBARRA | WEN YANG LIN | NHU NGUYEN

CELLULAR TRANSFORMATIONS

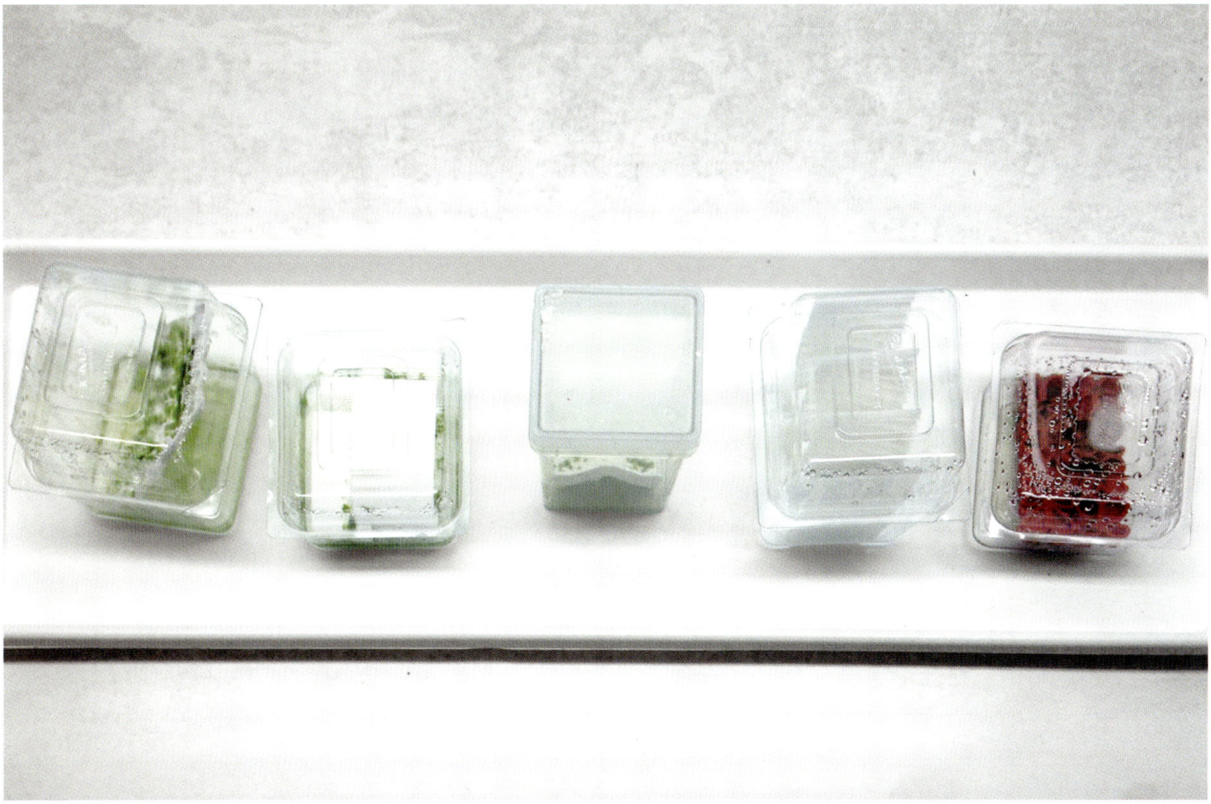

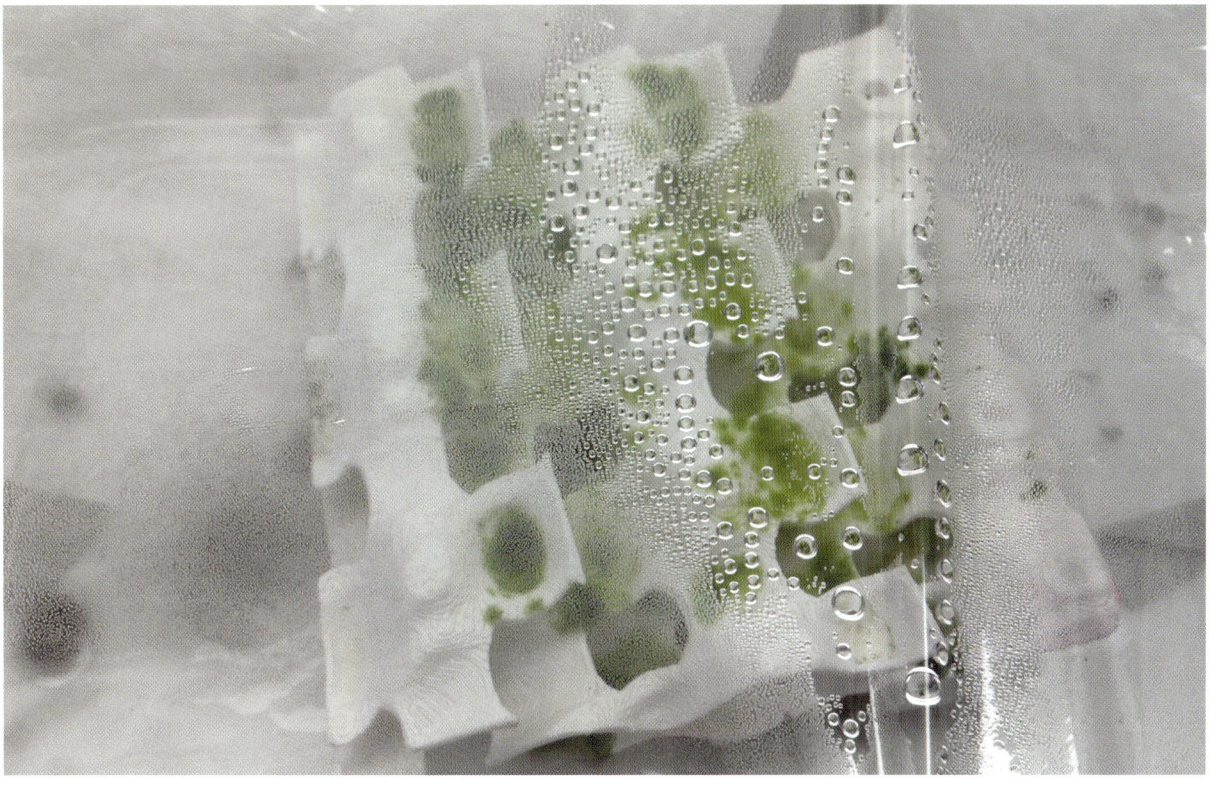

MICHAEL POLITTE | CAITLIN SANDERS | HARRISON WERNER | ERIN WONG | ZHAN YANG | KUAI YU

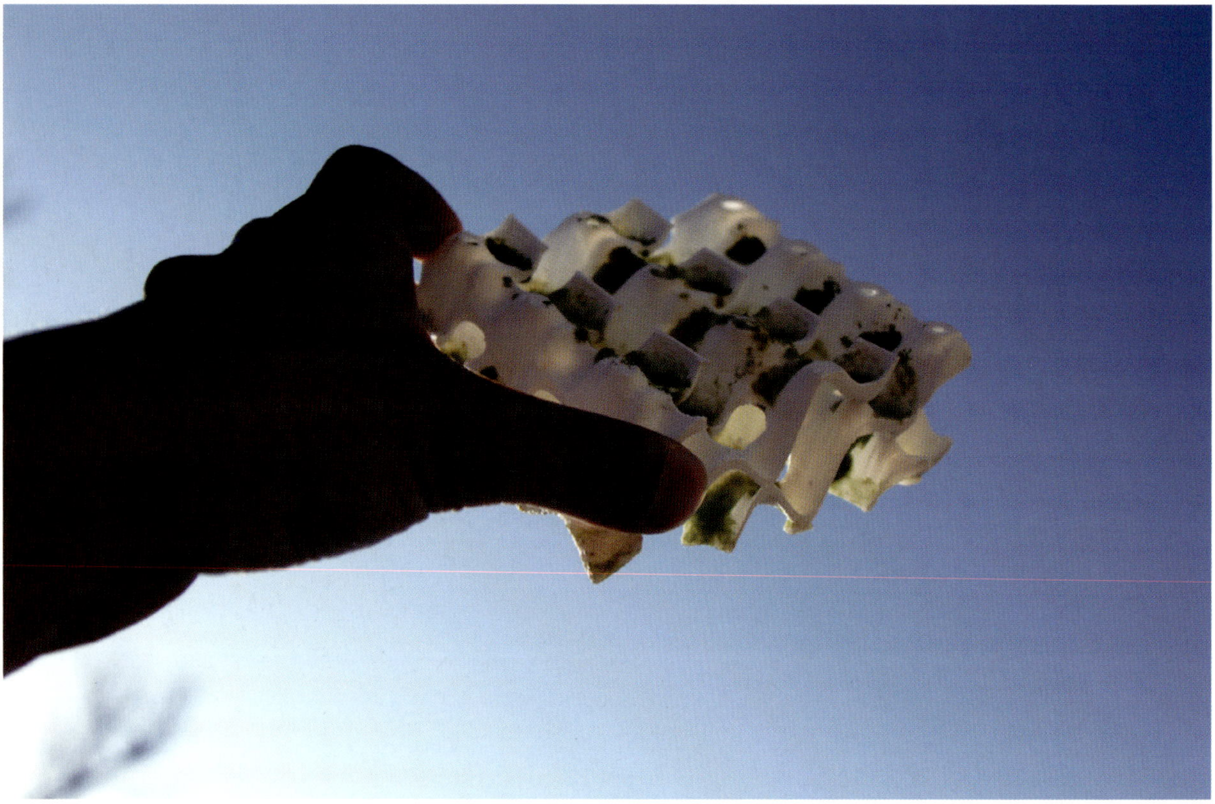

MENGYING BAI | ALLISON BERNETT | AMBER IBARRA | WEN YANG LIN | NHU NGUYEN

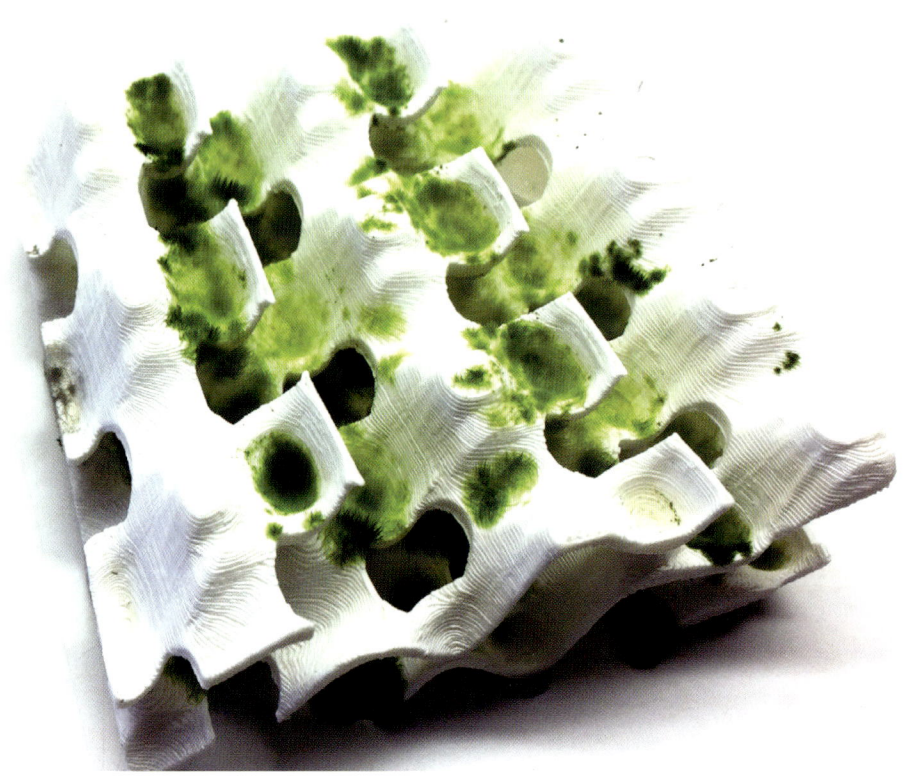

CELLULAR TRANSFORMATIONS

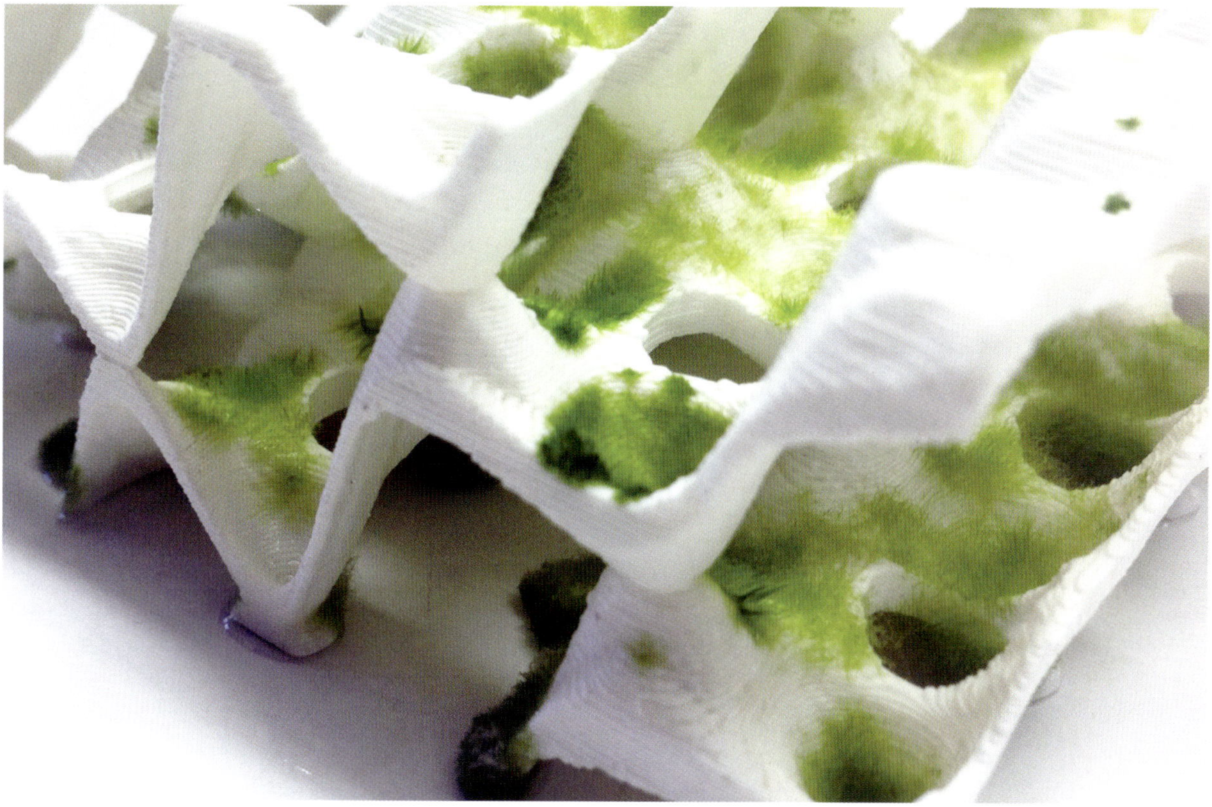

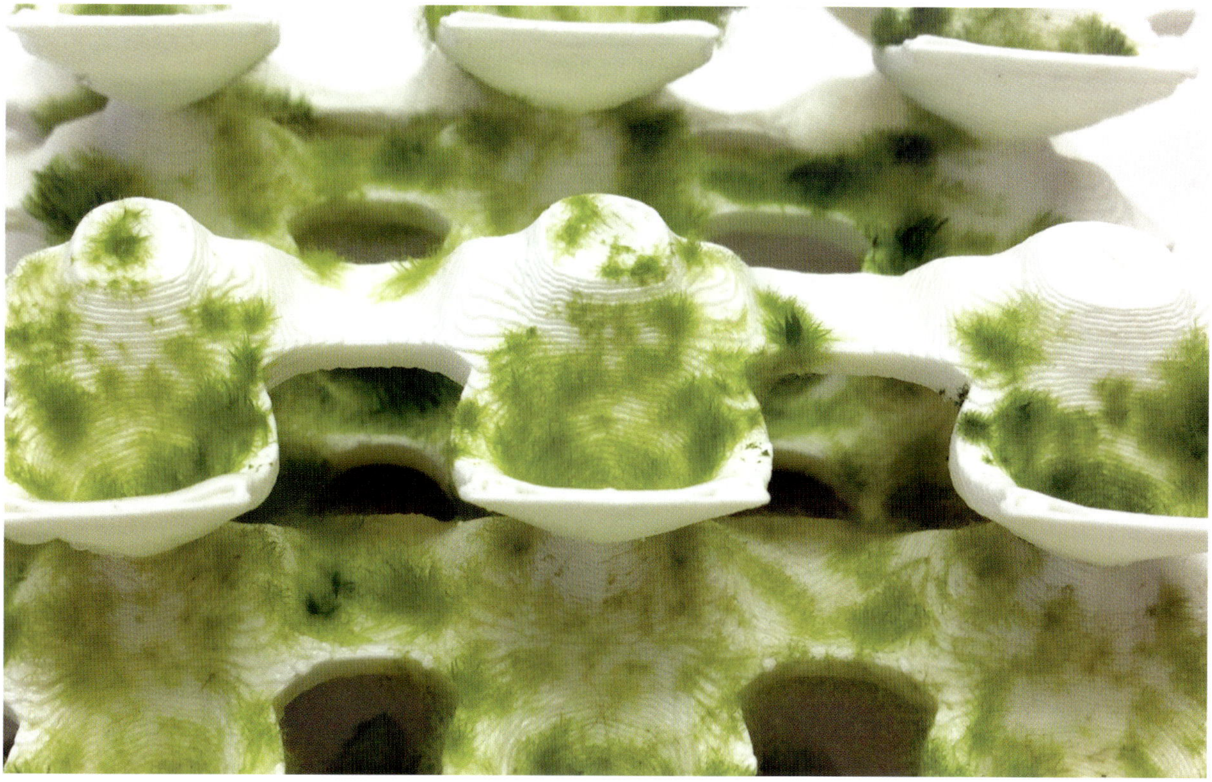

MICHAEL POLITTE | CAITLIN SANDERS | HARRISON WERNER | ERIN WONG | ZHAN YANG | KUAI YU

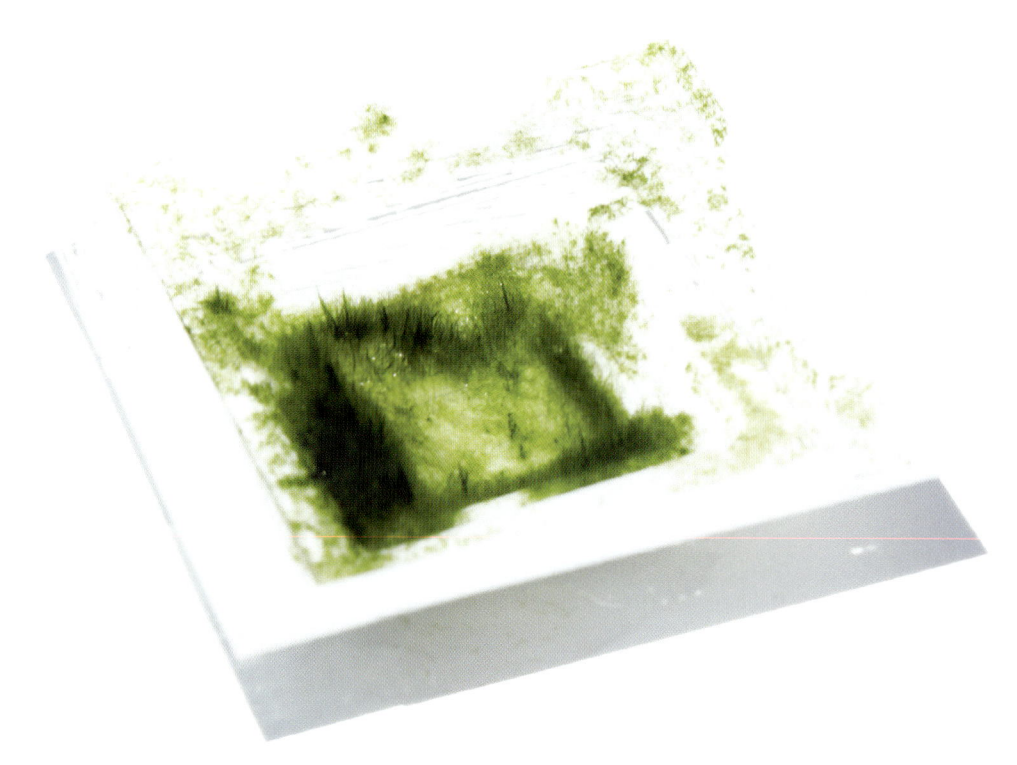

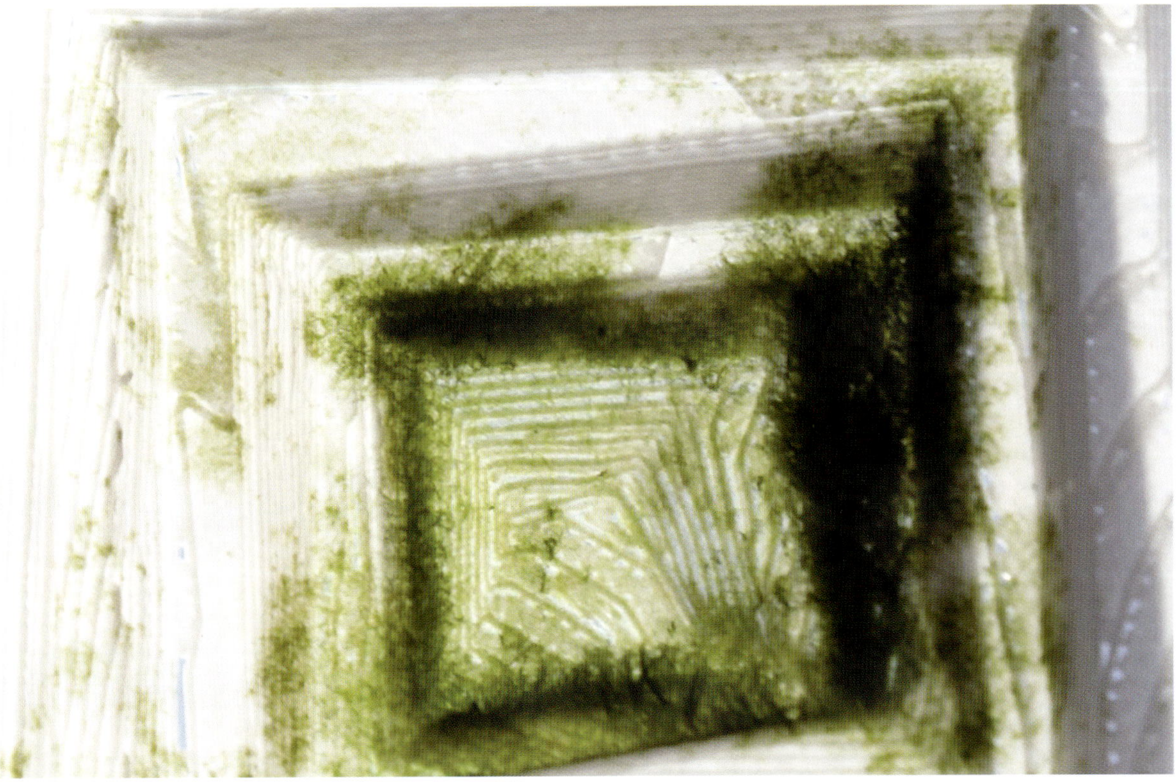

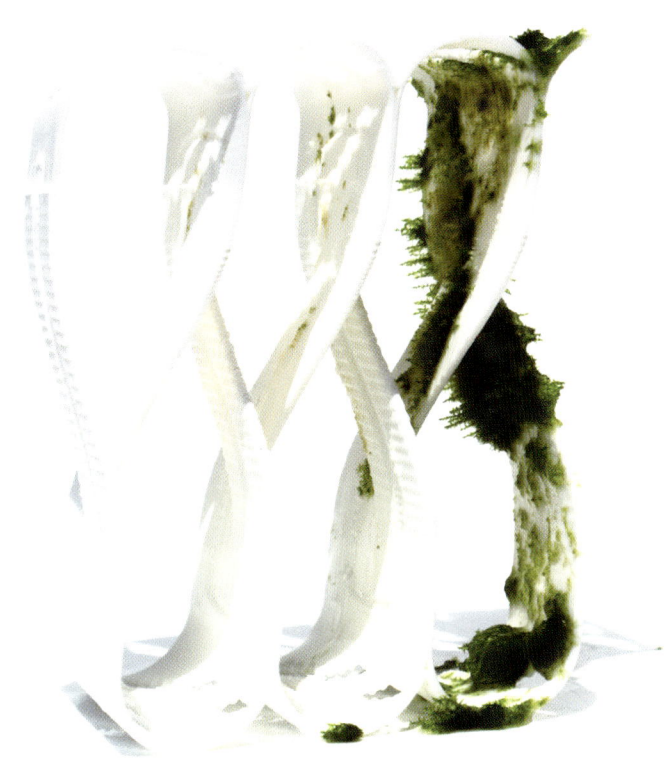

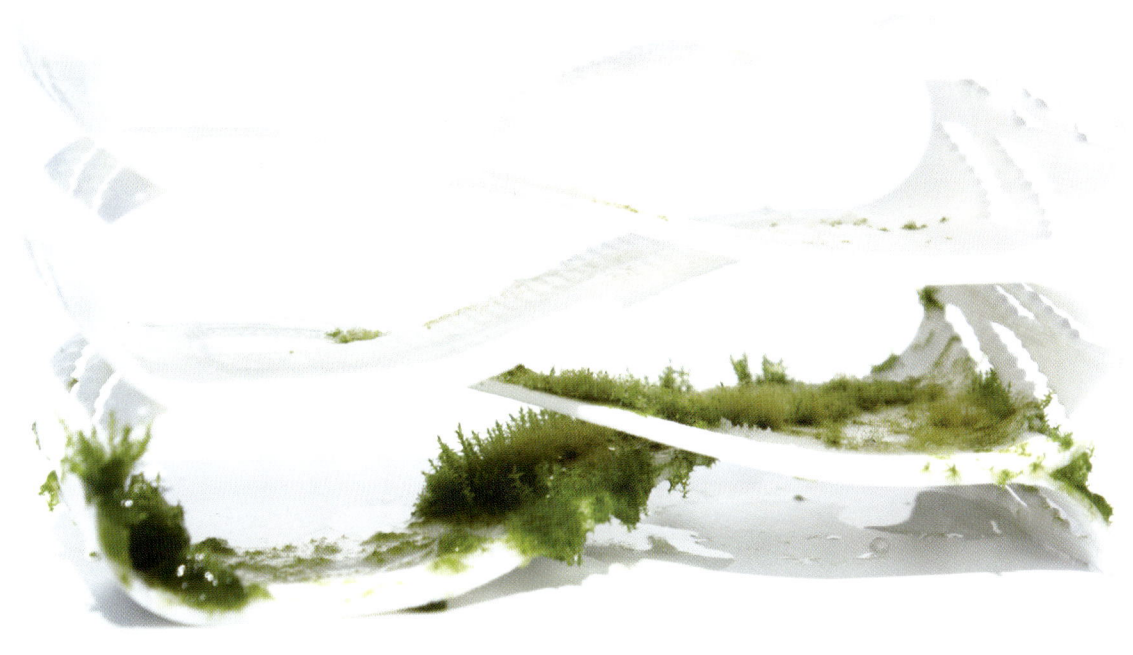

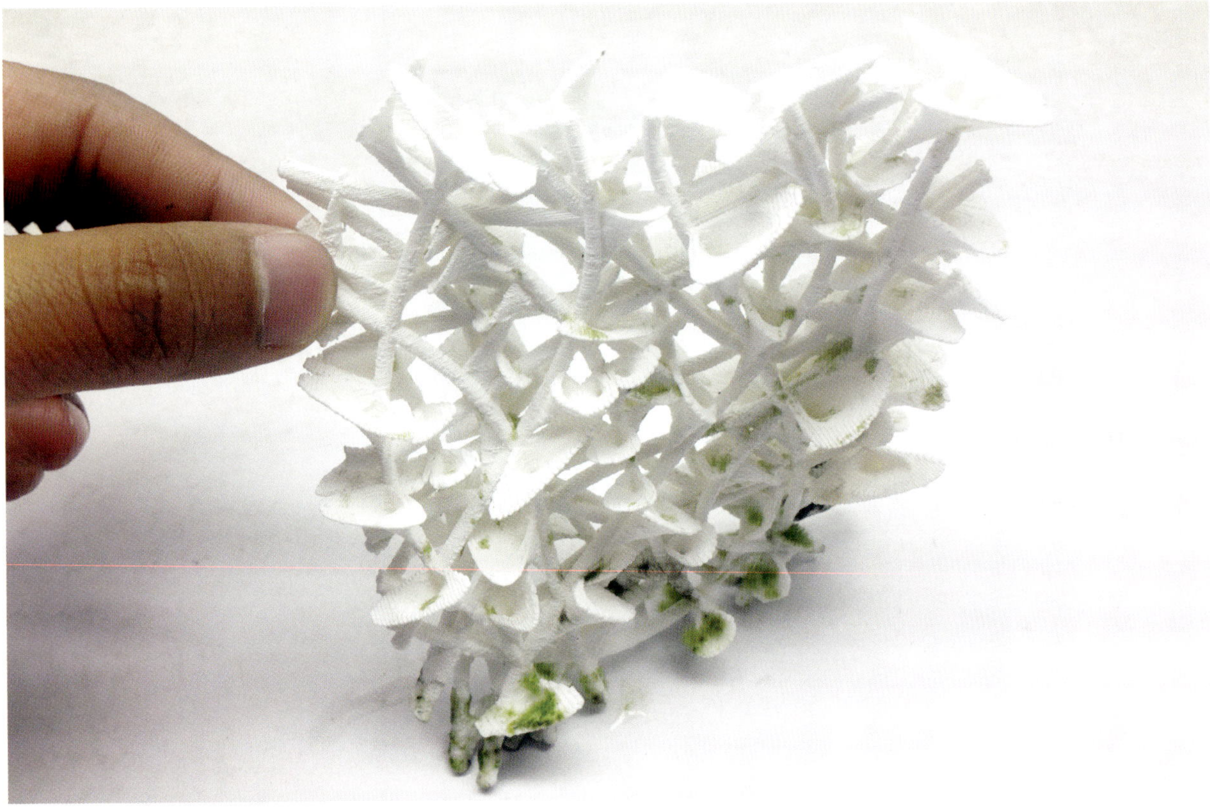

MENGYING BAI | ALLISON BERNETT | AMBER IBARRA | WEN YANG LIN | NHU NGUYEN

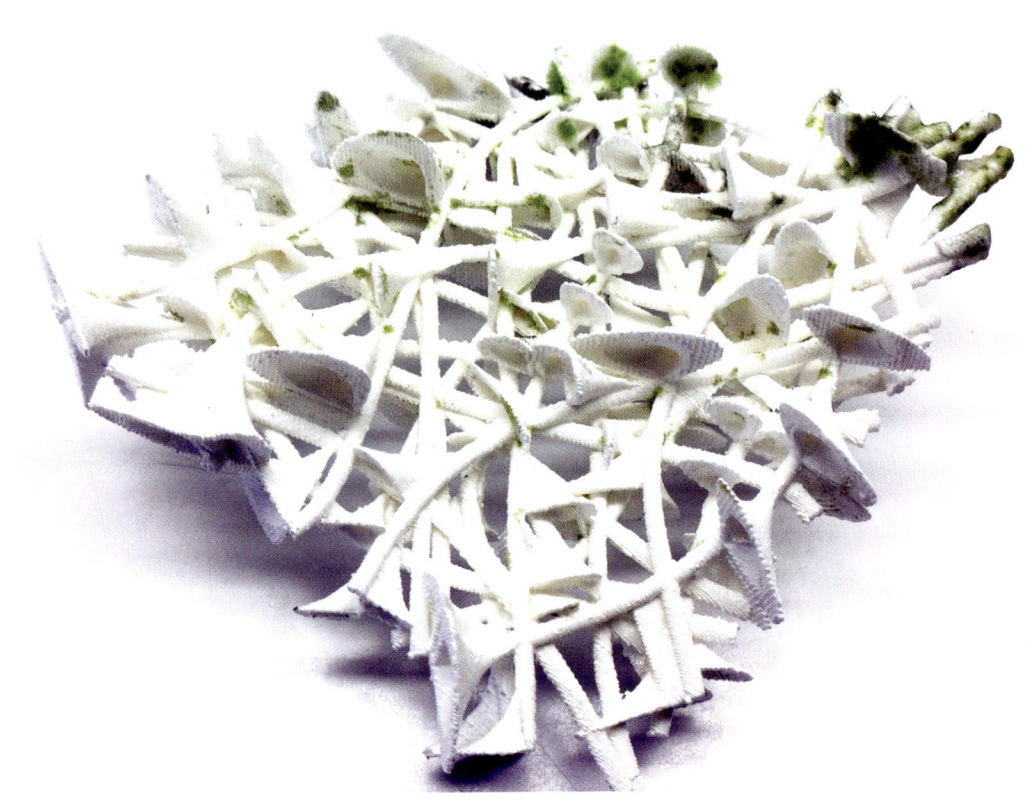

CELLULAR TRANSFORMATIONS

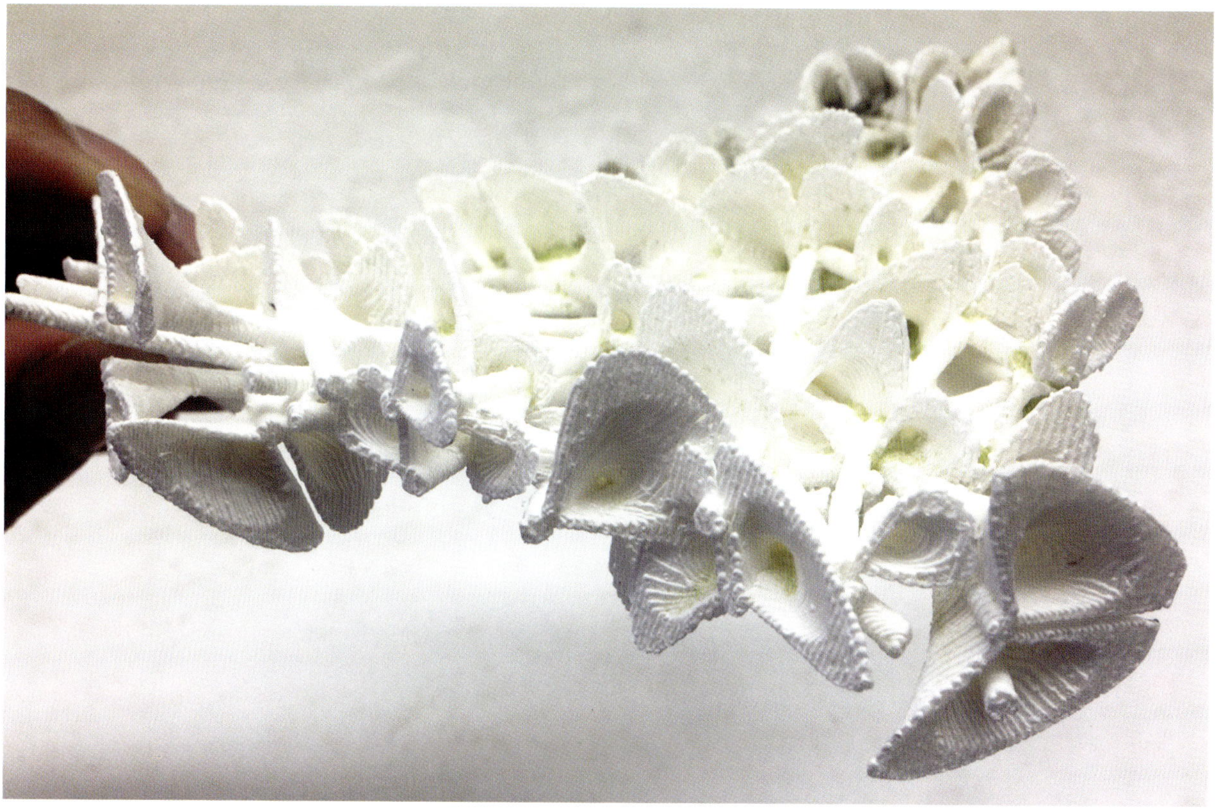

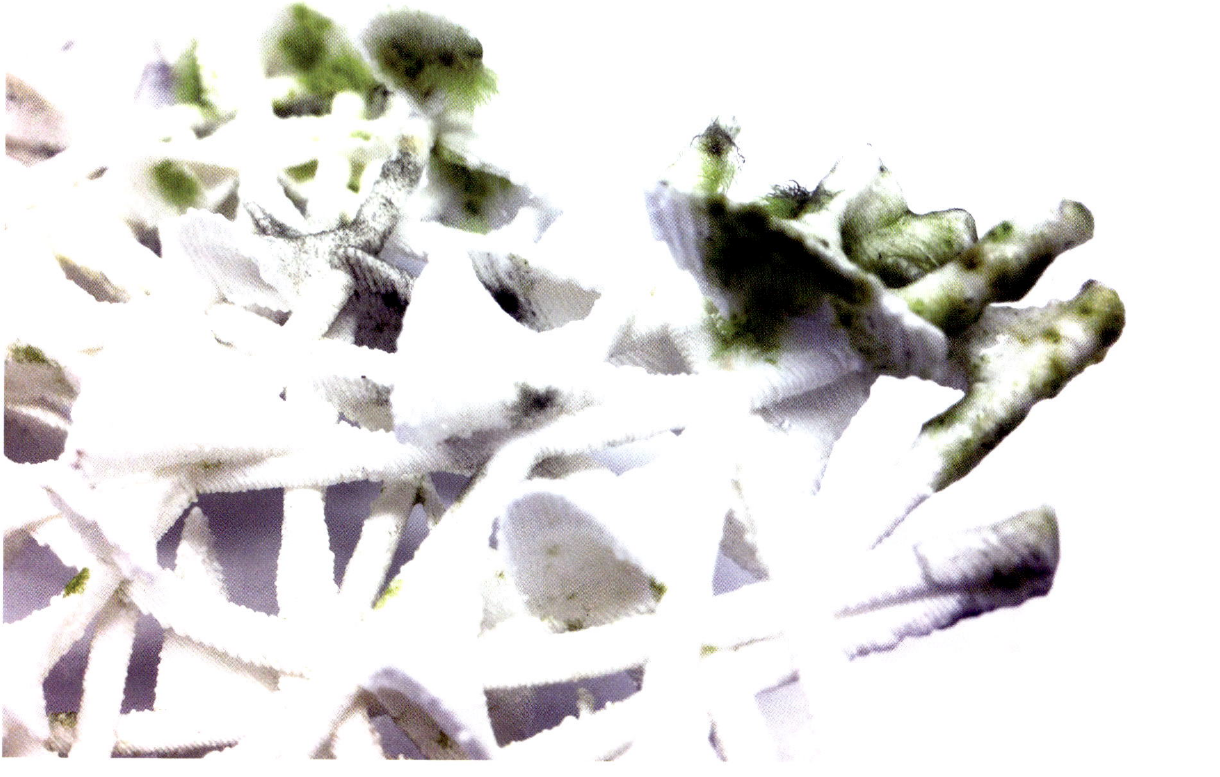

MICHAEL POLITTE | CAITLIN SANDERS | HARRISON WERNER | ERIN WONG | ZHAN YANG | KUAI YU

MICRO-ENVIRONMENTS

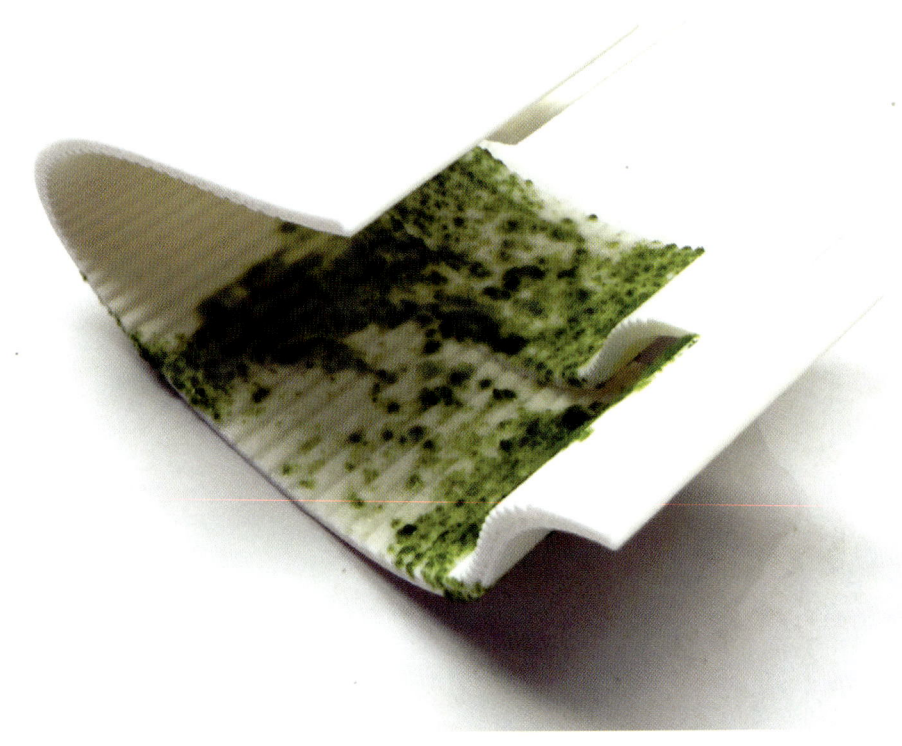

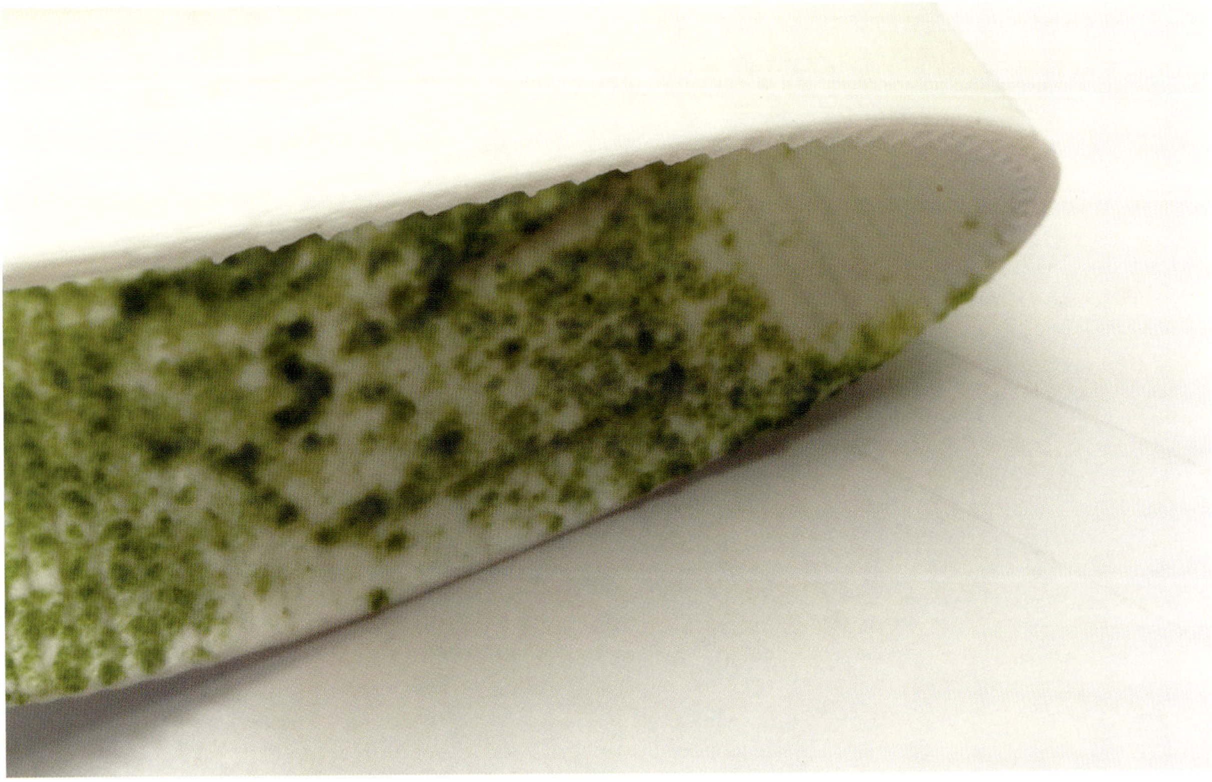

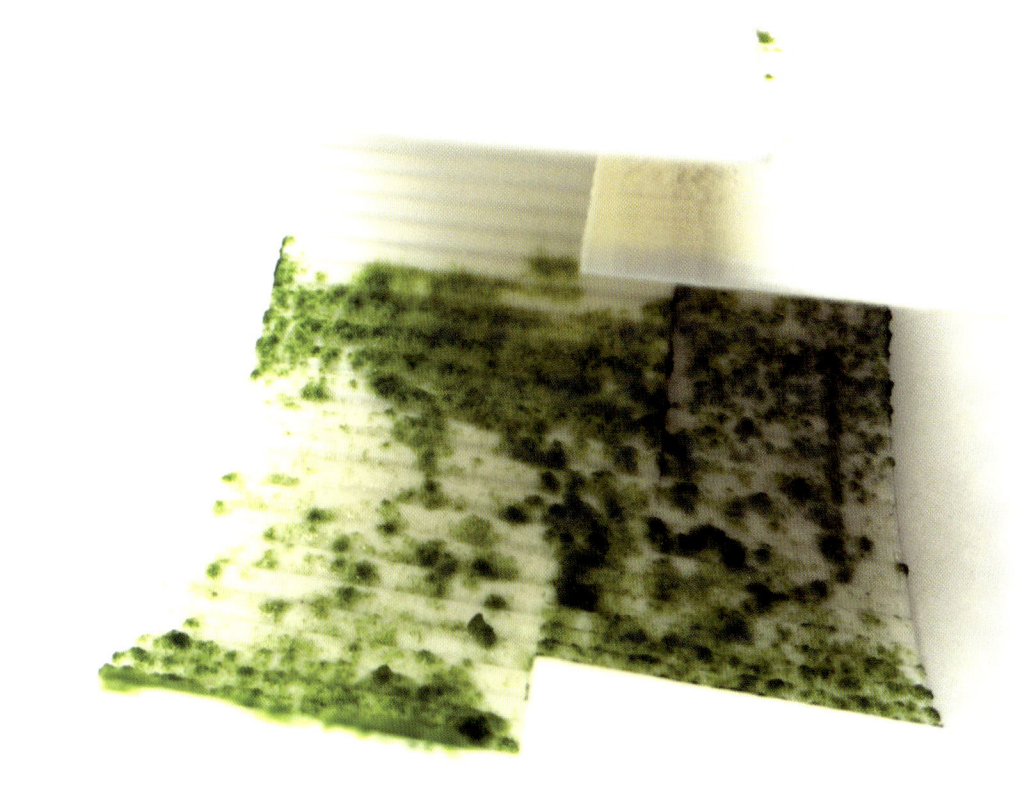

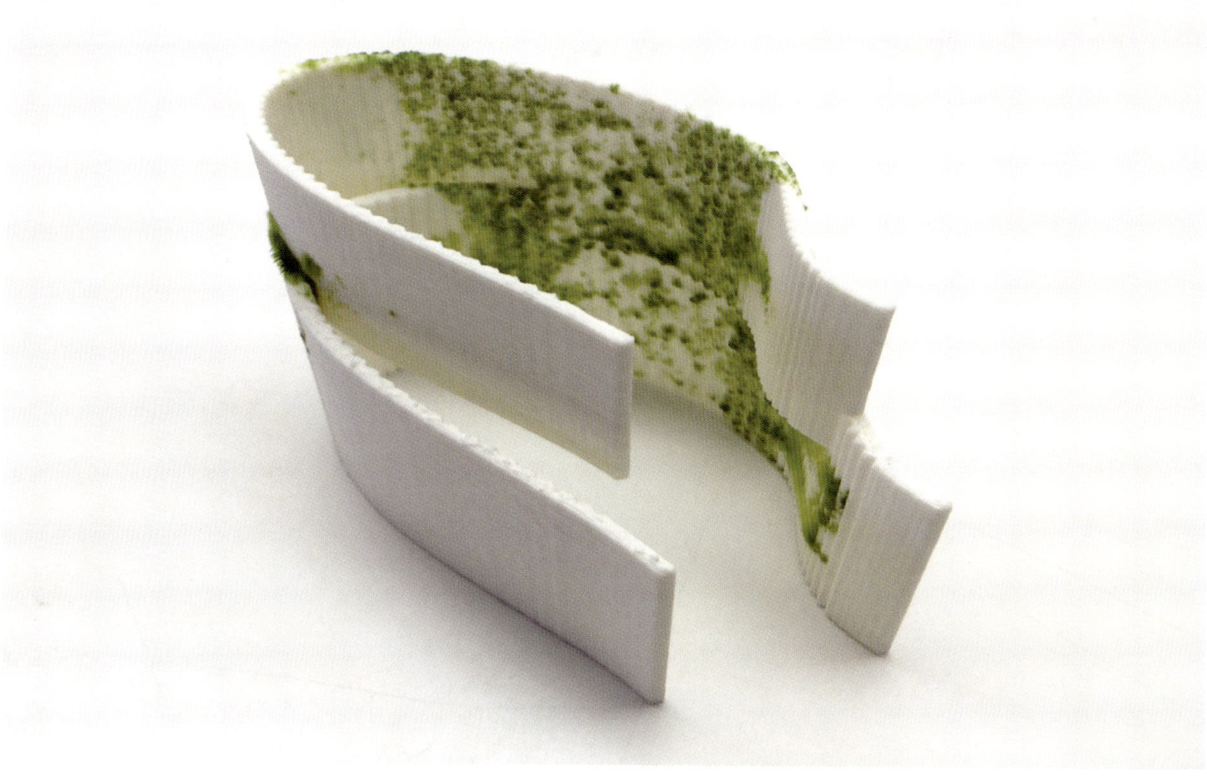

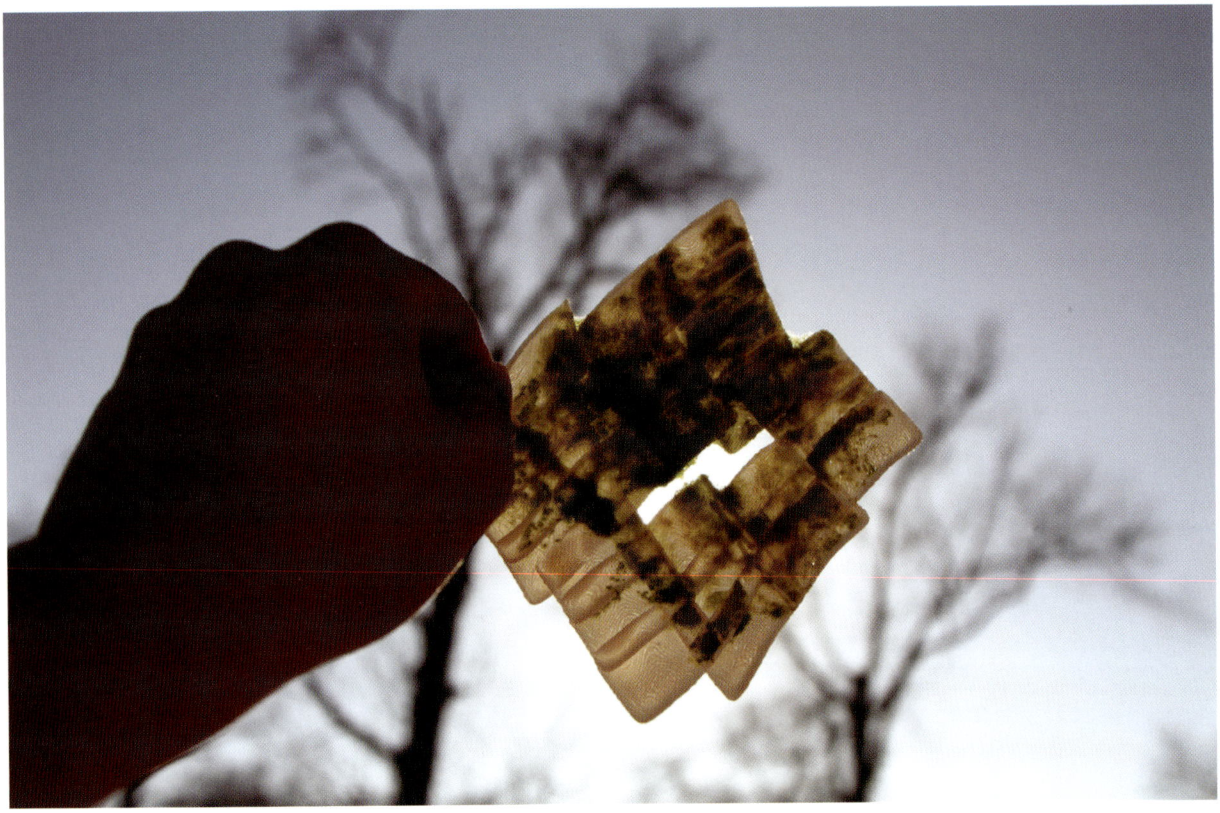

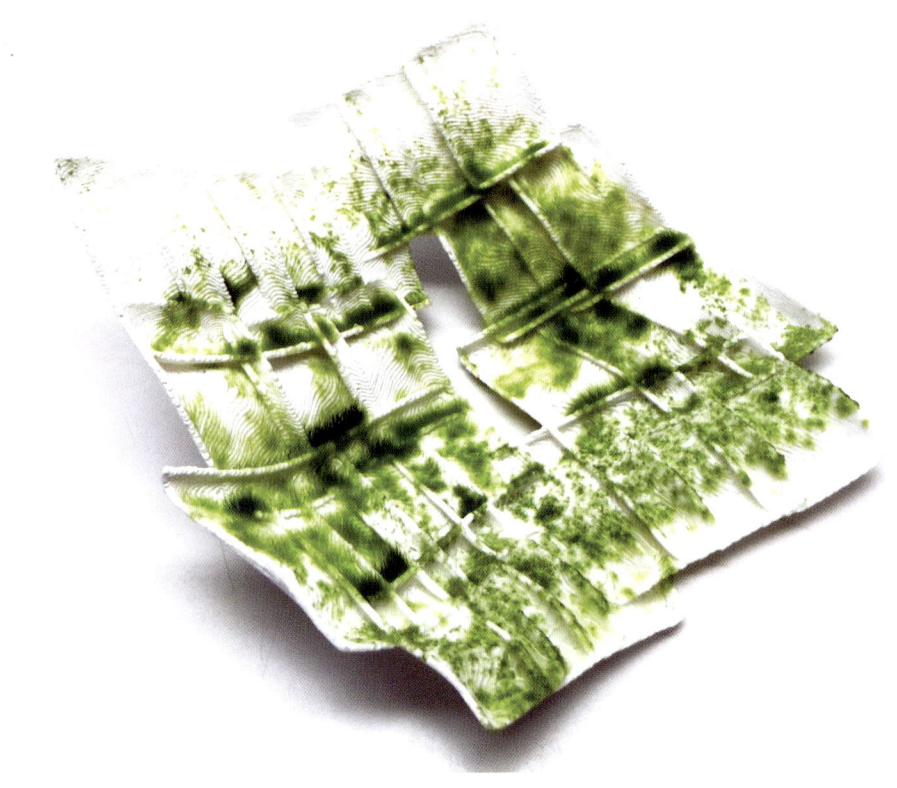

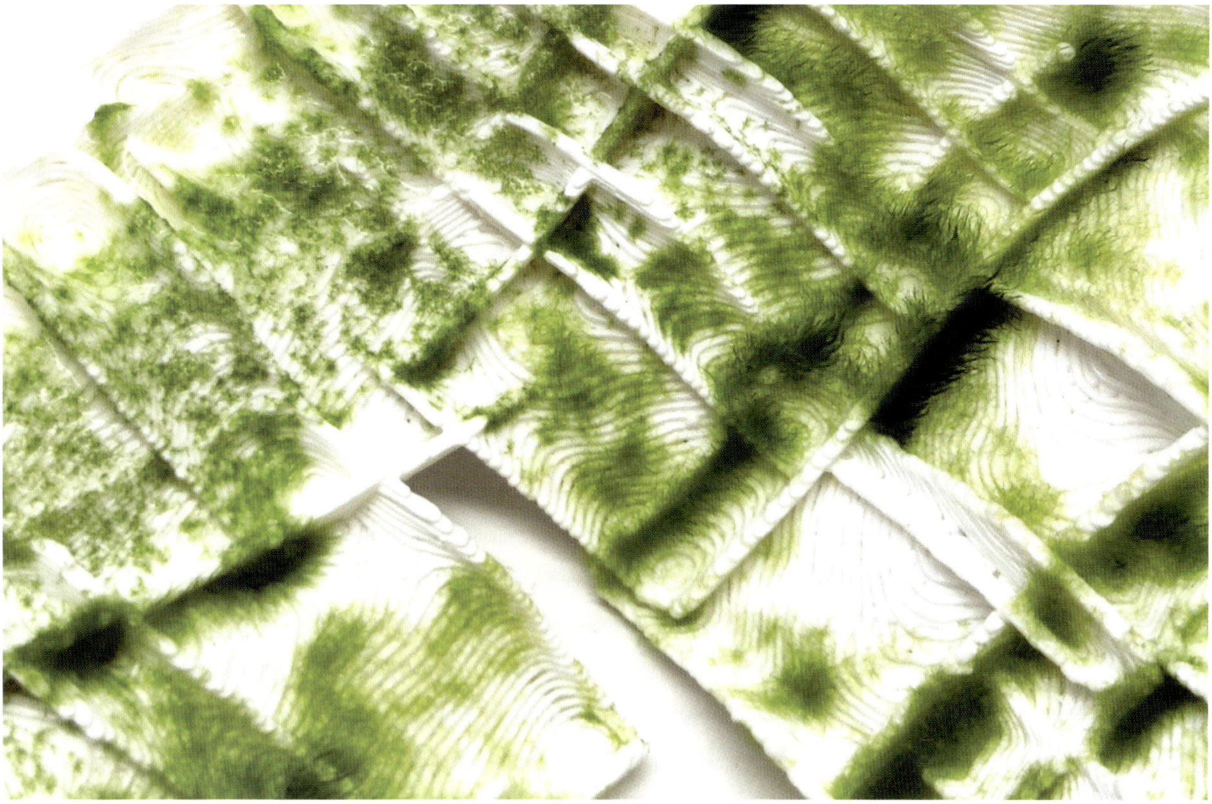

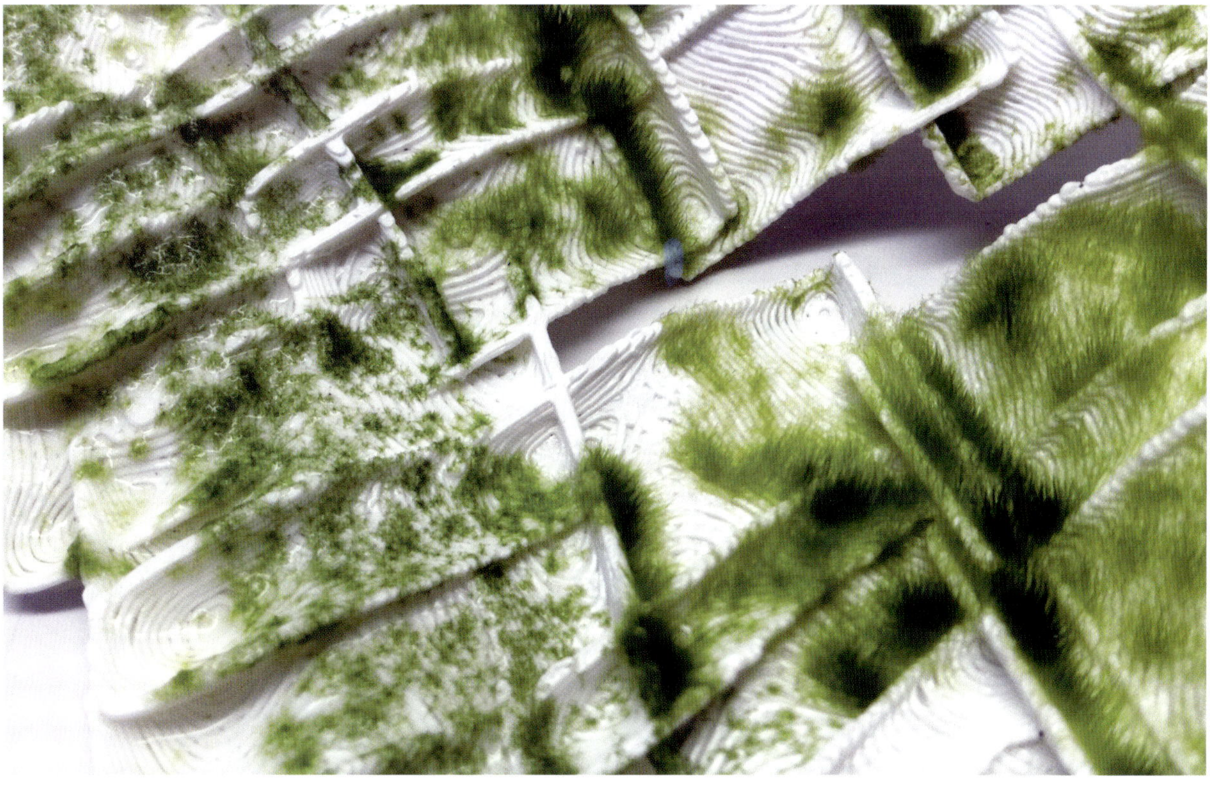

MICHAEL POLITTE | CAITLIN SANDERS | HARRISON WERNER | ERIN WONG | ZHAN YANG | KUAI YU

MICRO-ENVIRONMENTS

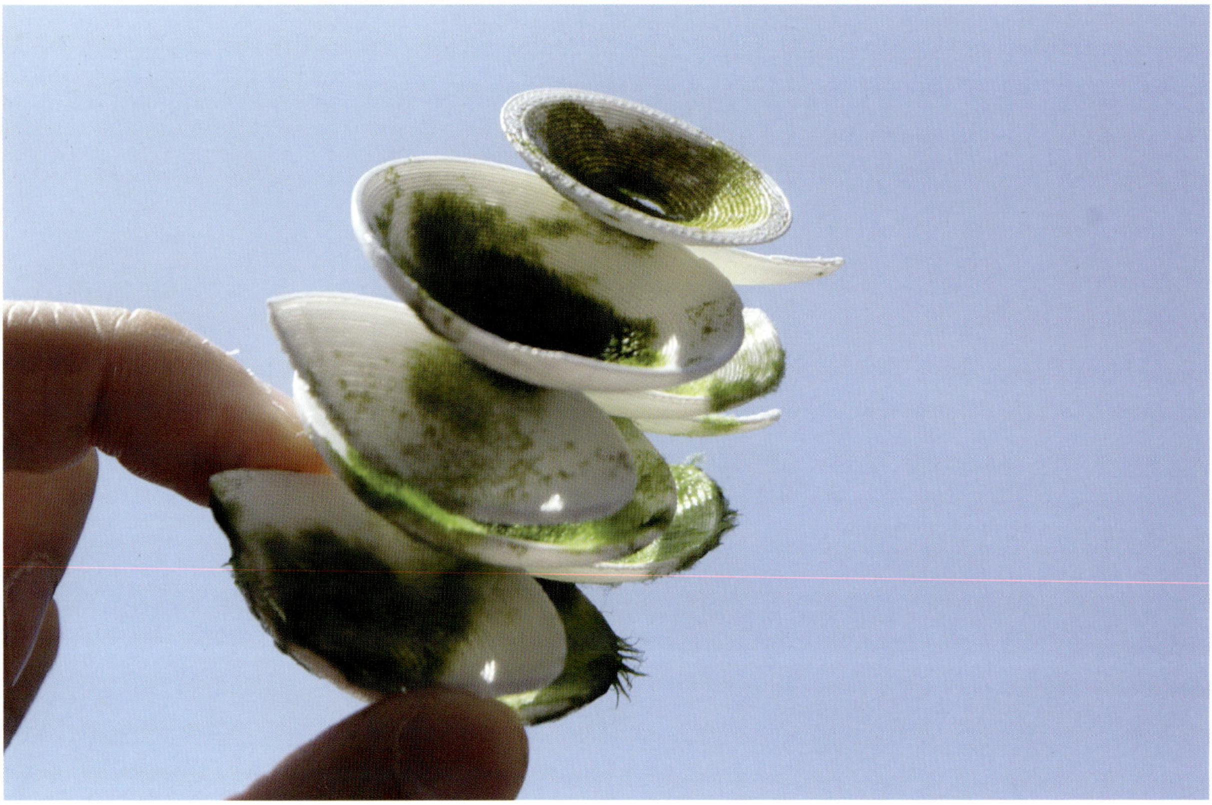

MENGYING BAI | ALLISON BERNETT | AMBER IBARRA | WEN YANG LIN | NHU NGUYEN

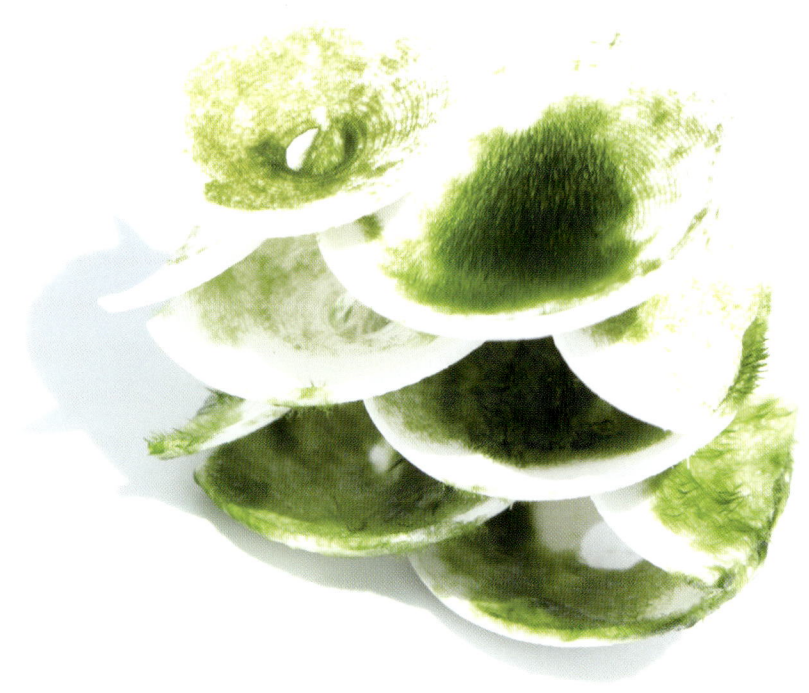

CELLULAR TRANSFORMATIONS

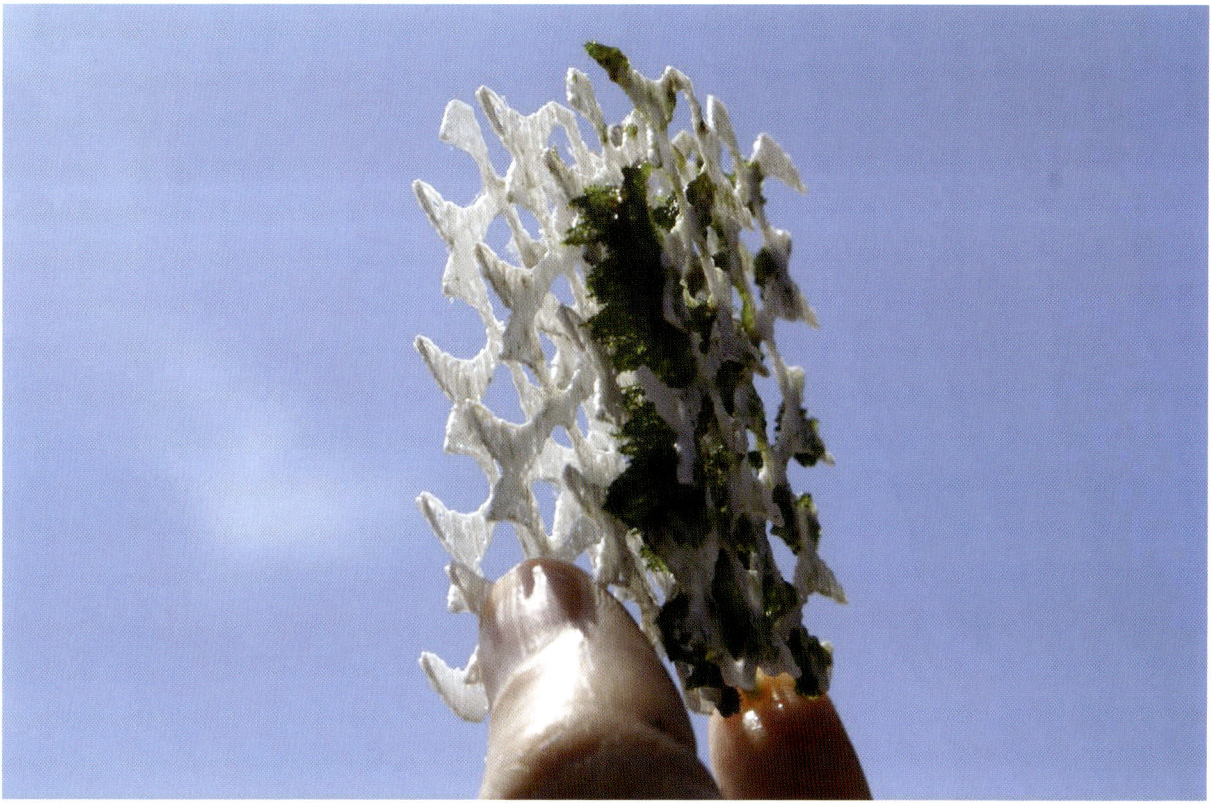

MICHAEL POLITTE | CAITLIN SANDERS | HARRISON WERNER | ERIN WONG | ZHAN YANG | KUAI YU

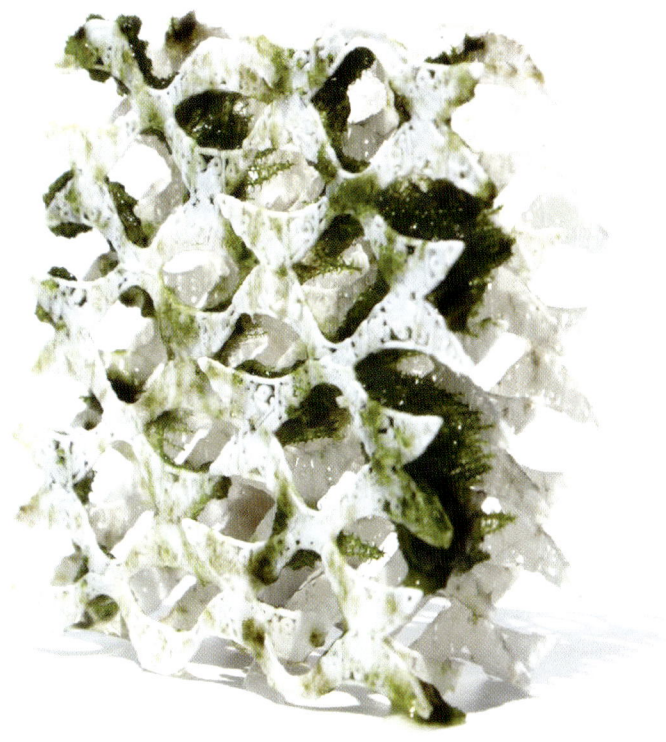

MICRO-ENVIRONMENTS

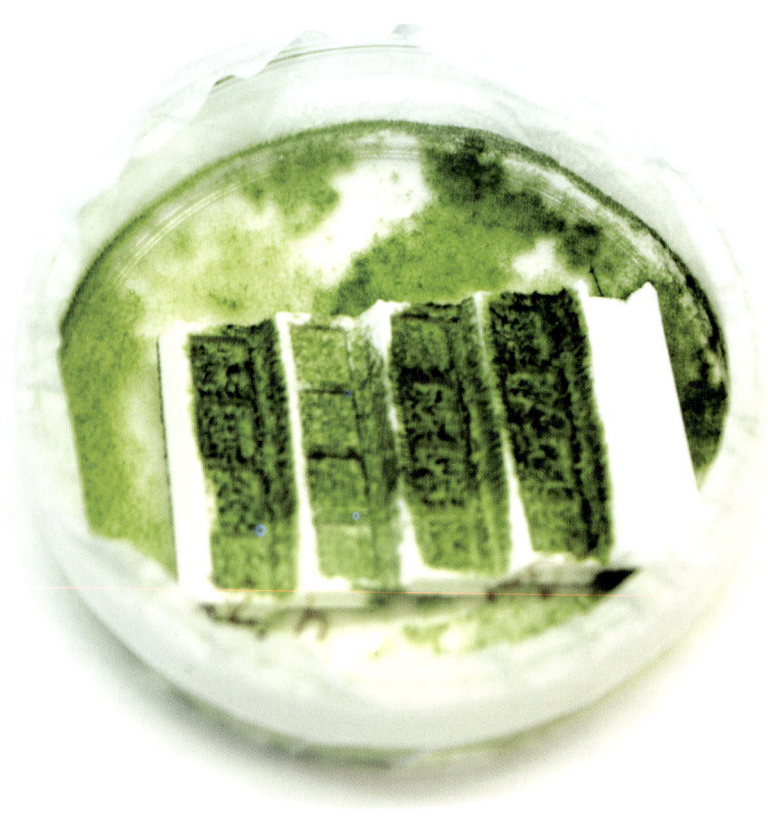

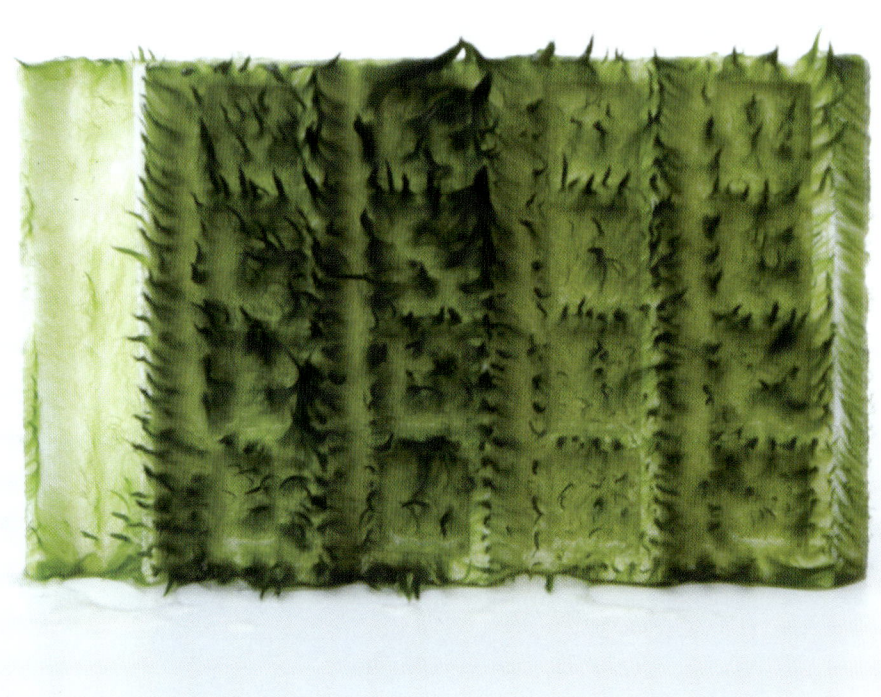

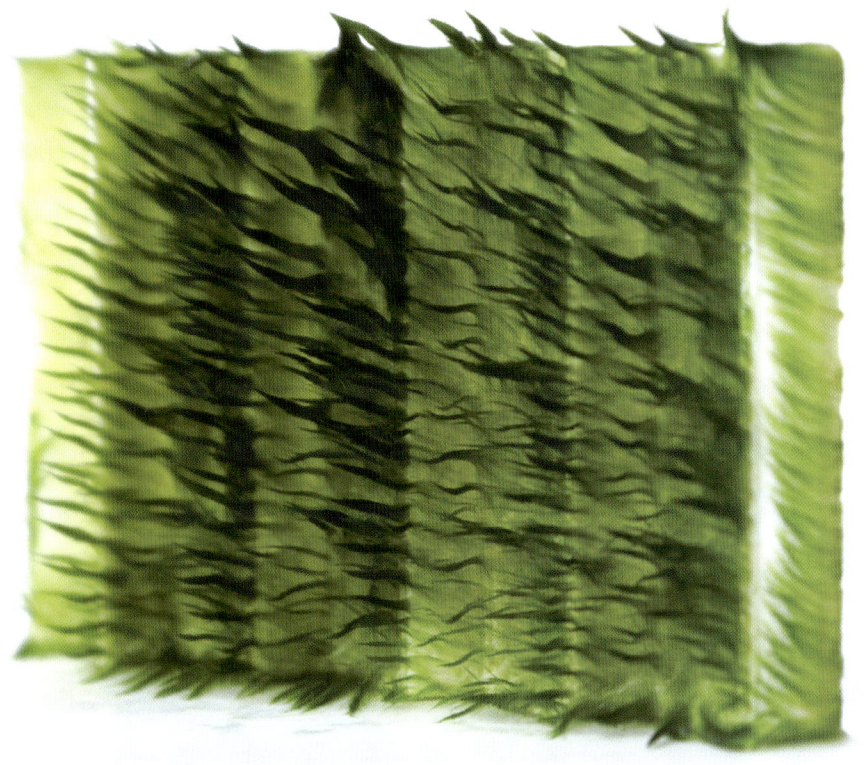

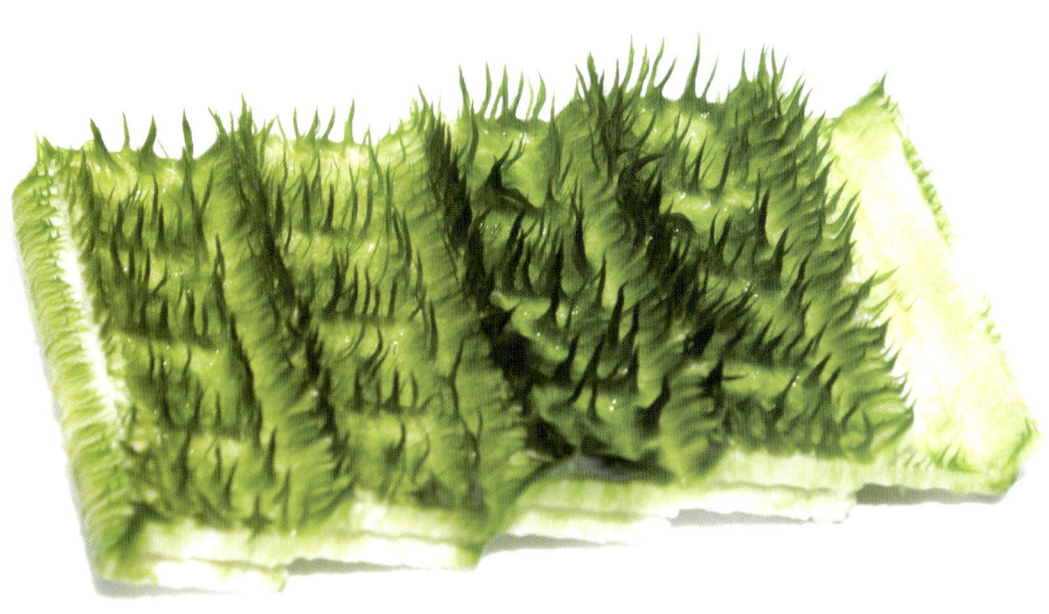

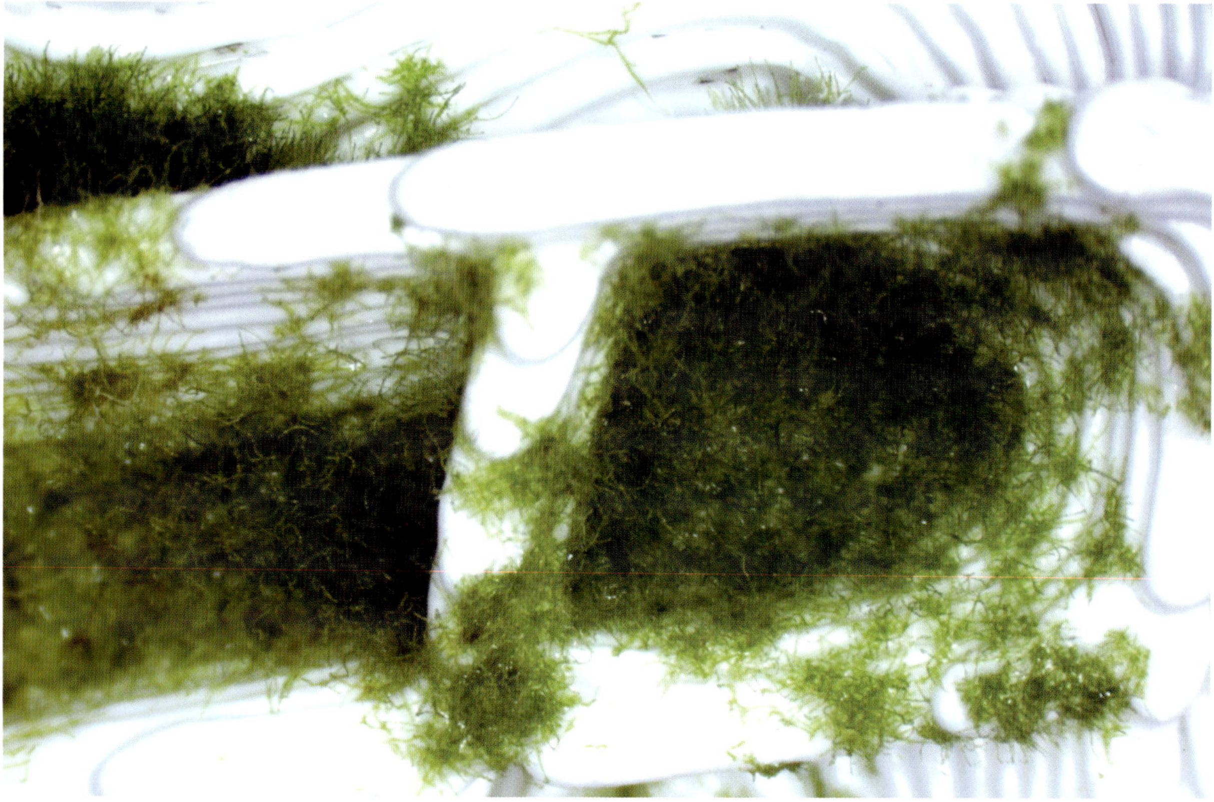

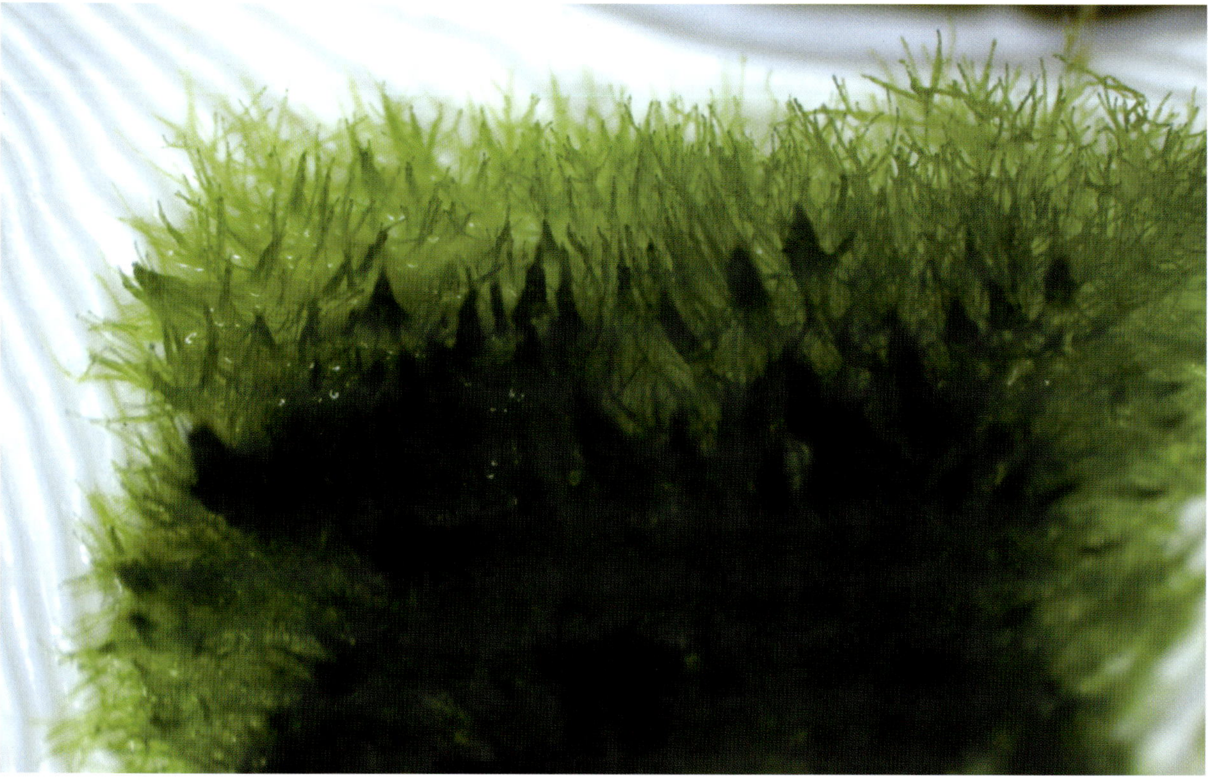

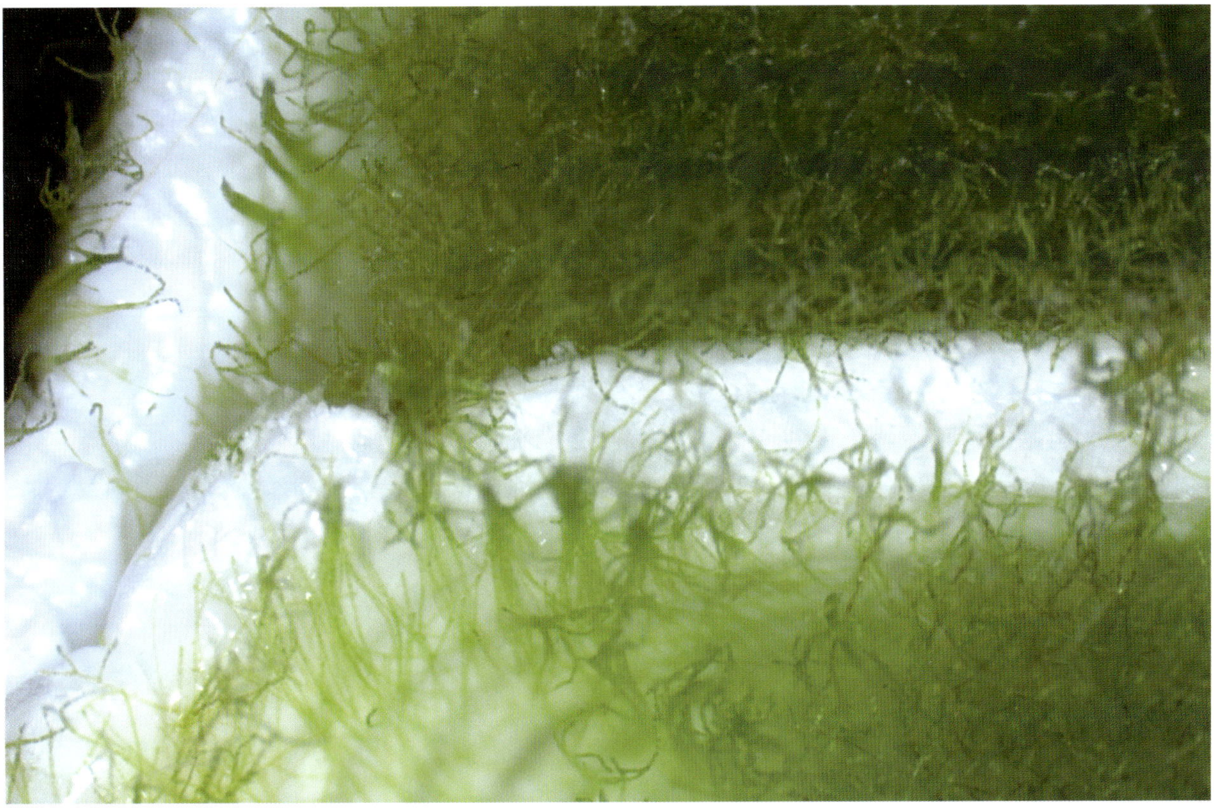

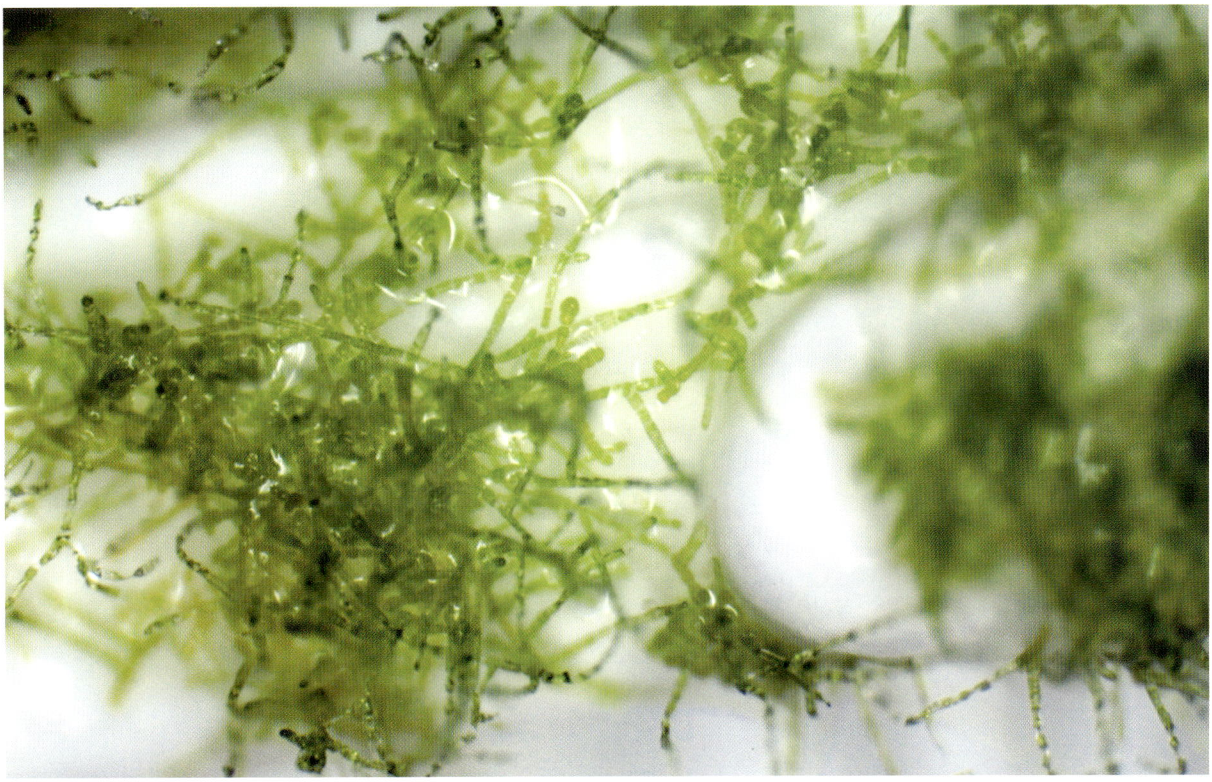

MICHAEL POLITTE | CAITLIN SANDERS | HARRISON WERNER | ERIN WONG | ZHAN YANG | KUAI YU

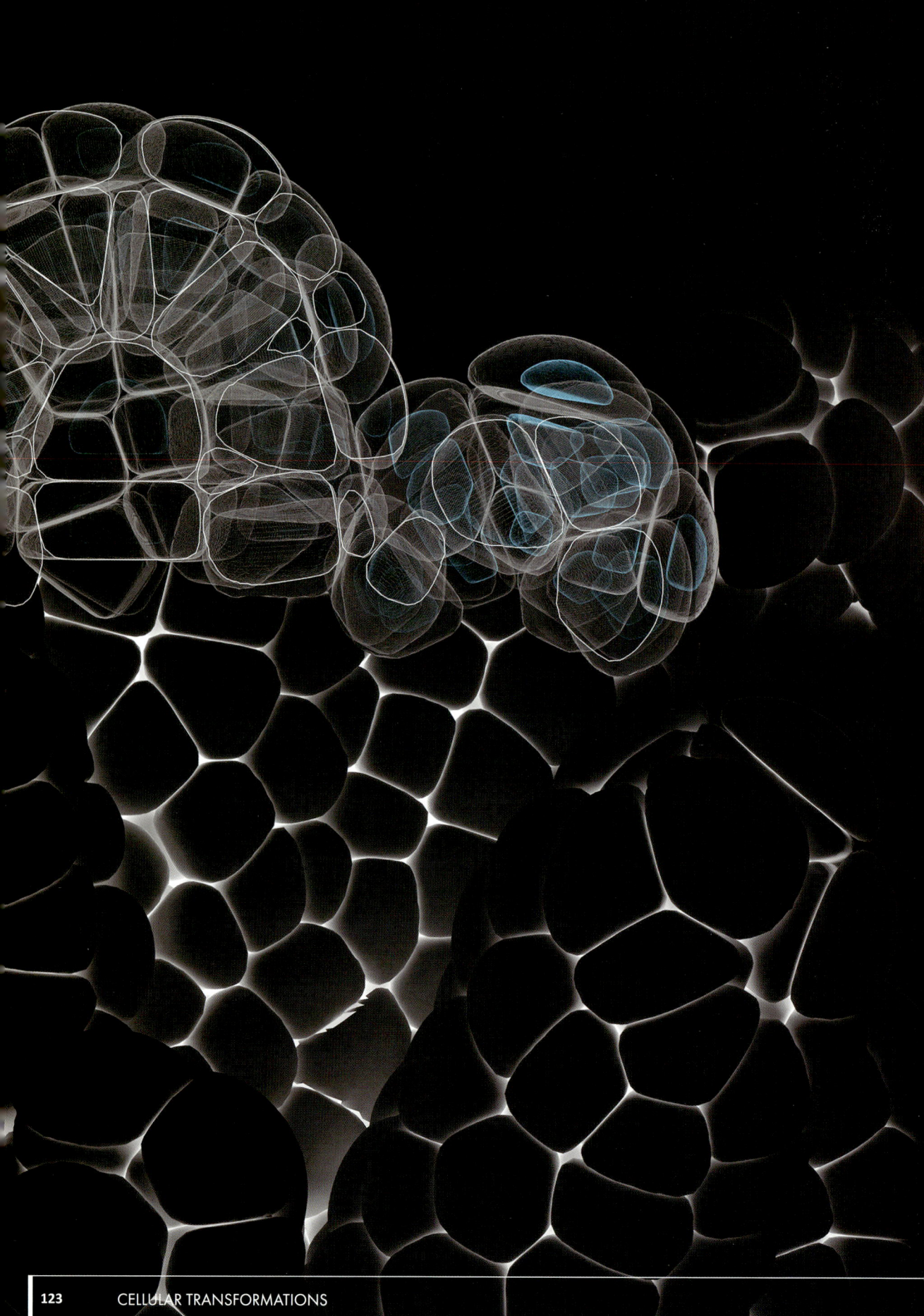

TRANSFORMATION: 2014
ADVANCED CELL ANALYSIS 01

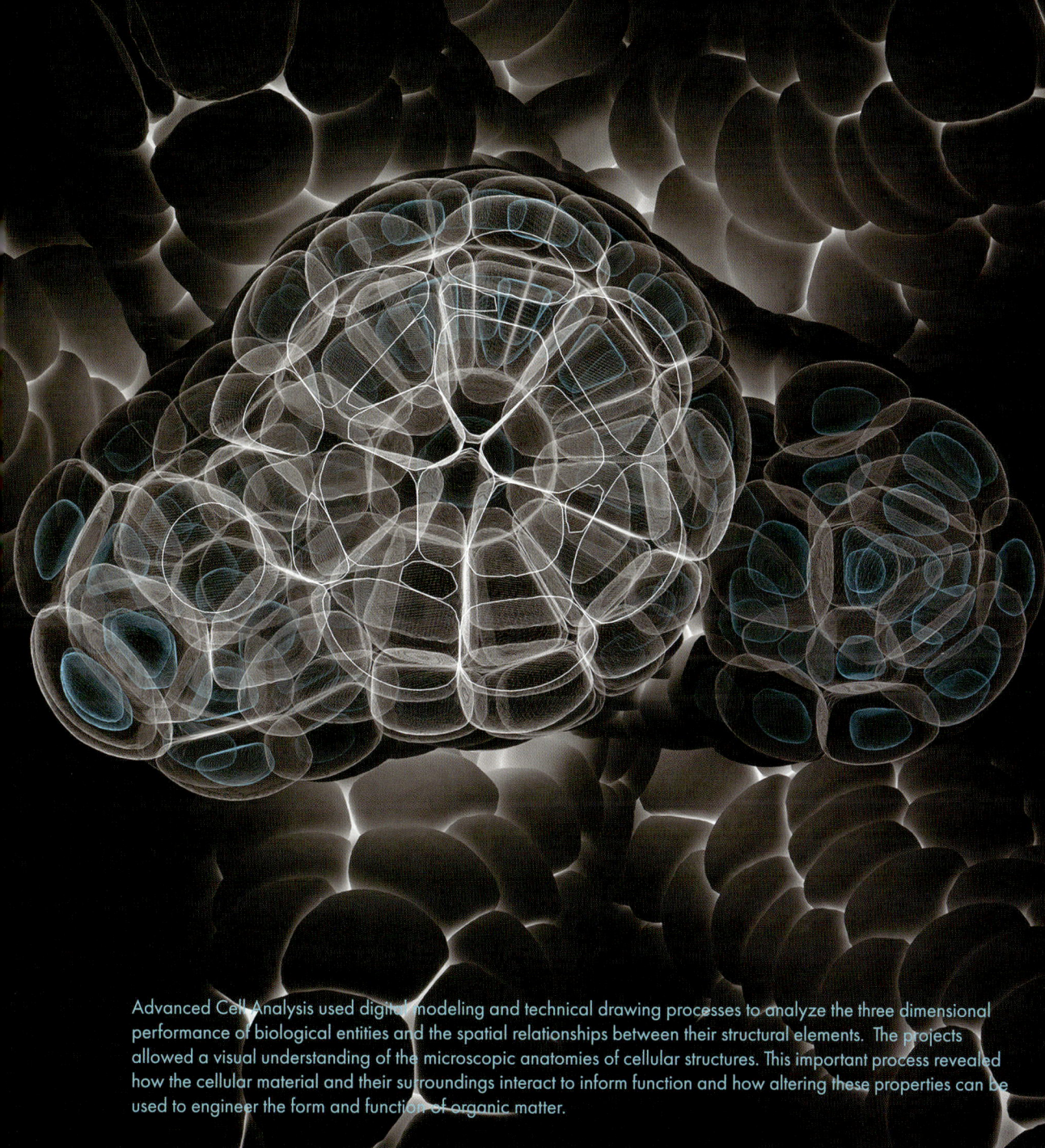

Advanced Cell Analysis used digital modeling and technical drawing processes to analyze the three dimensional performance of biological entities and the spatial relationships between their structural elements. The projects allowed a visual understanding of the microscopic anatomies of cellular structures. This important process revealed how the cellular material and their surroundings interact to inform function and how altering these properties can be used to engineer the form and function of organic matter.

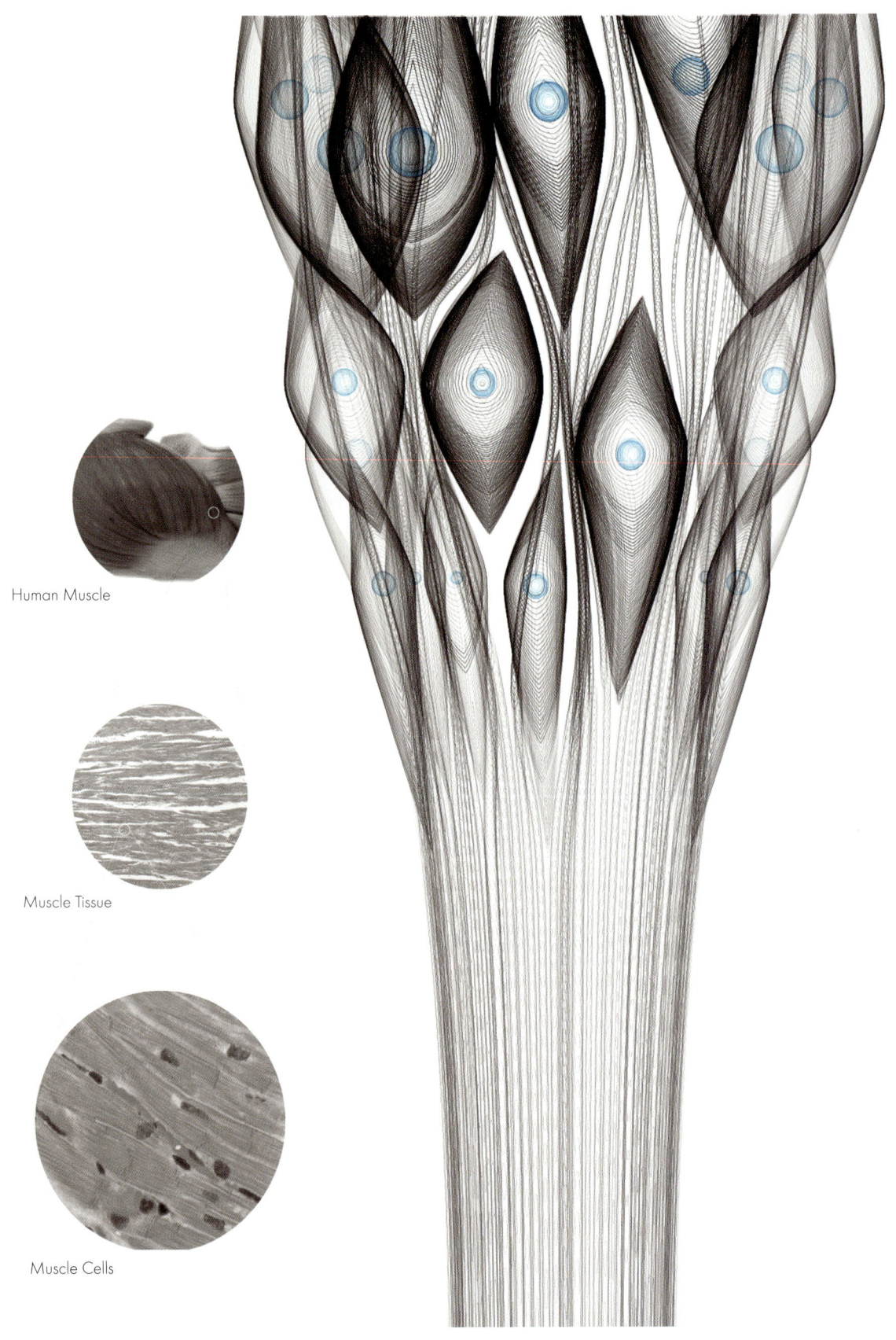

Human Muscle

Muscle Tissue

Muscle Cells

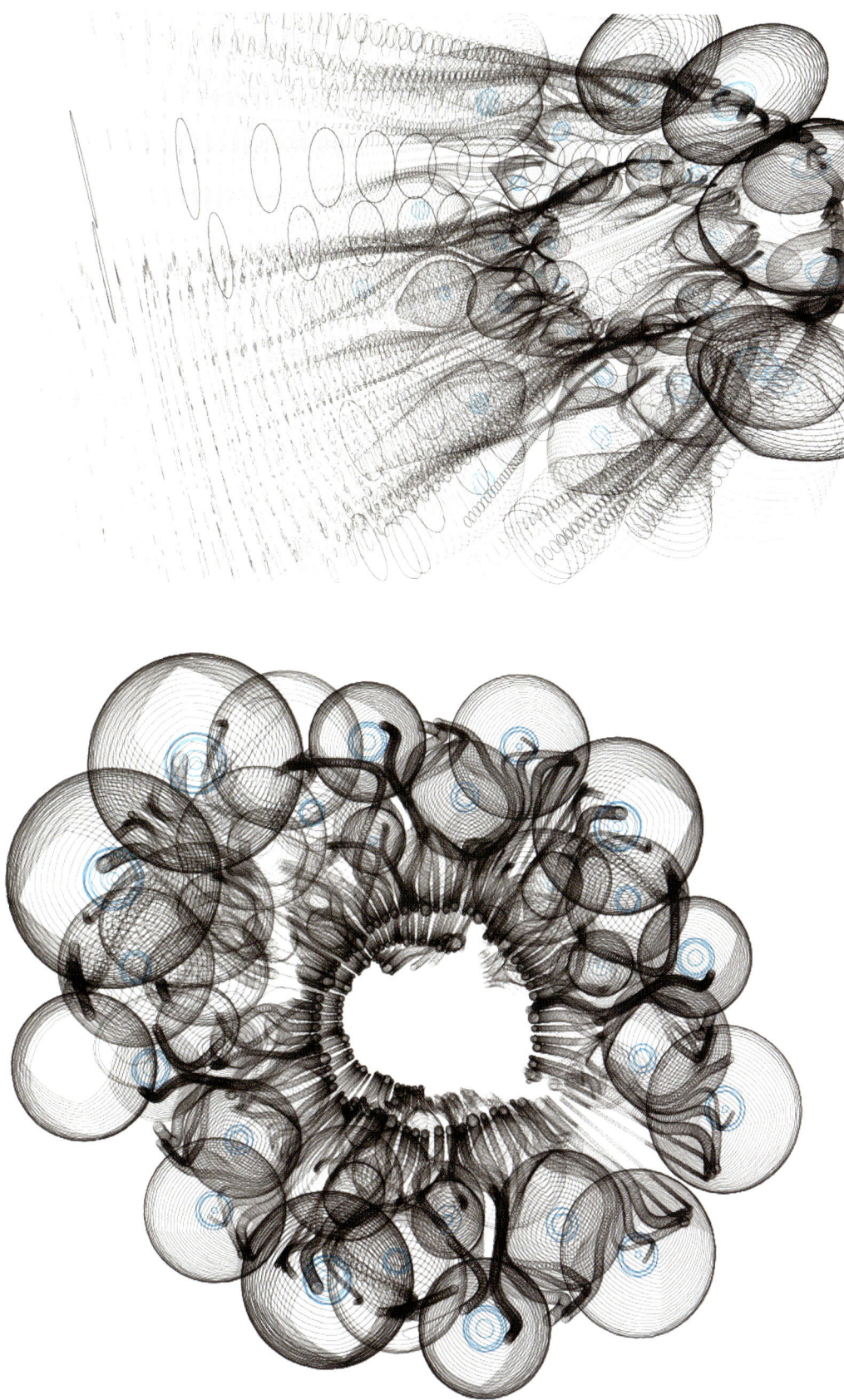

SHENG LI

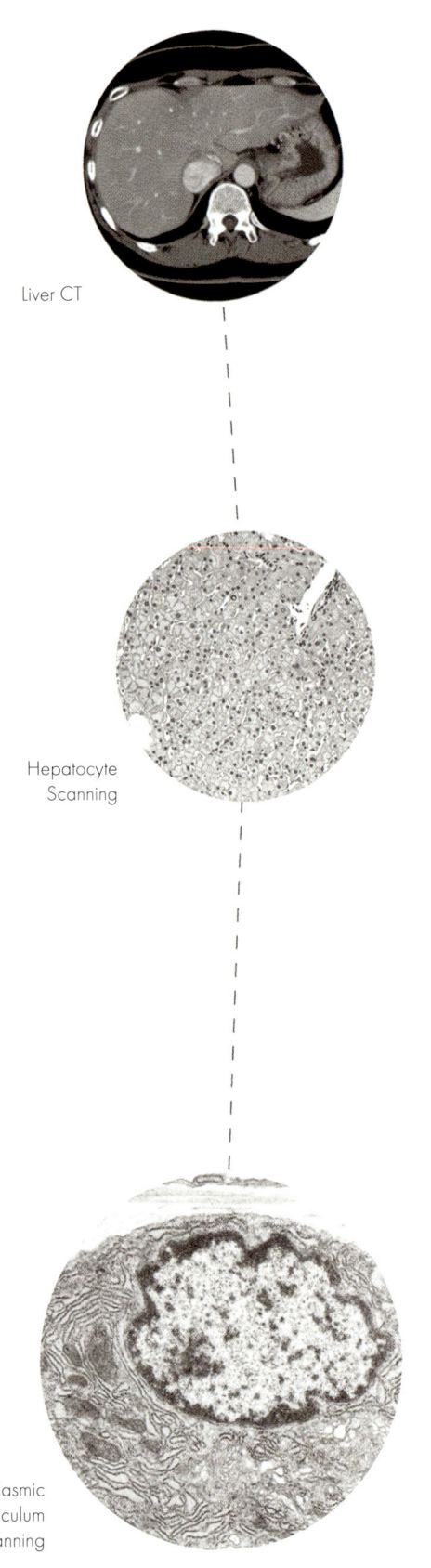

Liver CT

Hepatocyte Scanning

Endoplasmic Reticulum Scanning

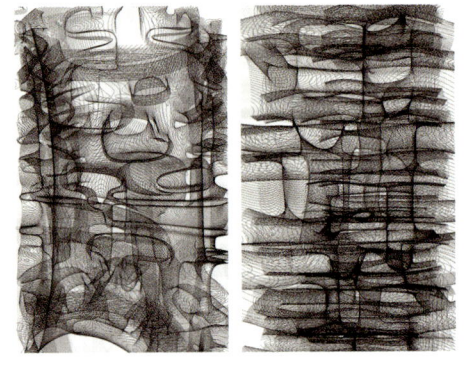

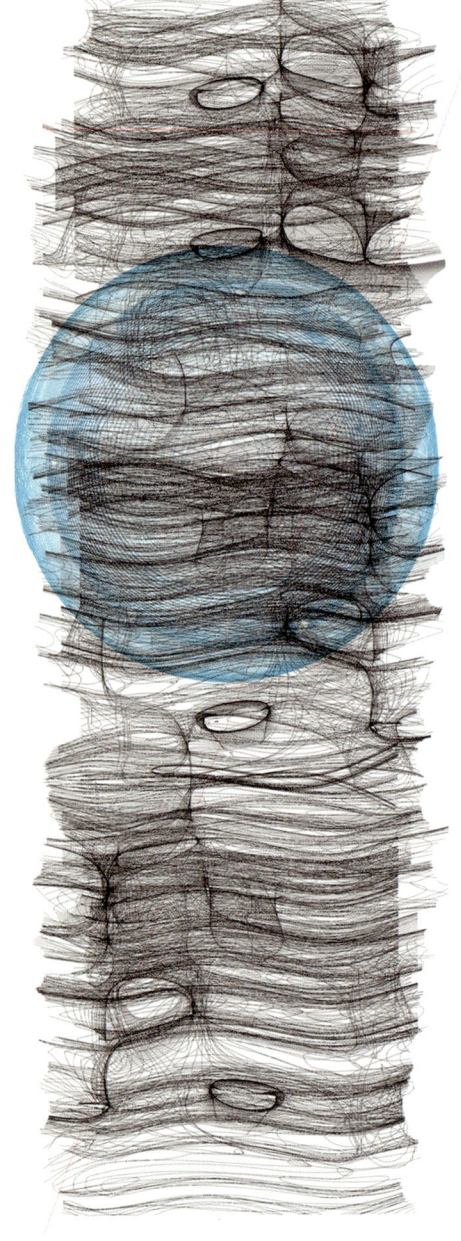

127 CELLULAR TRANSFORMATIONS

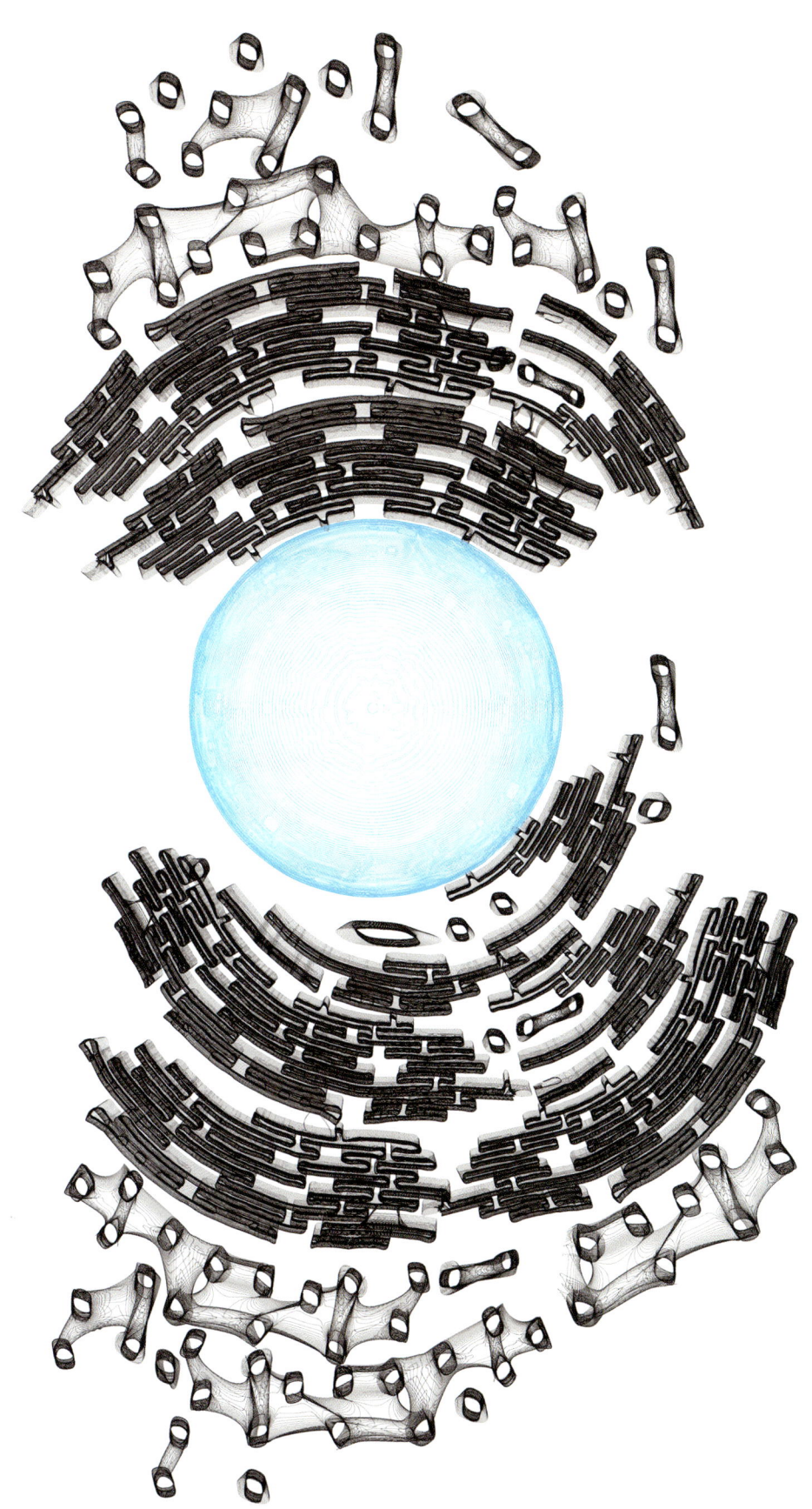

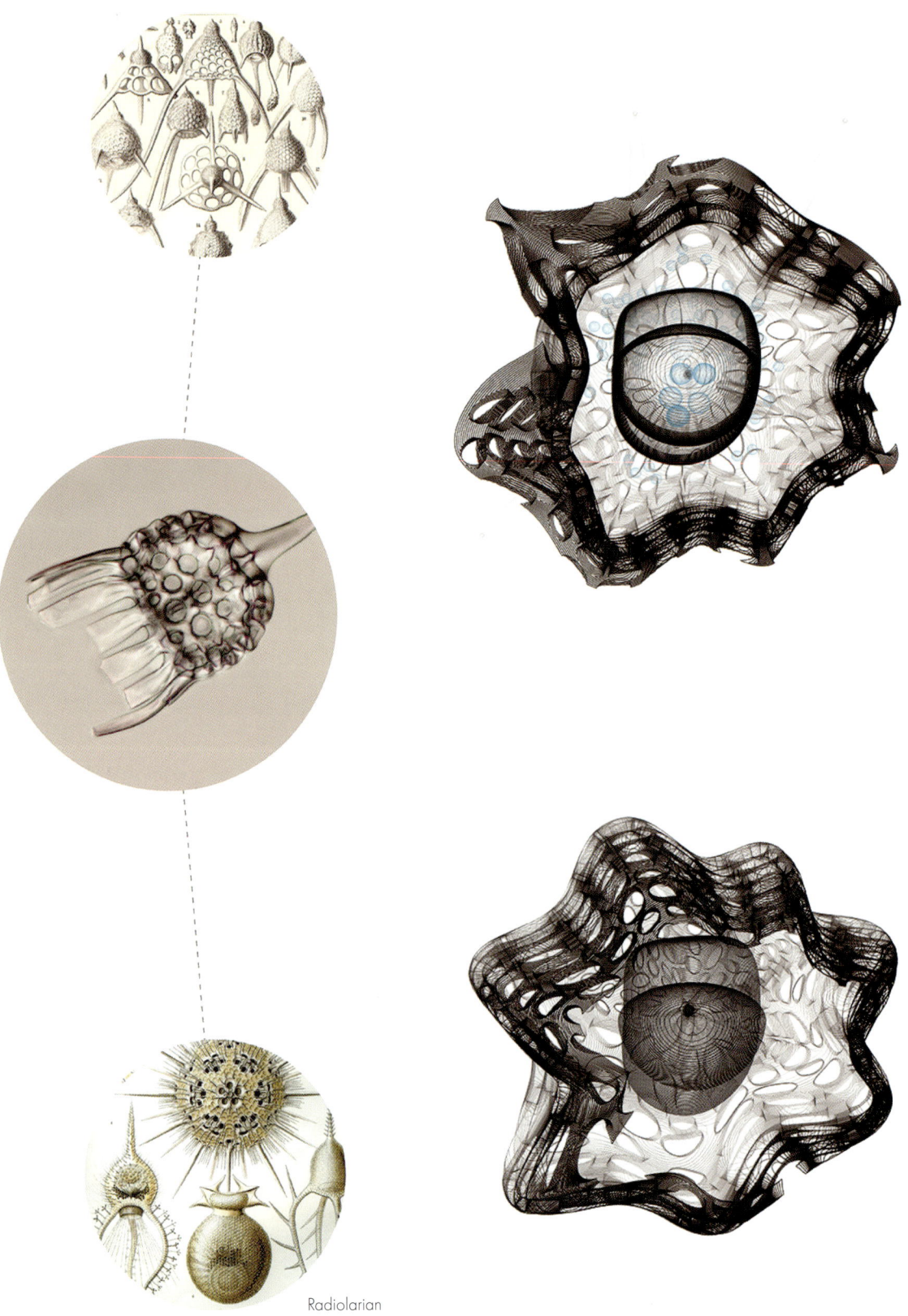

Radiolarian

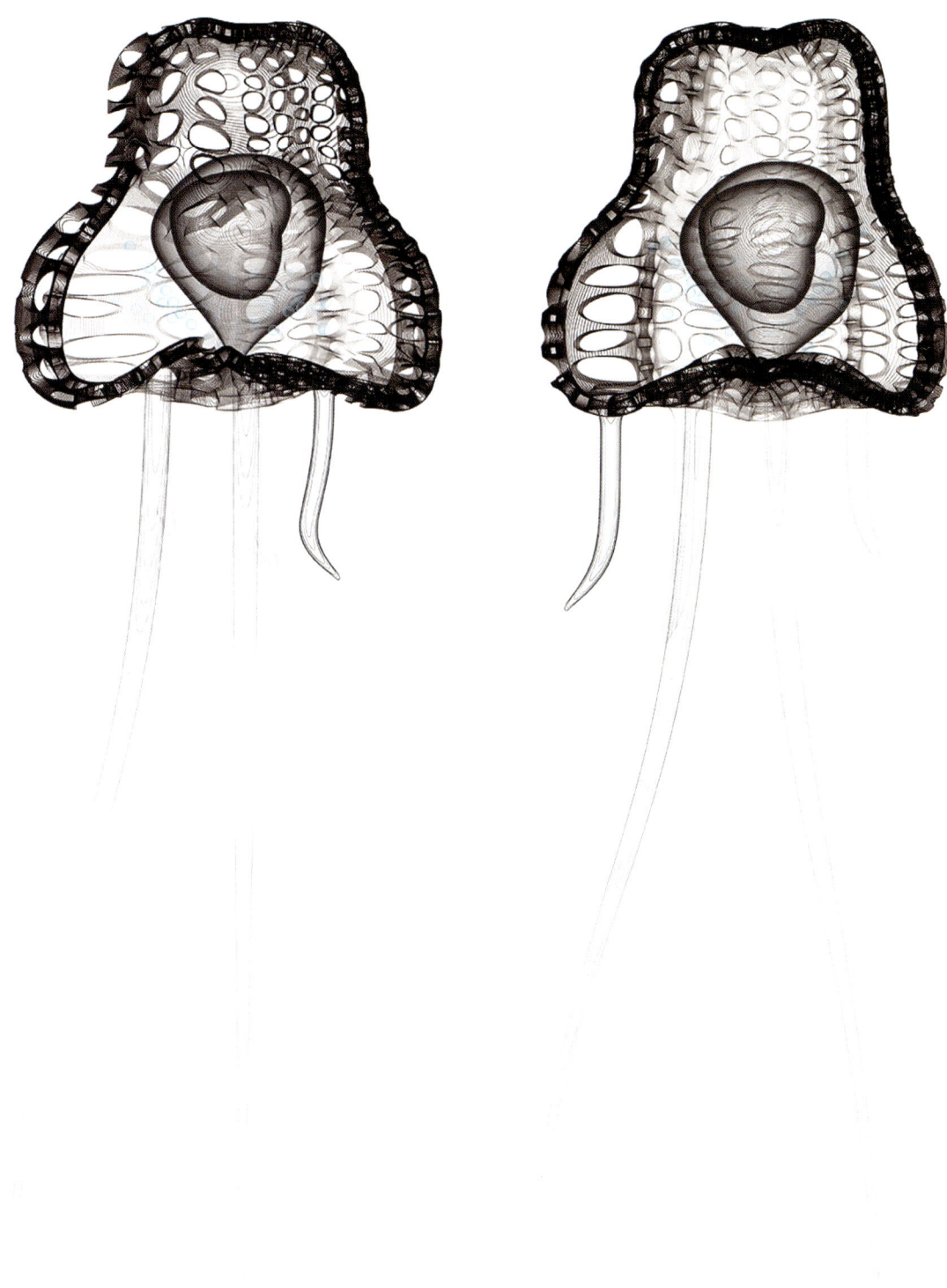

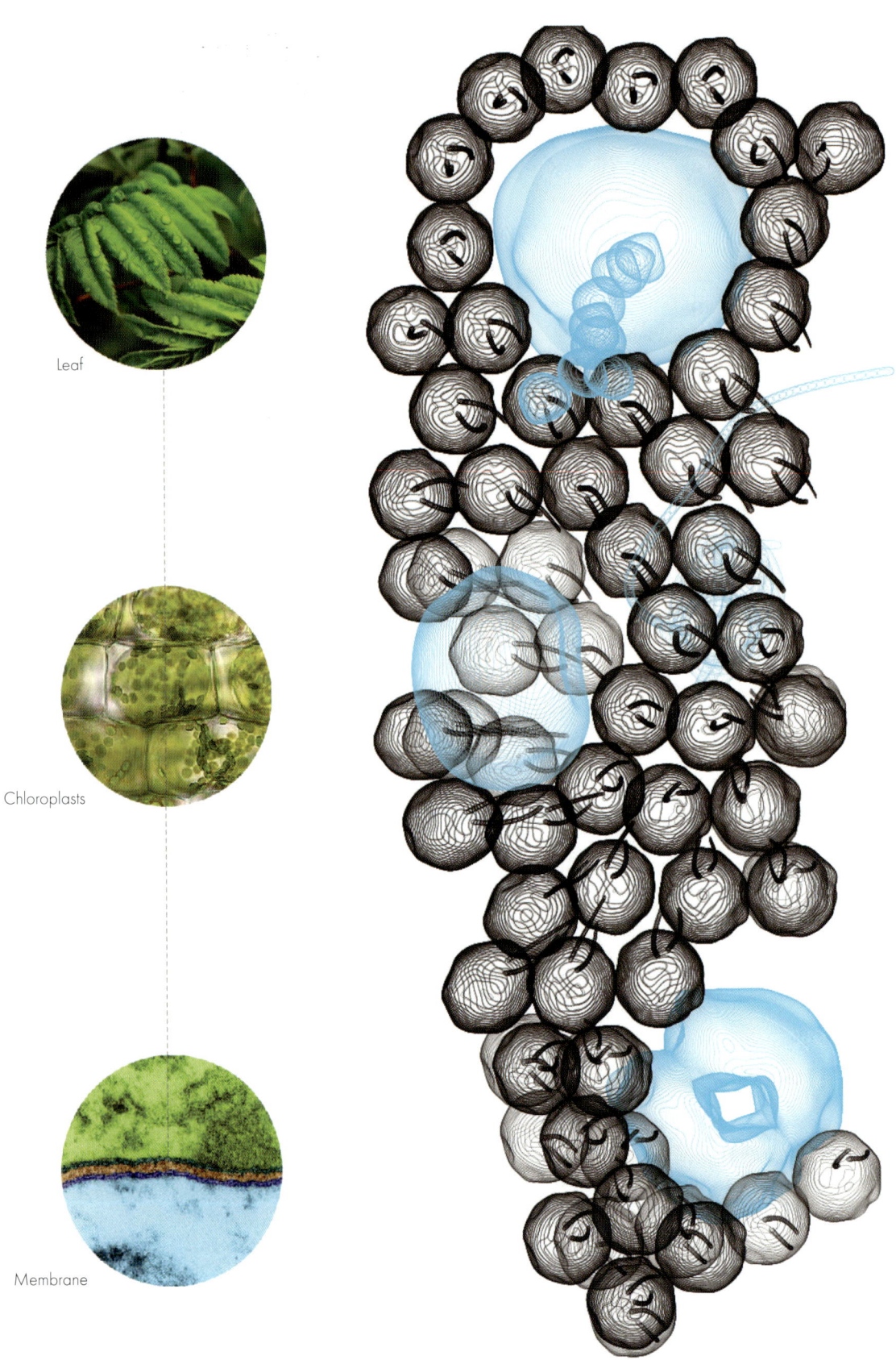

Leaf

Chloroplasts

Membrane

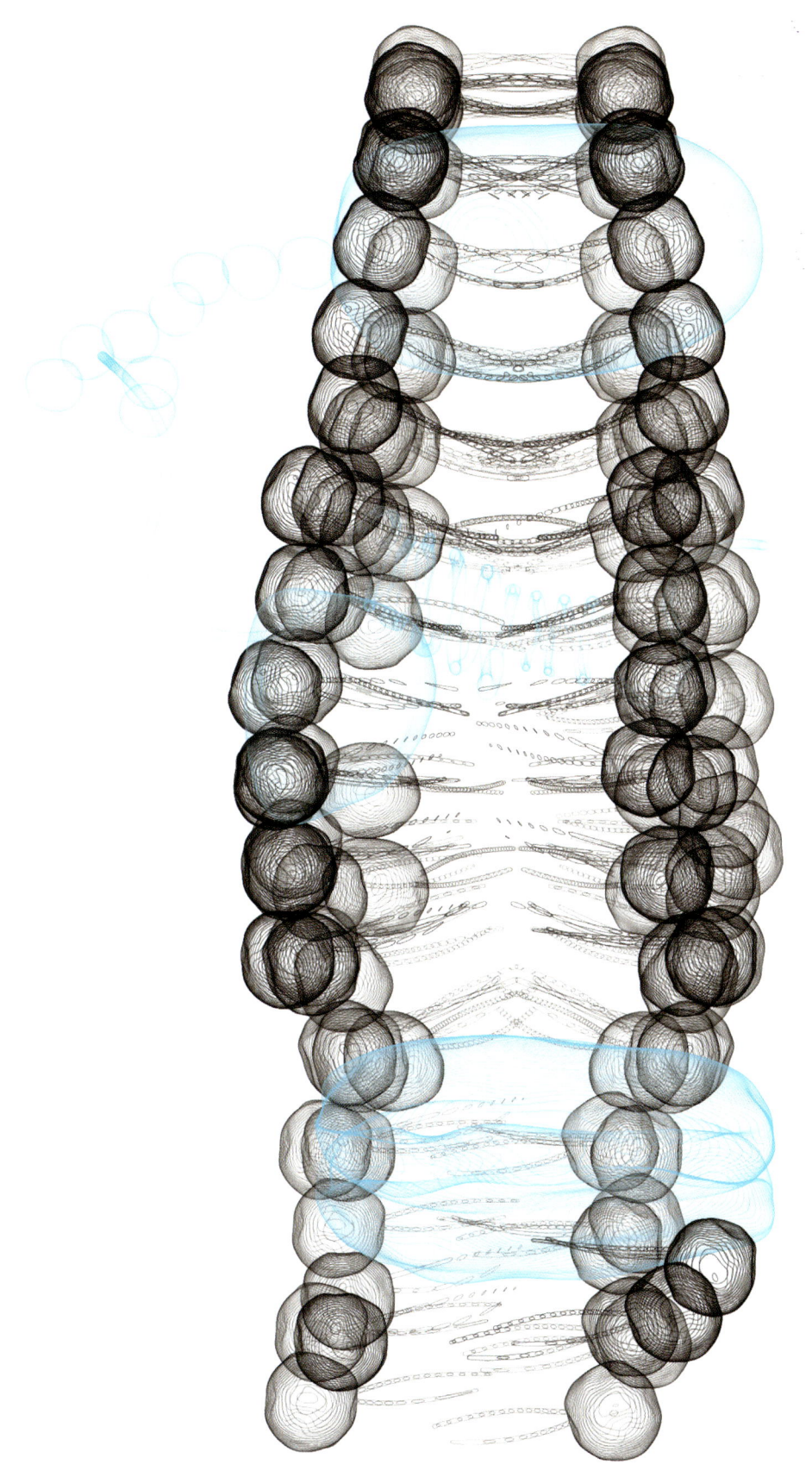

YINAN ZHU

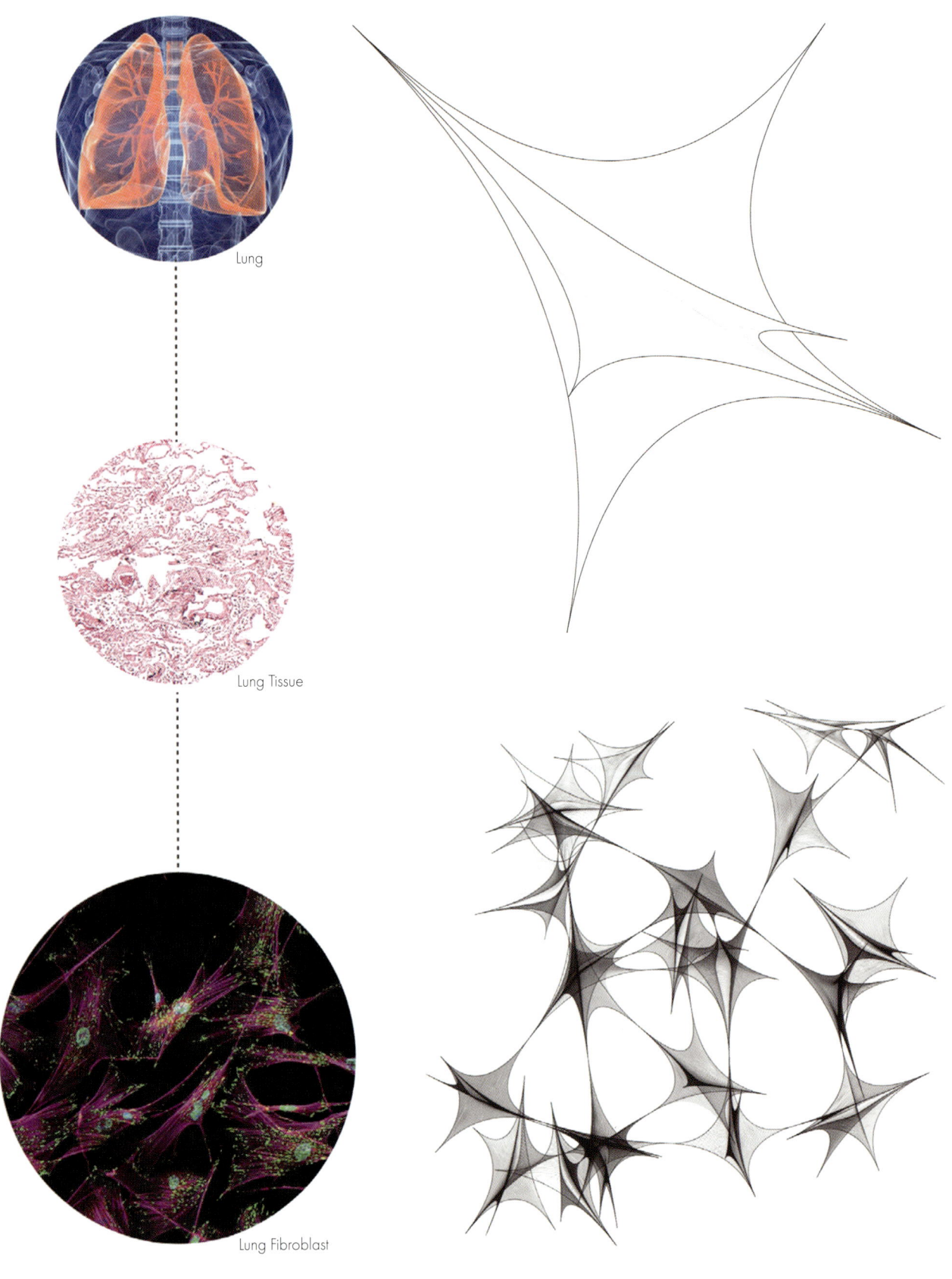

Lung

Lung Tissue

Lung Fibroblast

CELLULAR TRANSFORMATIONS

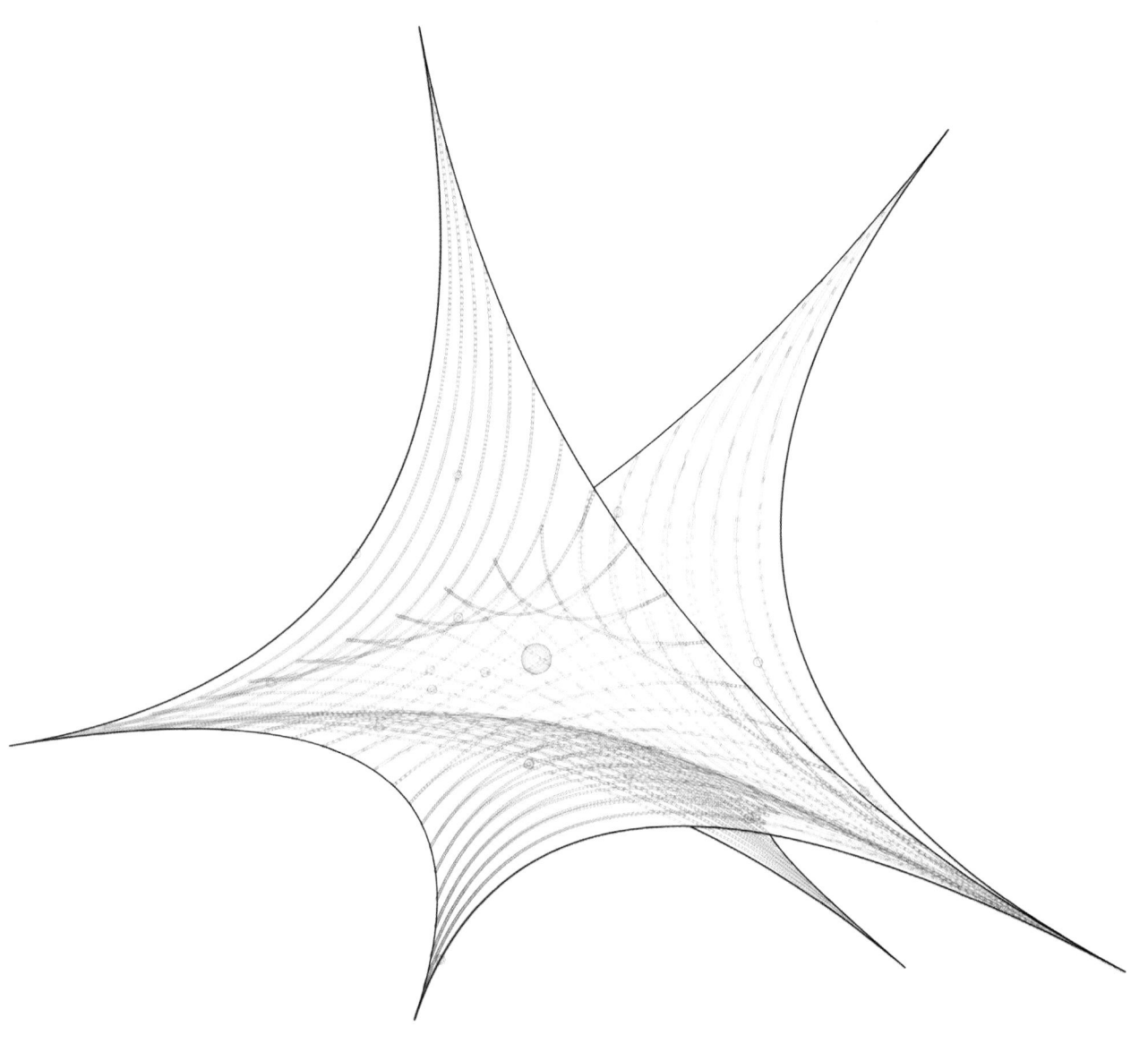

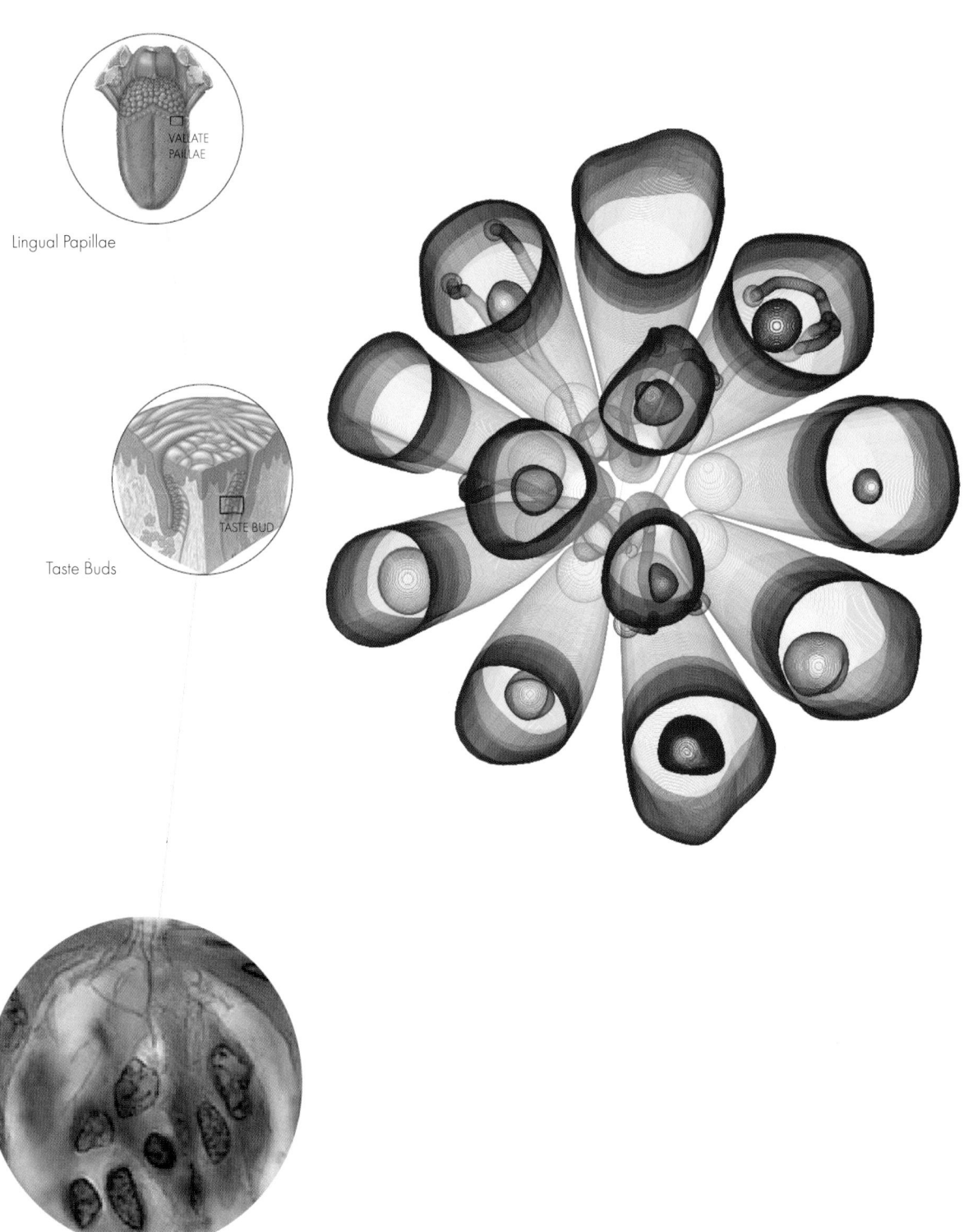

Lingual Papillae

Taste Buds

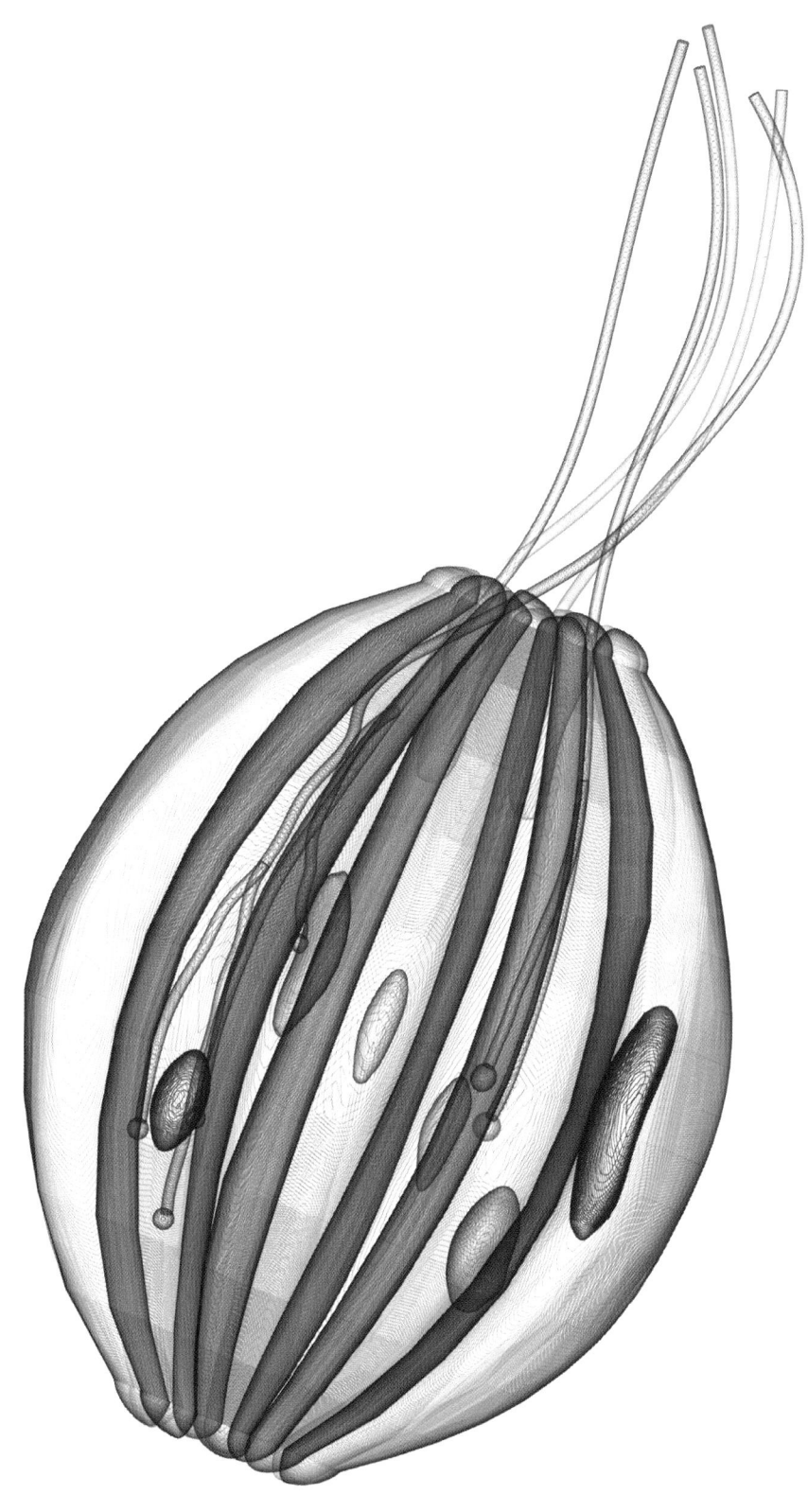

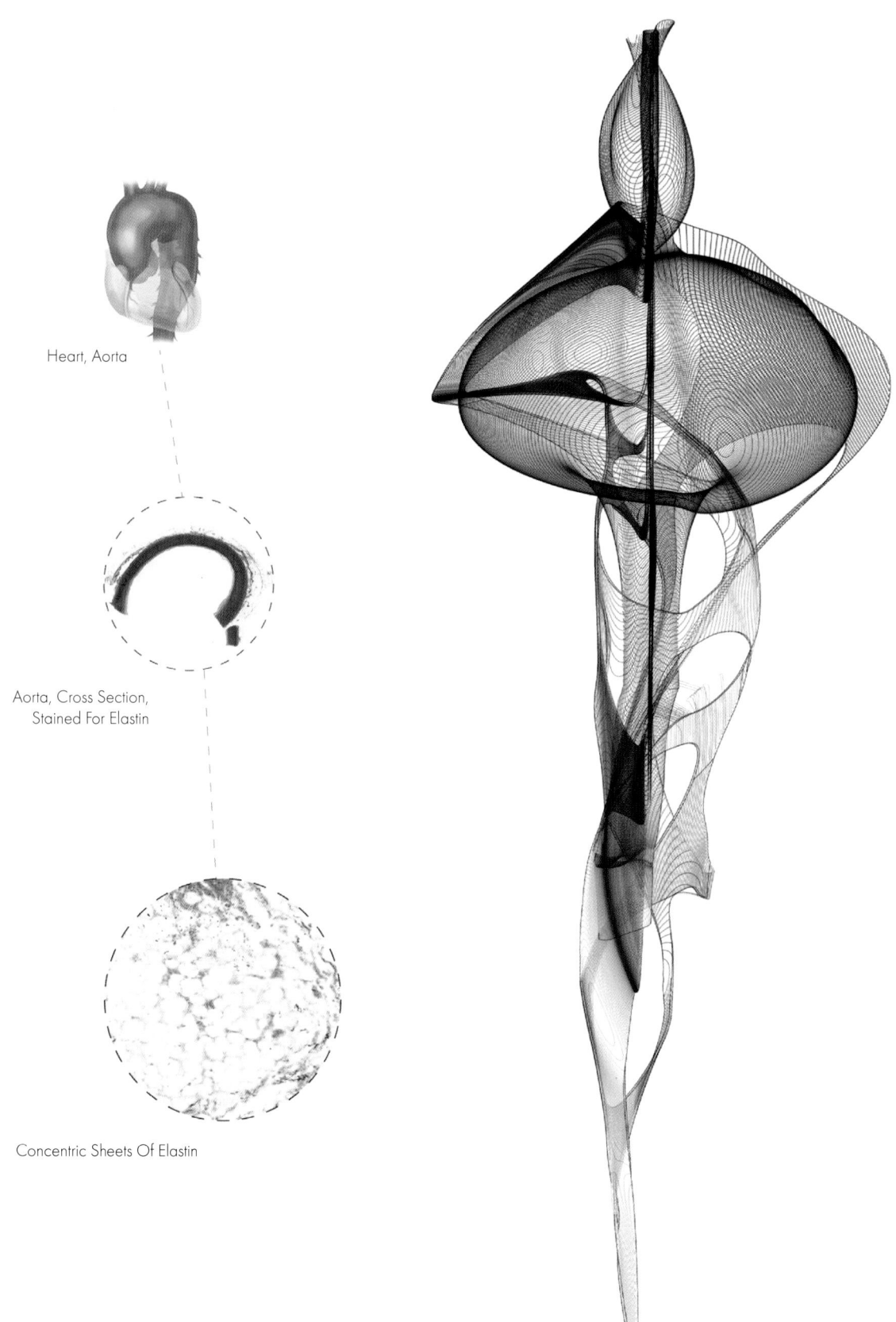

Heart, Aorta

Aorta, Cross Section, Stained For Elastin

Concentric Sheets Of Elastin

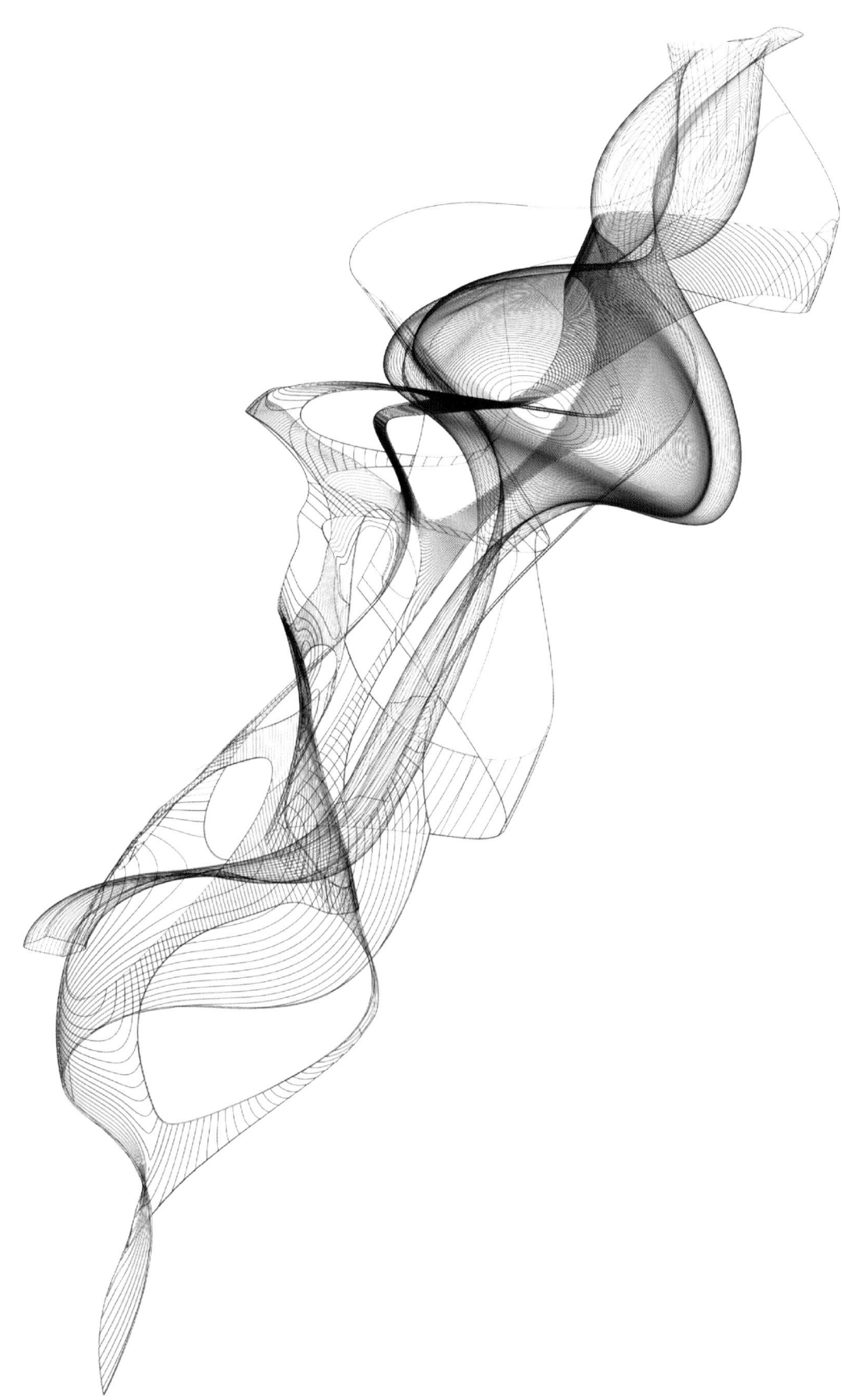

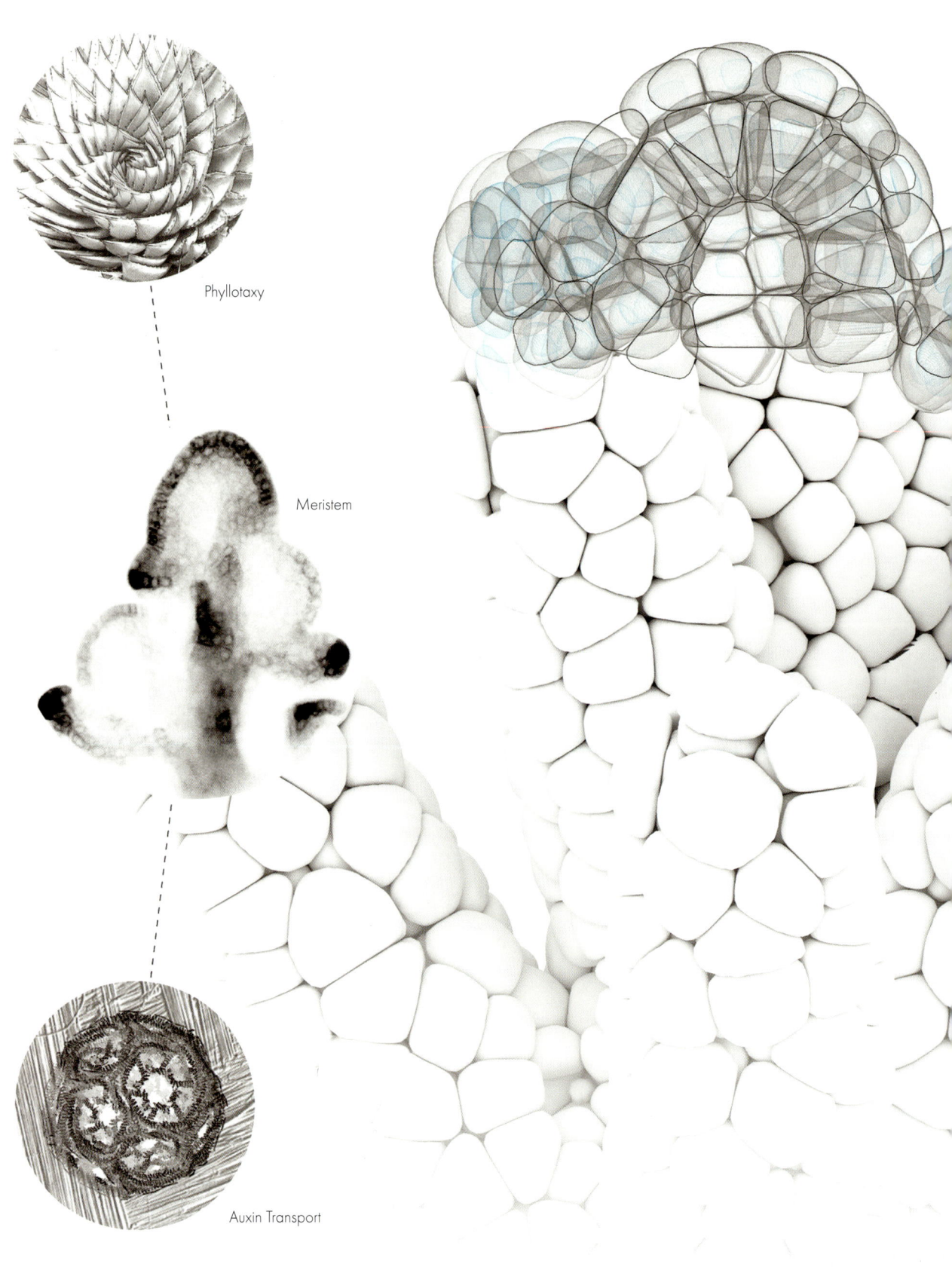

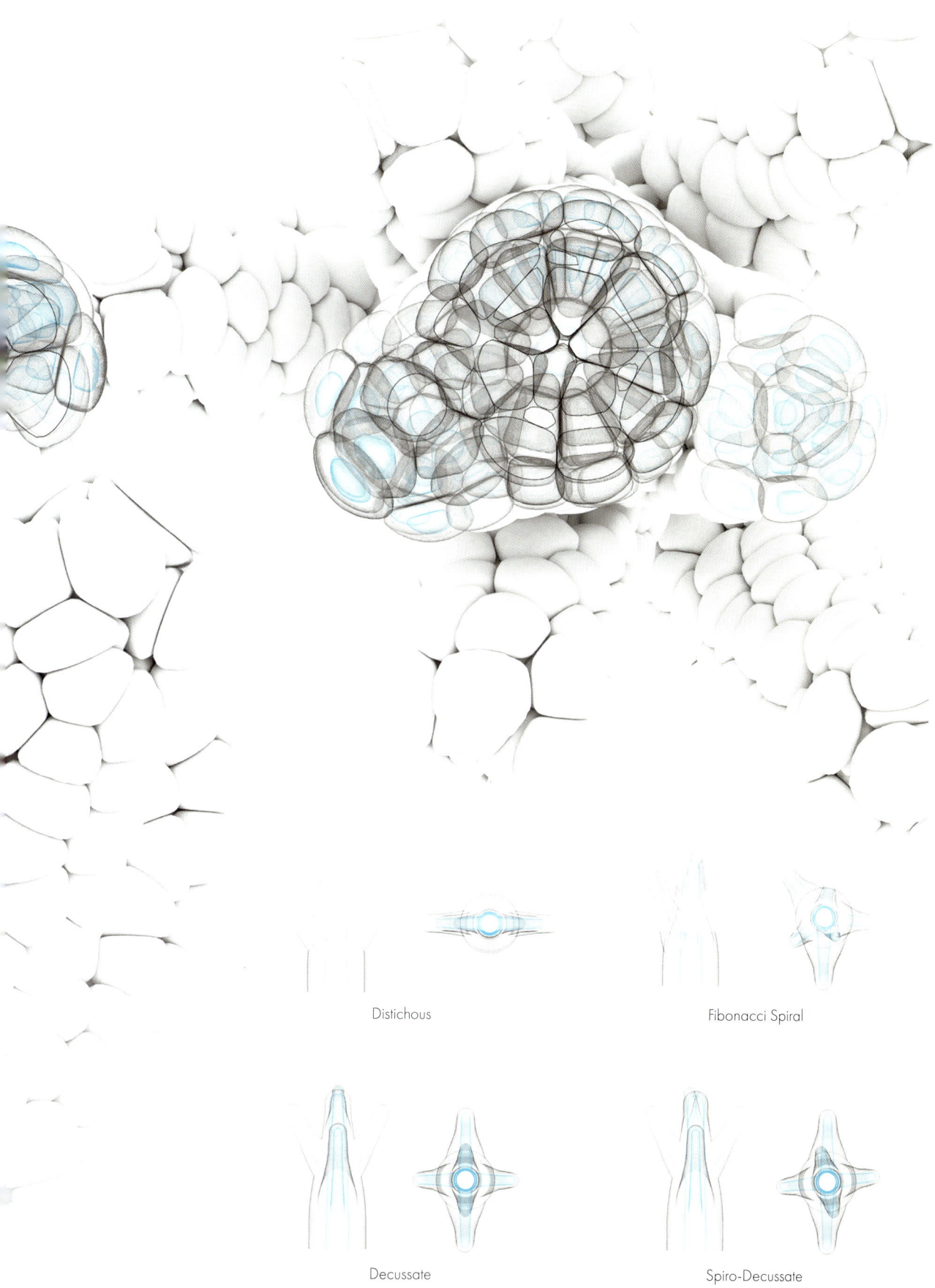

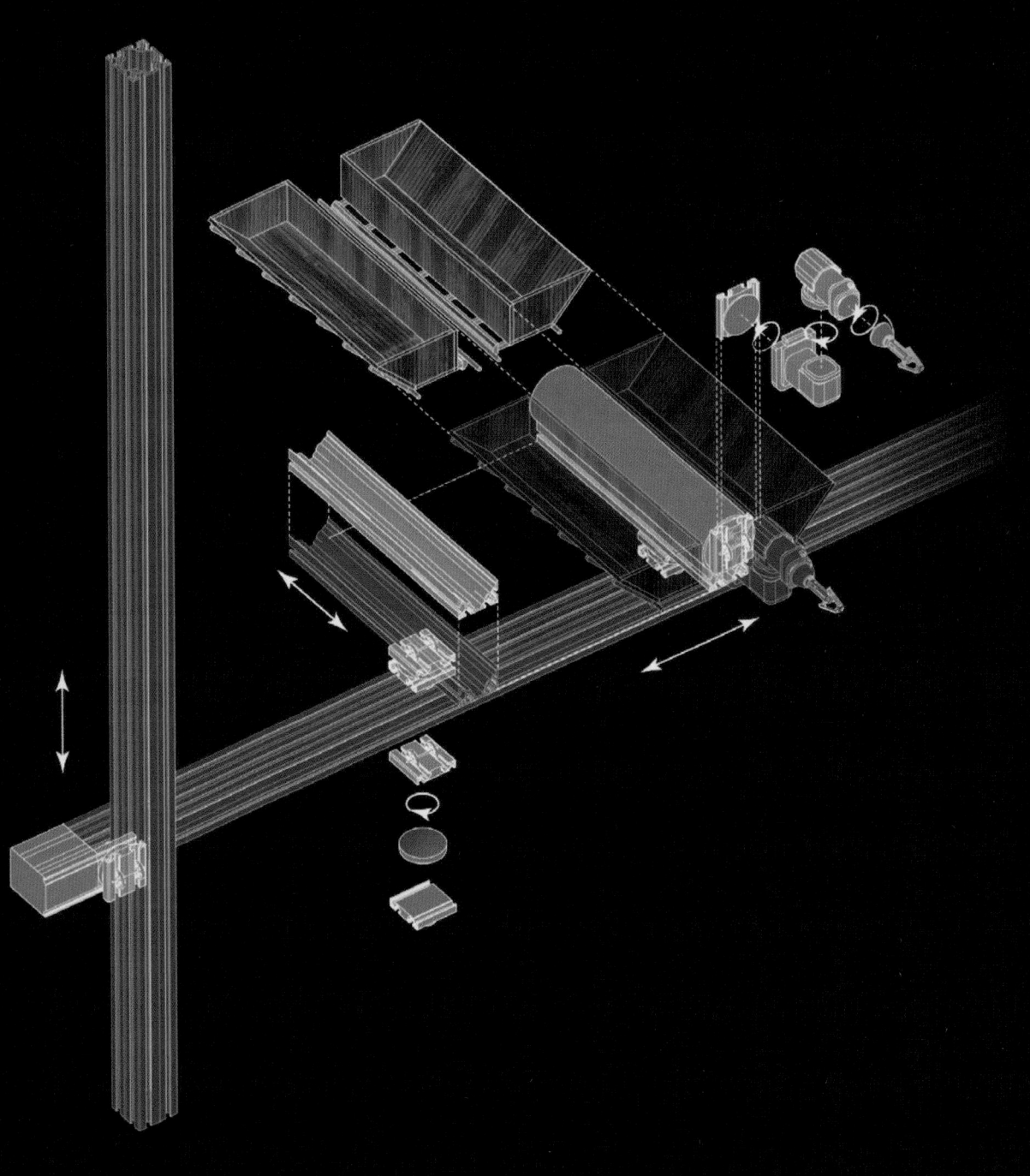

REMEDIATION: 2014
CHERNOBYL RESEARCH

The goal of the Chernobyl Research project was to propose bioremediation strategies for the contaminated surroundings following the disastrous accident in the Chernobyl Nuclear Power Plant, near the city of Pripyat in the north of Ukraine. It is considered the worst nuclear disaster in modern history. Projects used existing and engineered plants to decontaminate the air, water, soil and buildings at the Chernobyl site. They implemented specialized infrastructural design for the safe deployment, harvesting and removal of contaminated materials to return the environment to its original state.

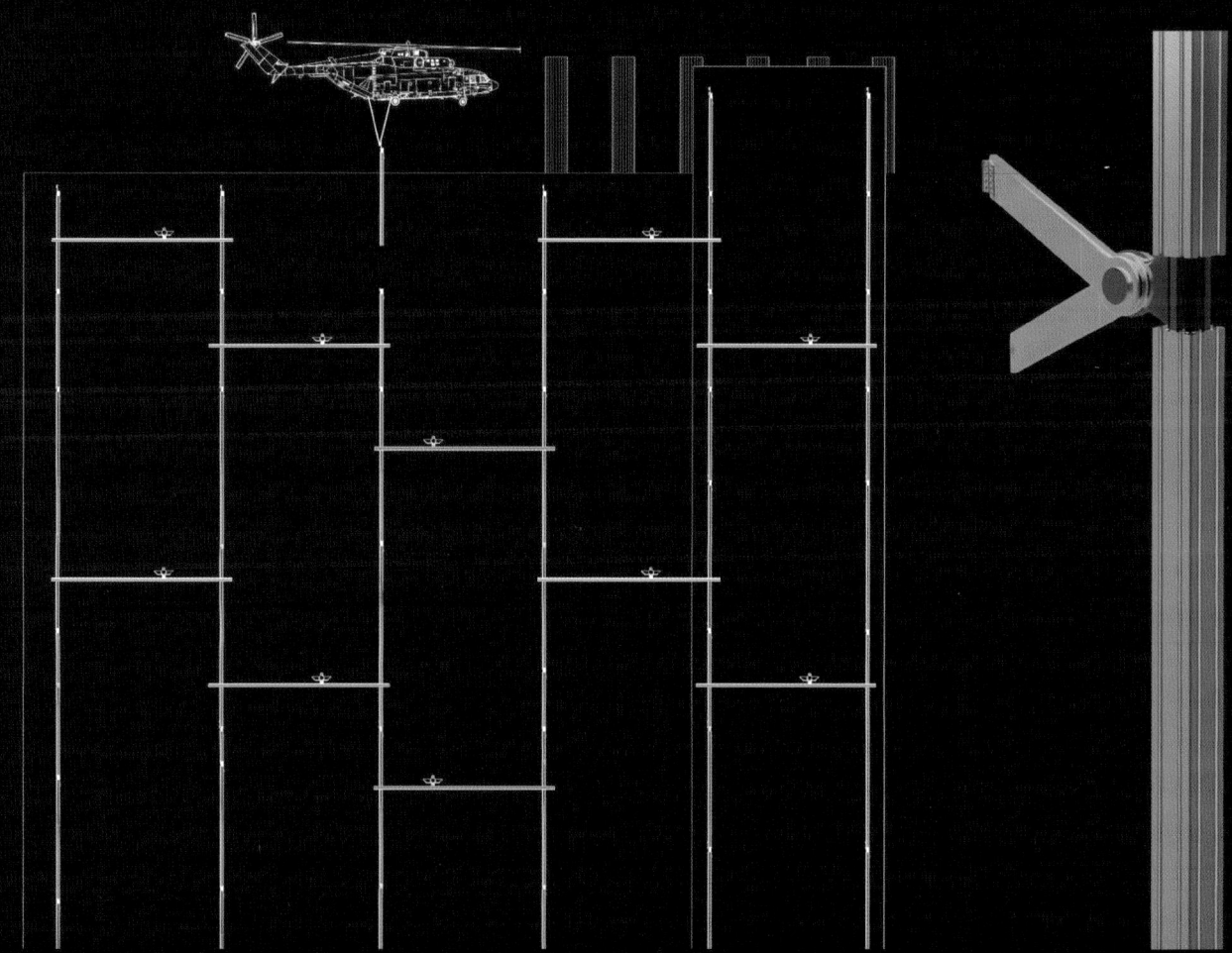

FLOWER OF LIFE

The Chernobyl disaster was a catastrophic nuclear accident that occurred on 26 April 1986 at the Chernobyl Nuclear Power Plant in Ukraine, which was under the direct jurisdiction of the central authorities of the Soviet Union. An explosion and fire released large quantities of radioactive particles into the atmosphere, which spread over much of the western USSR and Europe.

The Flower of Life is a machine to deal with the pollution in the air after the nuclear accident. The idea was inspired by kites. The machine incorporates radiotrophic fungus on the kite panels. The function of the fungus is to absorb radiation in the air. The machine provides nutrients and attachment sites for the fungus.

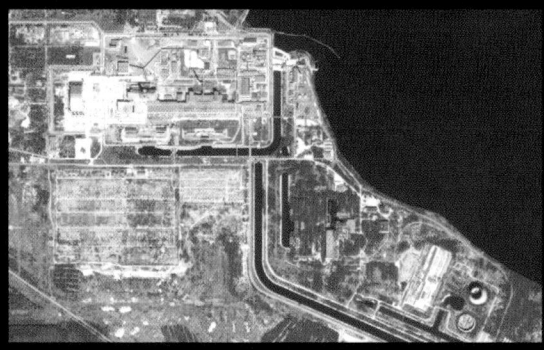

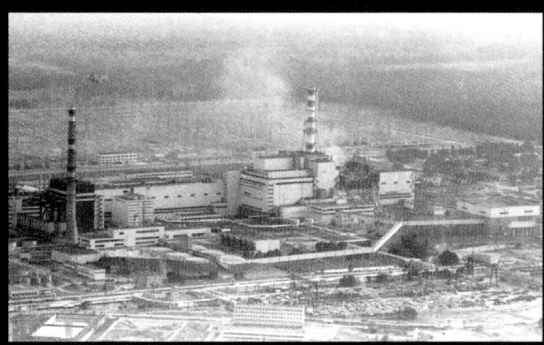

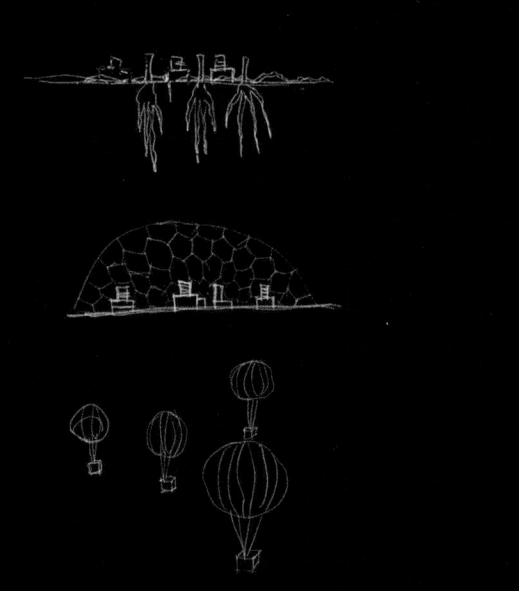

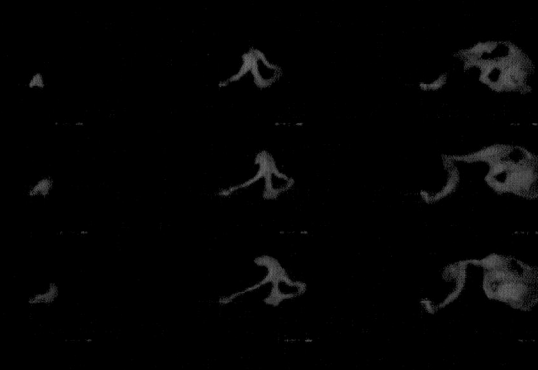

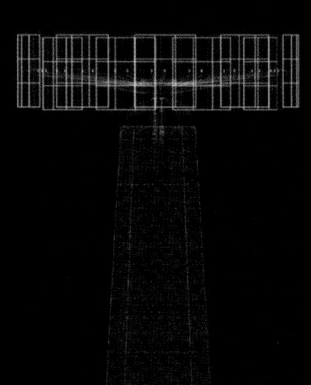

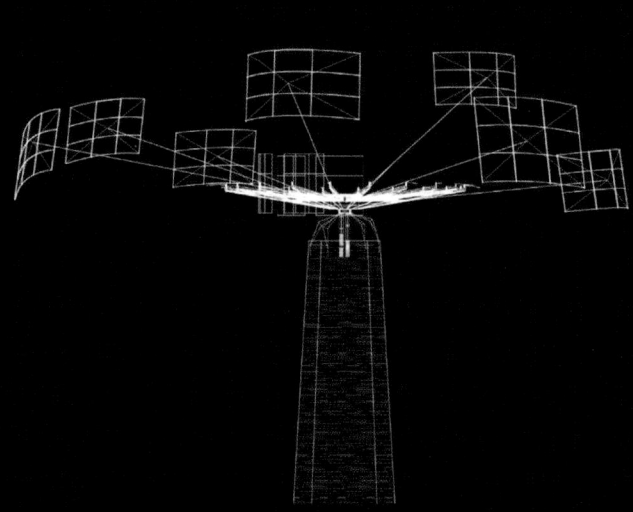

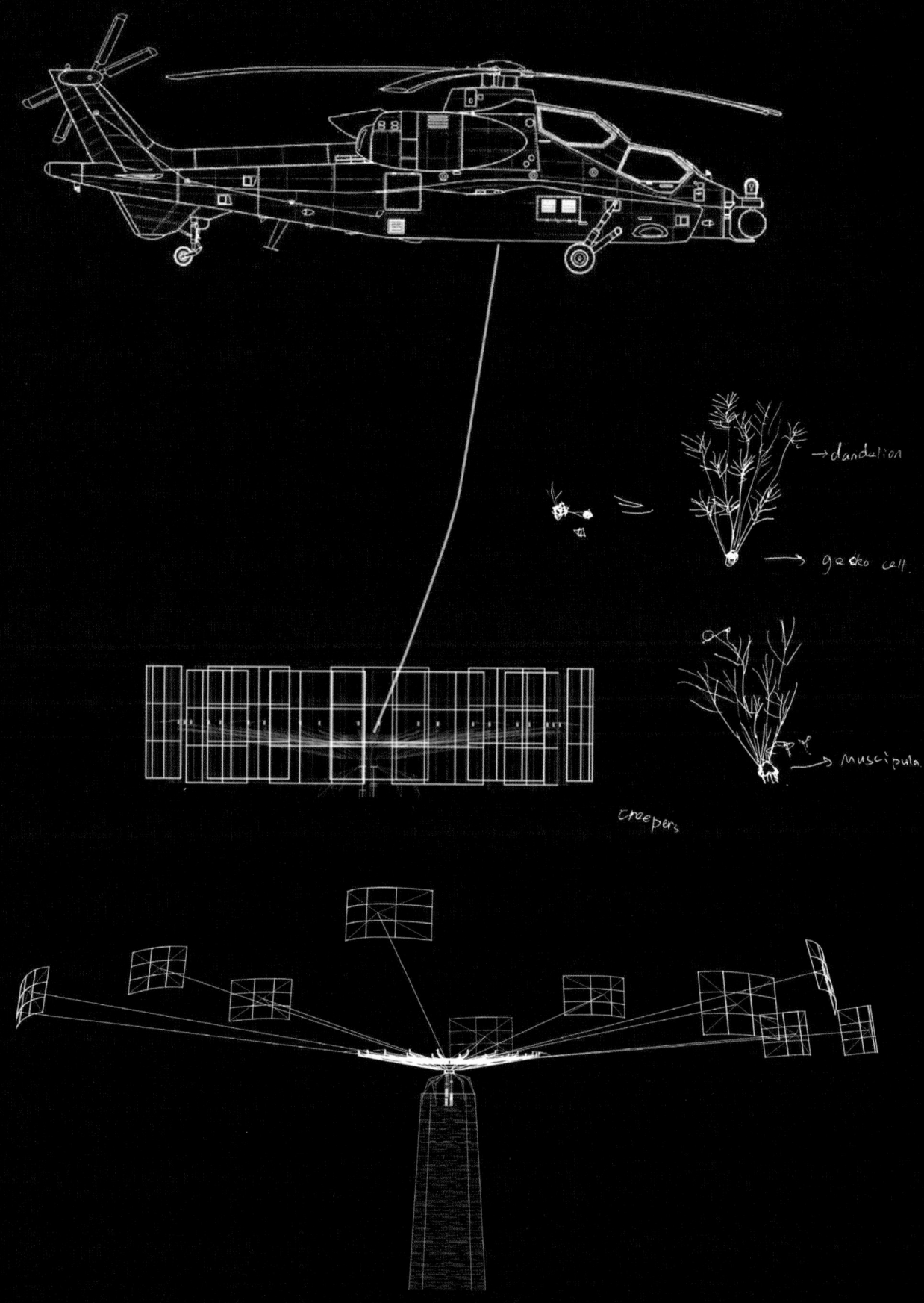

YAFENG LIU | SHENG LI

Radiotrophic fungi appear to use the pigment melanin to convert gamma radiation into chemical energy for growth. This proposed mechanism may be similar to anabolic pathways for the synthesis of reduced organic carbon (e.g., carbohydrates) in phototrophic organisms, which capture photons from visible light with pigments such as chlorophyll to power photosynthesis.

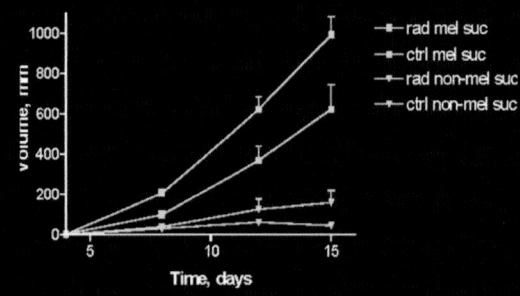

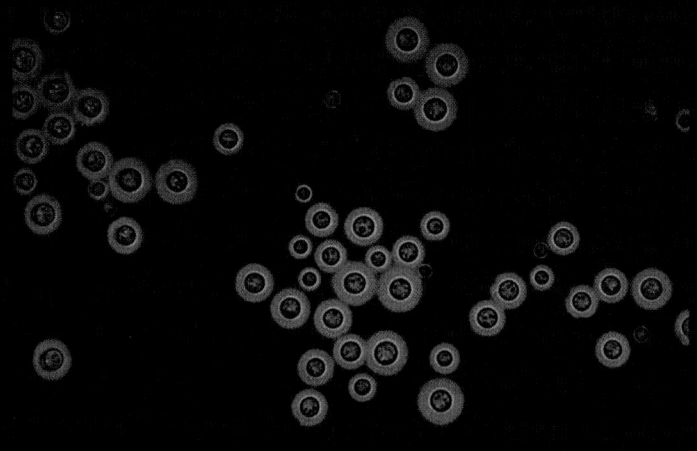

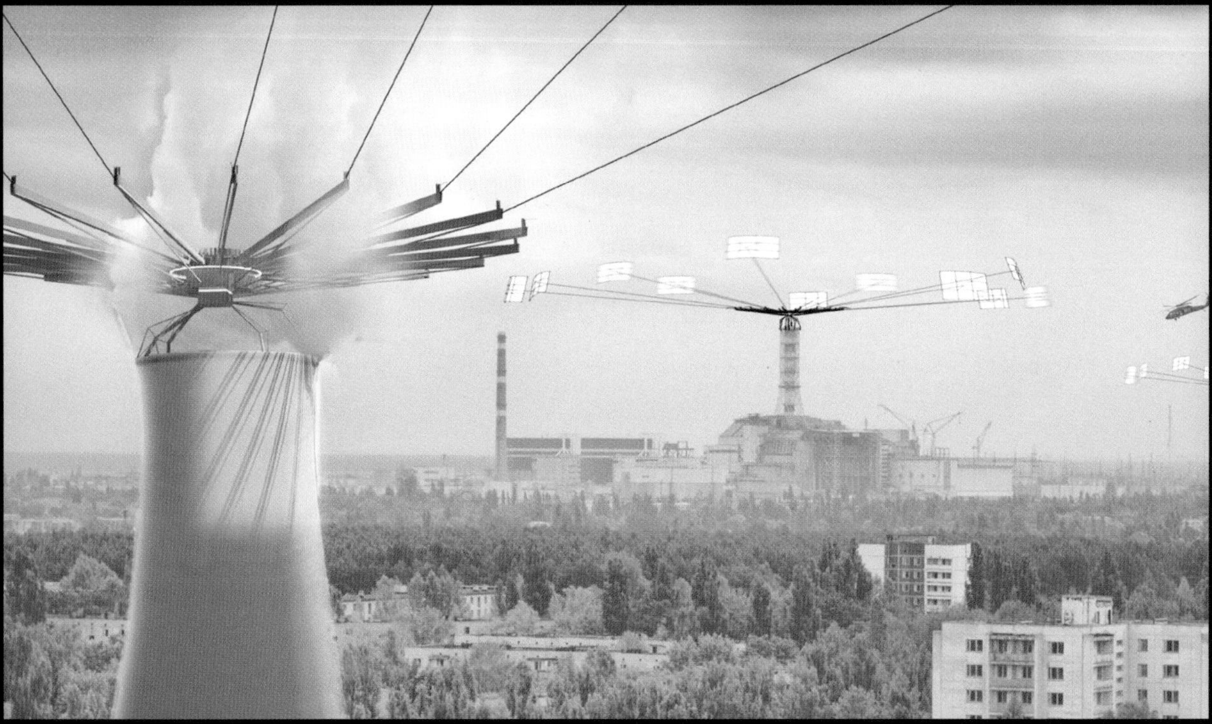

145   CELLULAR TRANSFORMATIONS

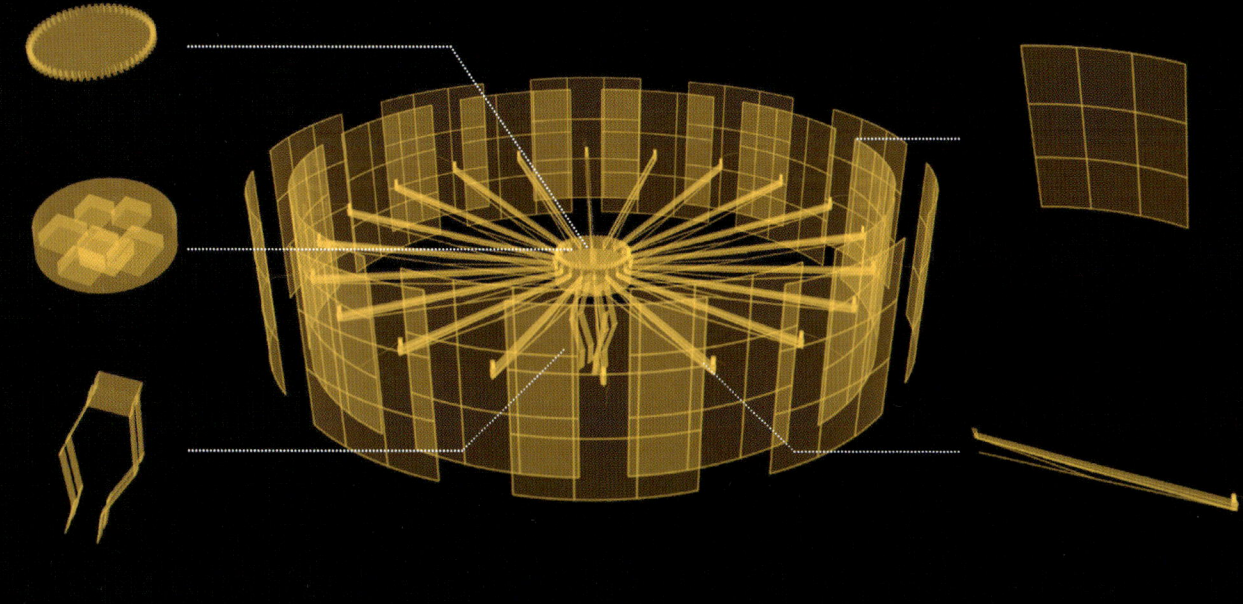
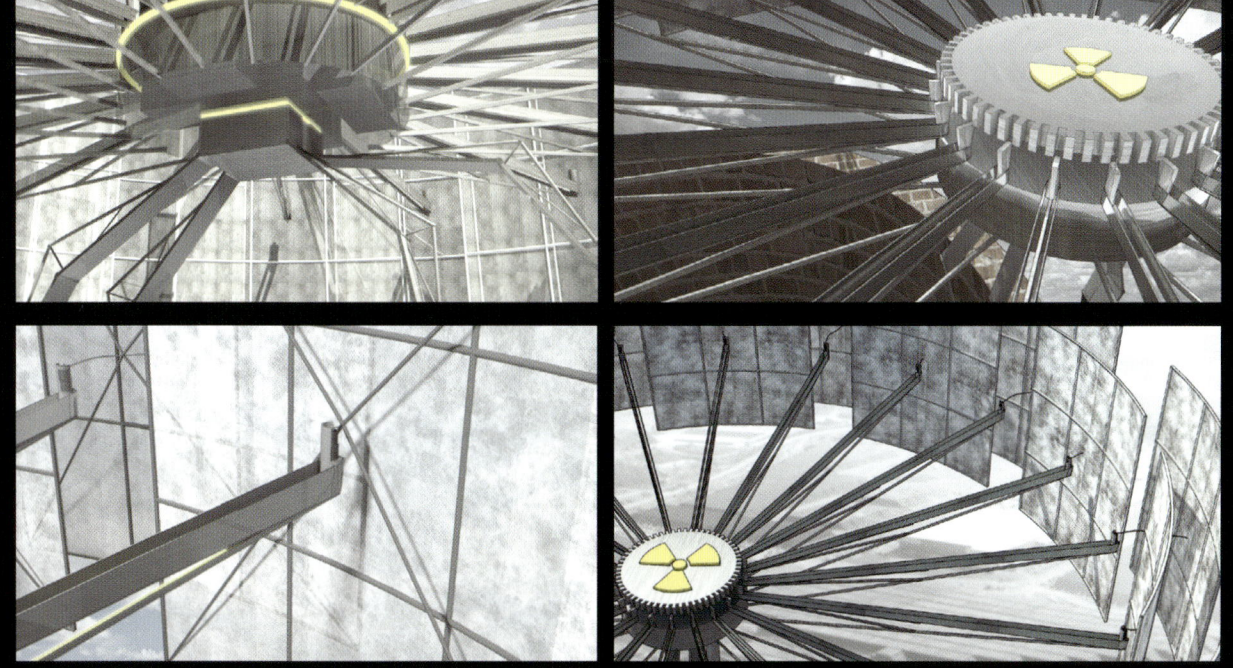

DANIEL ADAMS | YOUNGAH JUNG

CLEANSING THE HARDSCAPE

Symbiotic Encapsulation System

Kudzu is a highly invasive vining plant that reproduces vegetatively without the need for seeds or spores and not requiring a connection to the soil, making it extremely capable of climbing vertical surfaces.

Radiotrophic fungi spores would germinate within domatia engineered into Kudzu plants. When the spores detect radiation, they would affect auxin gradients within the plant, causing it to grow toward stronger sources of radiation.

Fungal colonies would grow into the concrete walls and encapsulate radioactive clusters. A melanin shield would reduce the radioactivity so additional spores will be more drawn to untouched hotspots.

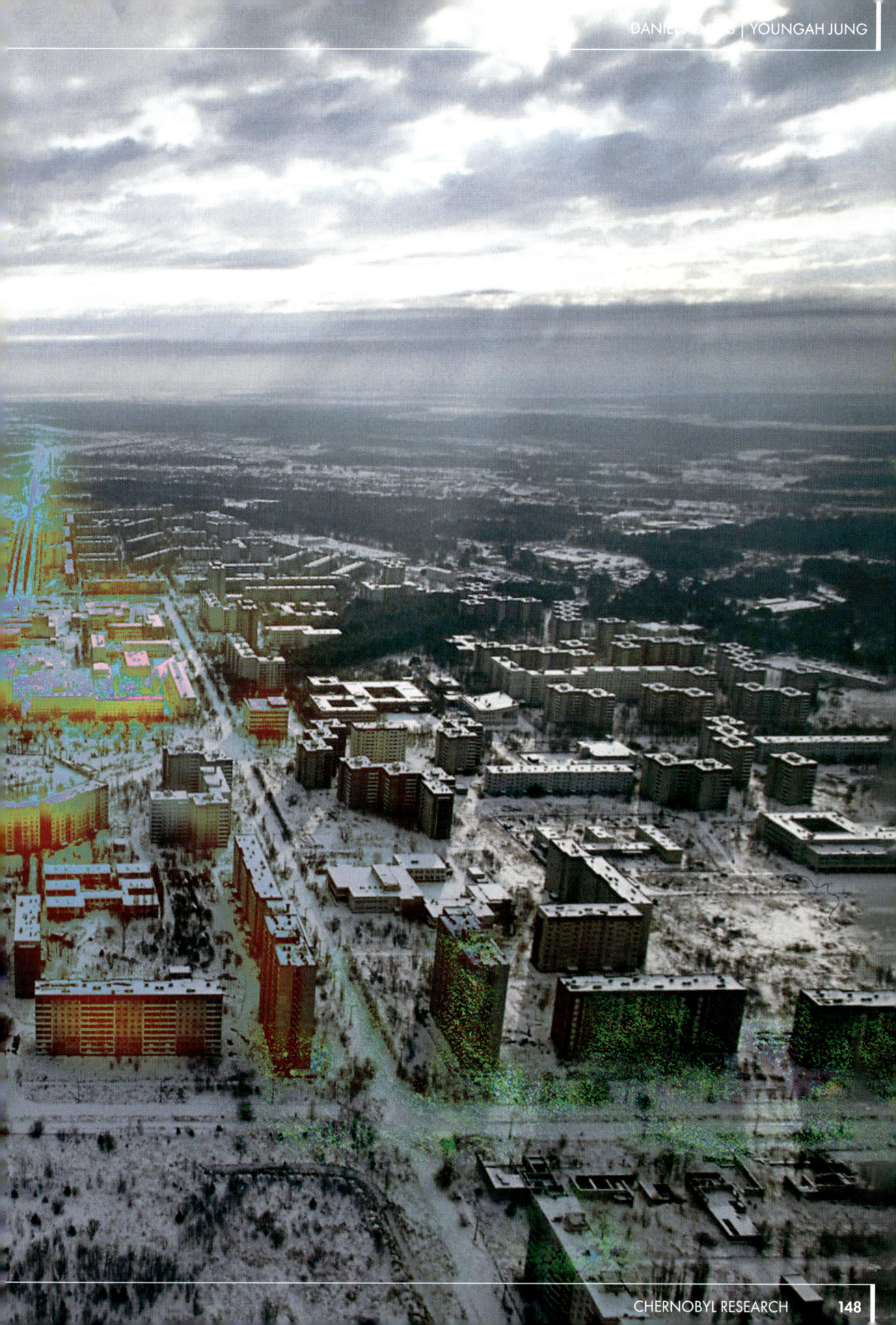

DANIEL ADAMS | YOUNGAH JUNG

The Russian Mi-26 is the largest helicopter ever put into production. A modified version, the Mi-26S was used after the Chernobyl disaster to measure radiation and to drop insulating material on the damaged reactor. Their large carrying capacity makes them ideal as a primary means of deployment and extraction: including frames and retrofitted tanks.

The Russian T-55 tank is the most prolifically produced tank in history, with many retrofitted models still in use today. Production ceased and they were considered obsolete by the Soviet army five years before the Chernobyl disaster. Models have been fitted with a large scale robot arm system in order to freely cover roads, parking lots, and other systems close to the ground.

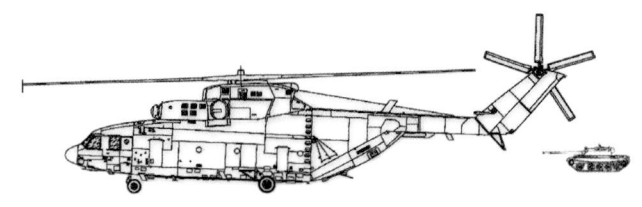

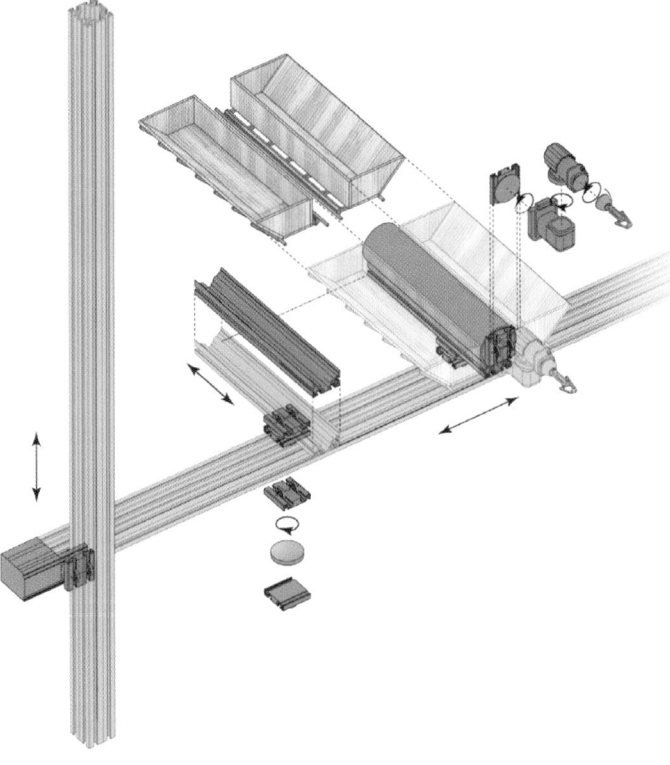

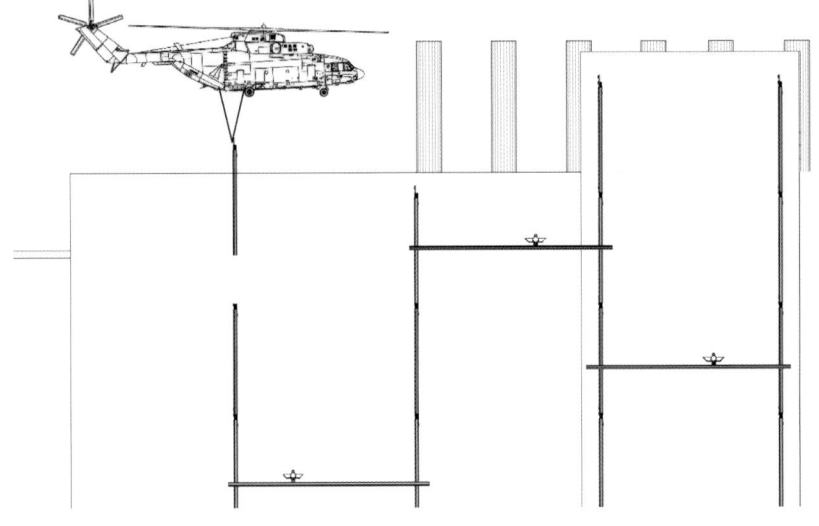

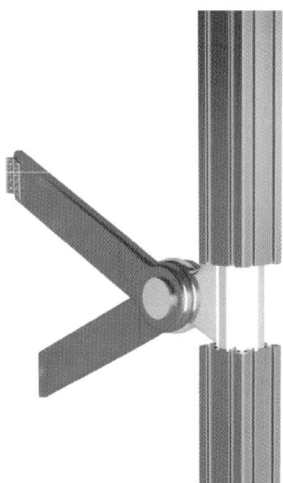

CELLULAR TRANSFORMATIONS

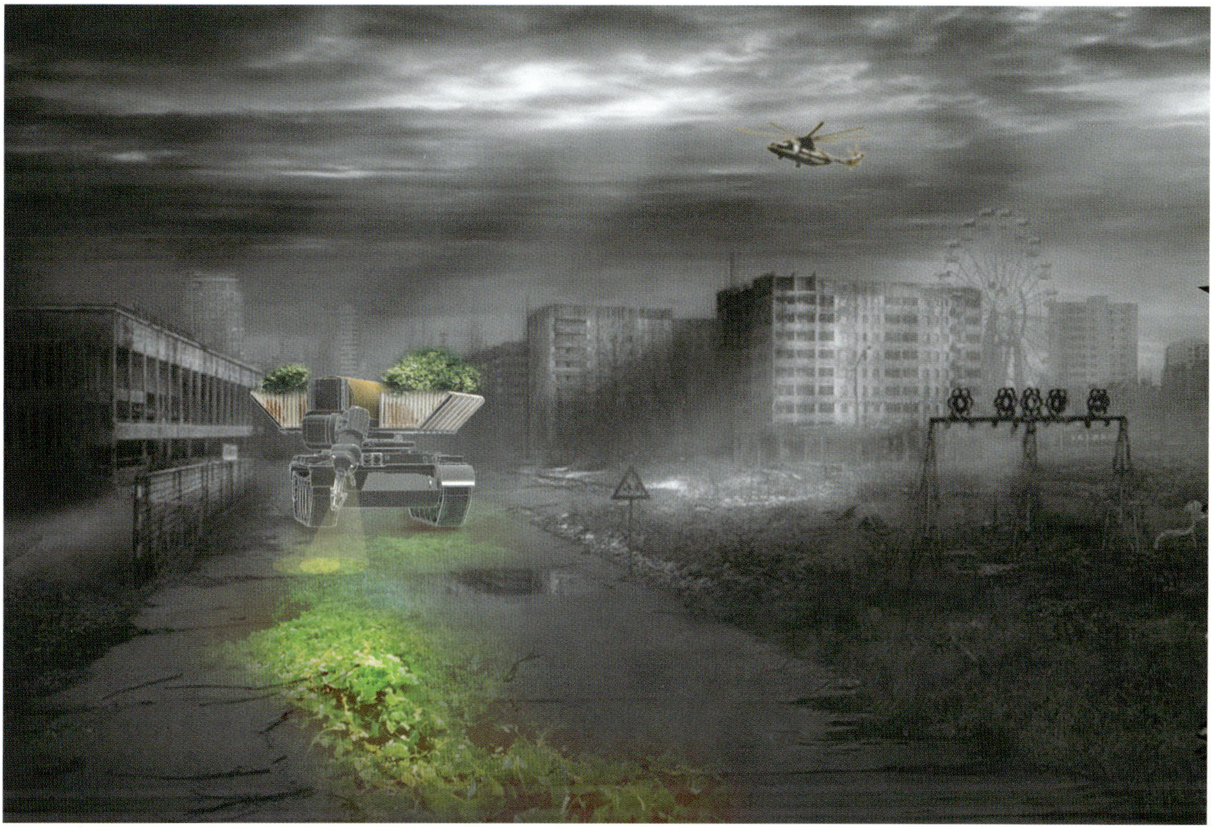

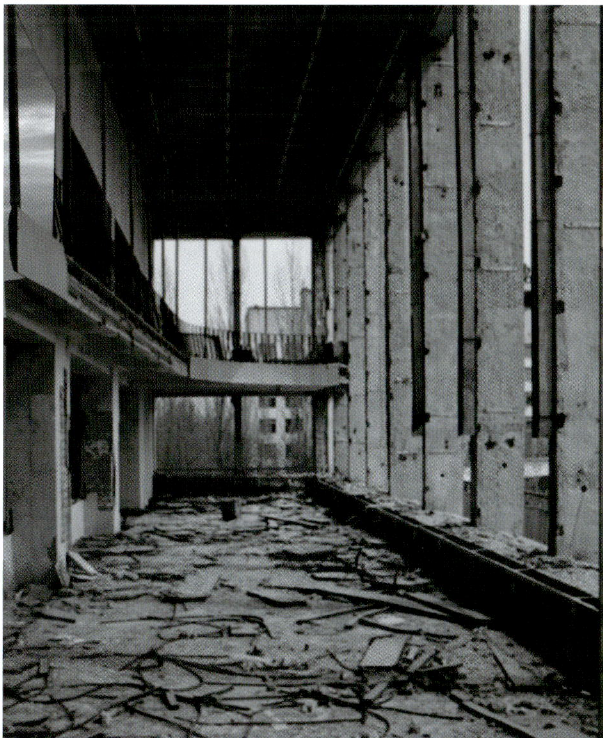

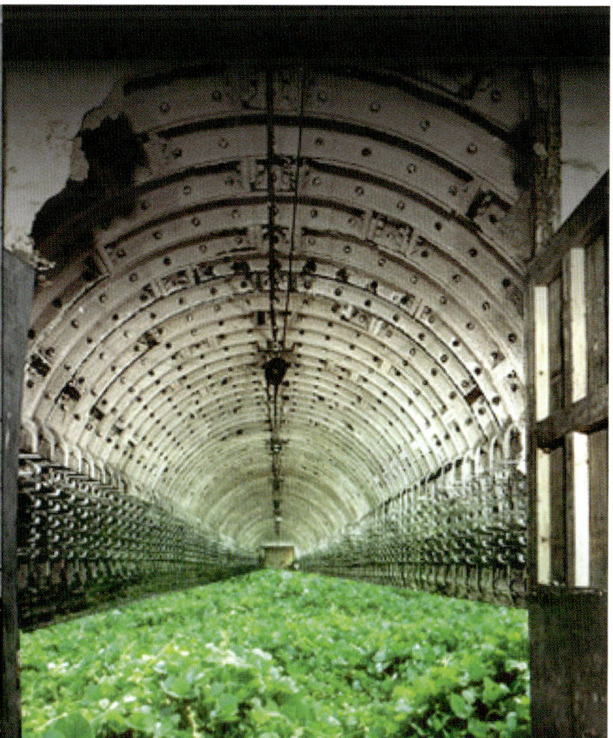

RADIATION DOOMBRINGER

This project aims to cure the Chernobyl landscape using plants that absorb radioactive elements. The machine is designed to not only set plantings but also to harvest them to dispose the nuclear waste.

A sunflower's root plays an important role in absorbing heavy metals, including radioactive elements. They have been wildly used in Fukushima, where nuclear radiation also leaked during the Japanese earthquake.

Similar to sunflowers, Silphium laciniatum can also absorb nuclear radiation according to some scientists. But they differ from sunflowers in their process of bioremediation. Whereas sunflowers are thought to absorb and store radioactive elements in their roots, Silphium laciniatum are thought to store radioactive elements primarily in their shoots.

Since it is easier to harvest shoots rather than roots after plants have absorbed radioactive elements, a new kind of plant is designed by combining the traits of sunflowers and Silphium laciniatum. As young plants are more efficient in bioremediation, they will be planted on the site after they are grown in a lab.

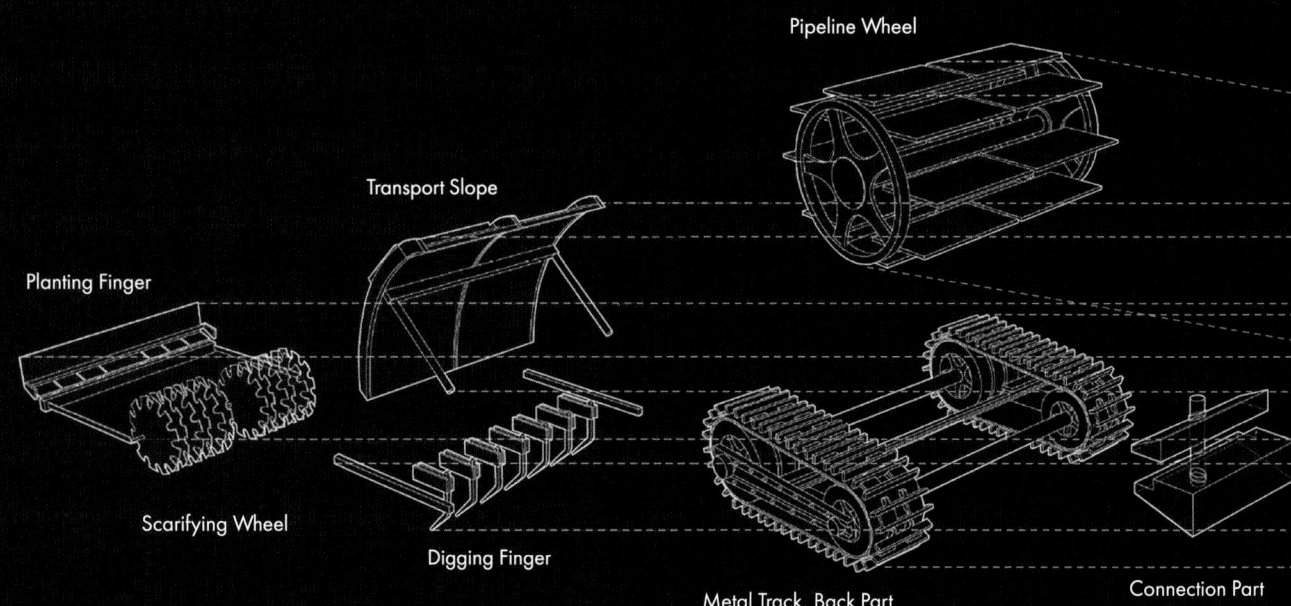

Shoot from
Silphium laciniatum
Root from sunflowers
Silphium laciniatum

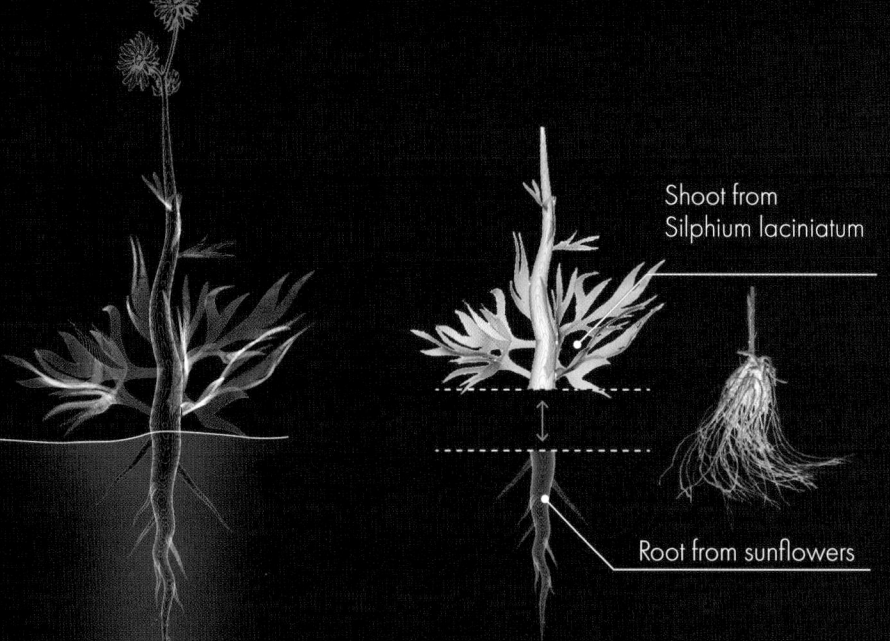

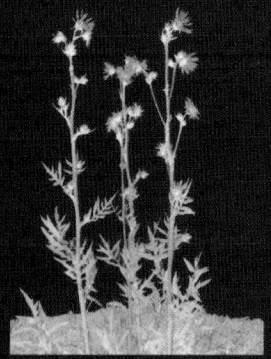

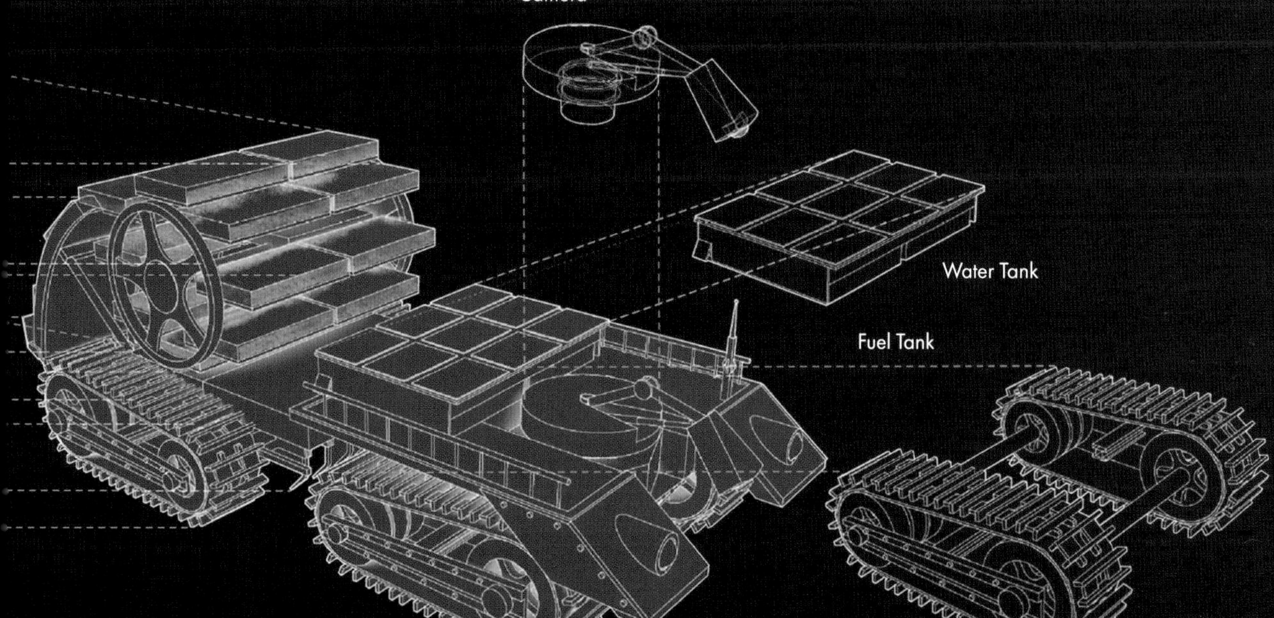
Camera
Water Tank
Fuel Tank
Metal Track, Front Part

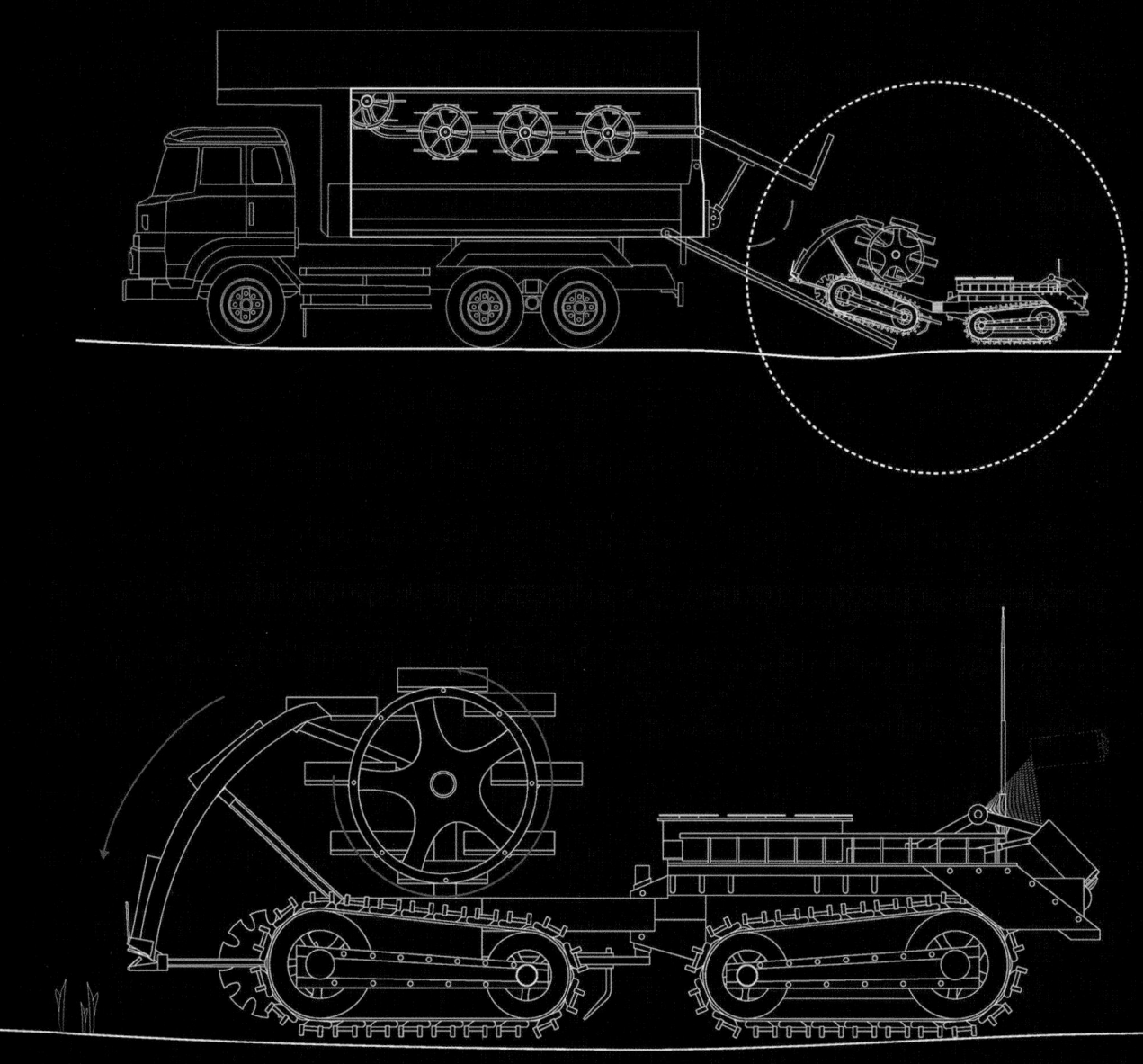

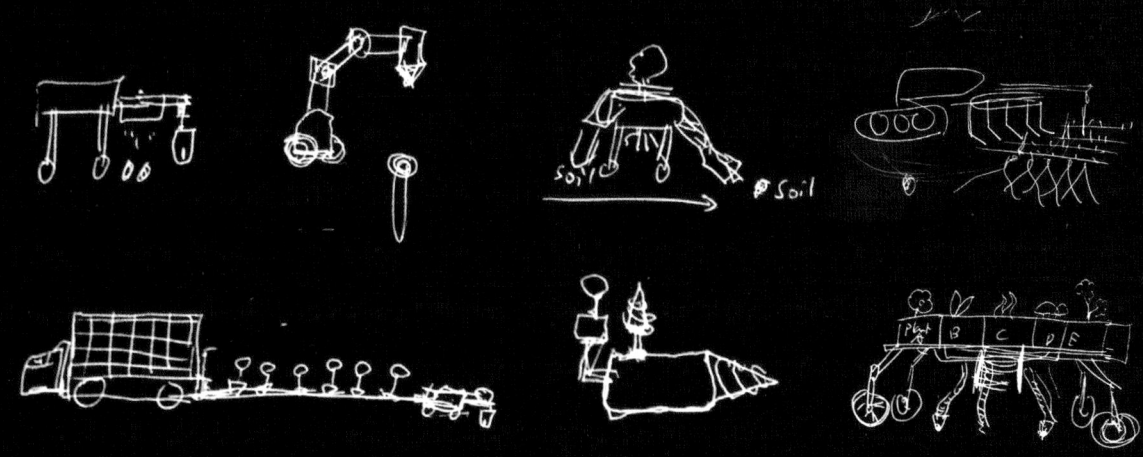

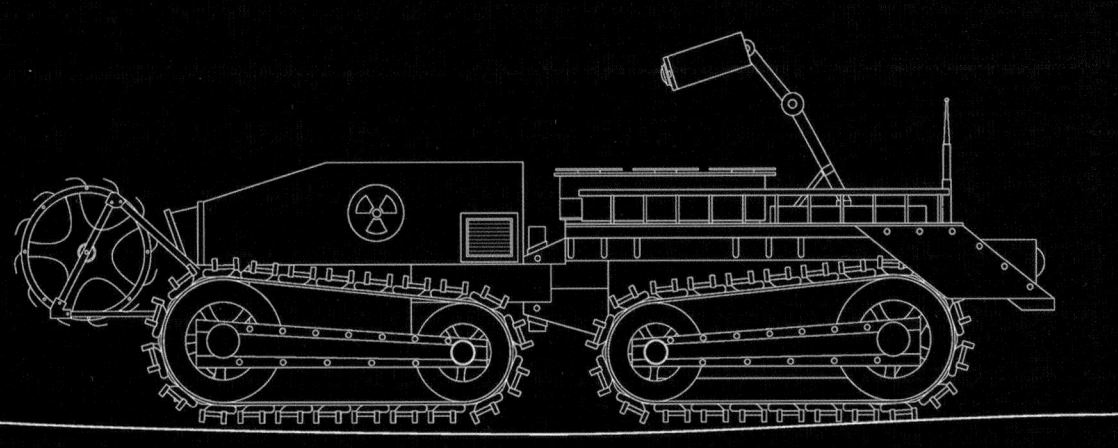

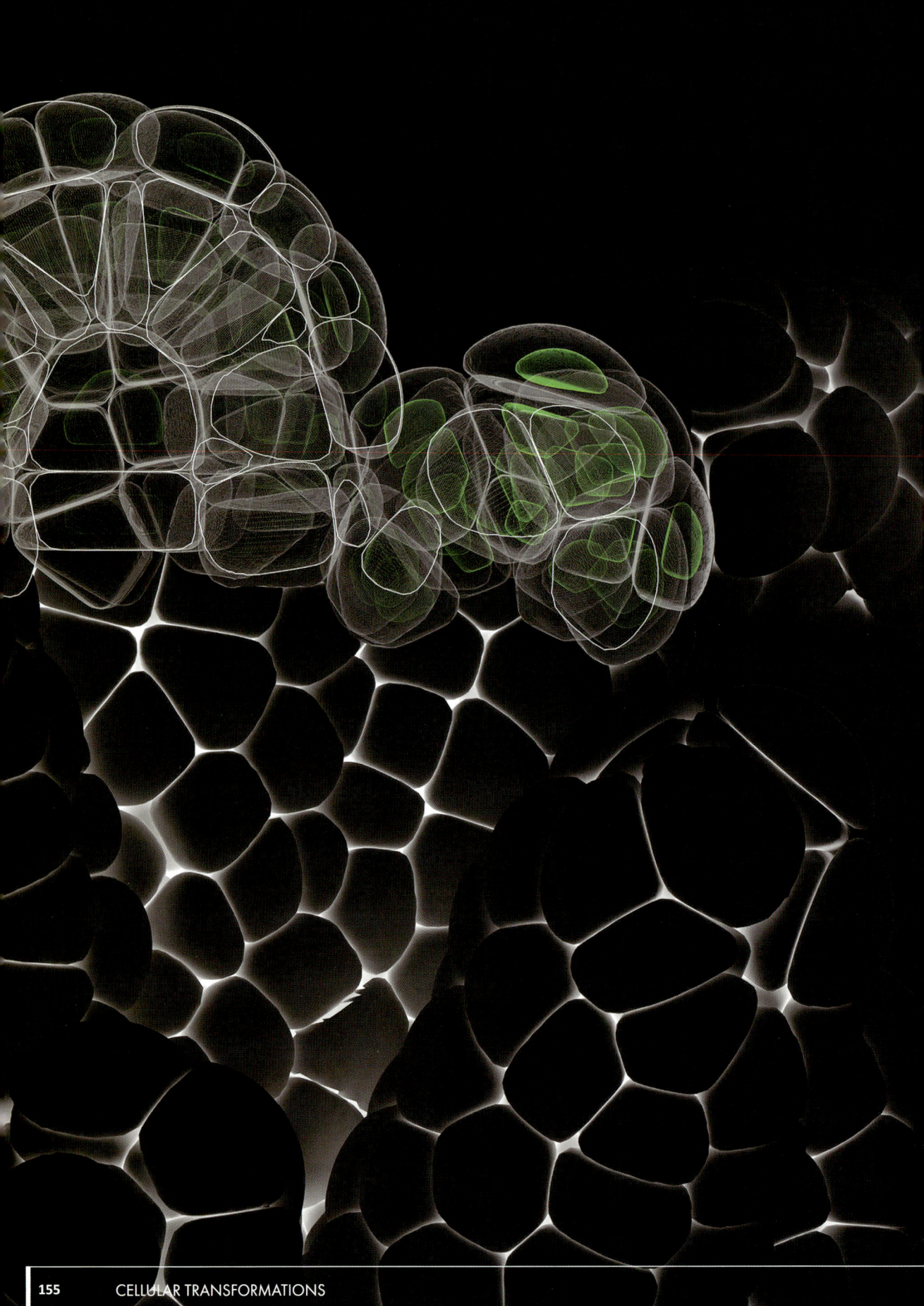

TRANSFORMATION: 2015
ADVANCED CELL ANALYSIS 02

Advanced Cell Analysis used digital modeling and technical drawing processes to analyze the three dimensional performance of biological entities and the spatial relationships between their structural elements. The projects allowed a visual understanding of the microscopic anatomies of cellular structures. This important process revealed how the cellular material and their surroundings interact to inform function and how altering these properties can be used to engineer the form and function of organic matter.

ASTROCYTE AND THE BLOOD BRAIN BARRIER

Astrocyte is one type of glial cell in the brain, which serves as a "glue" to hold the neurons and blood vessels in place. These star-shaped spiky cells take up to 20%-40% of all glia. Astrocytes' main task is to envelope synapses and blood vessels, to protect them from unwanted molecules. Besides their connectivity to themselves and other neurons, astrocytes also makes the blood brain barrier, which only exists in the brain. This barrier is permeable to certain types of molecules while inhibiting others from entering the blood vessels in the brain.

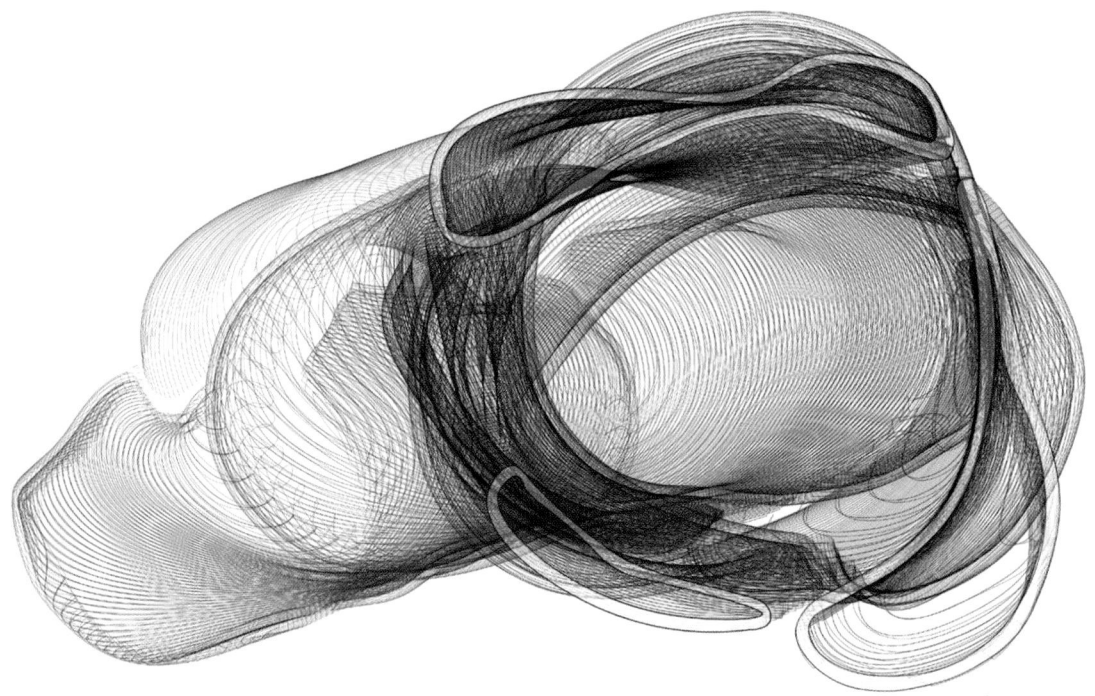

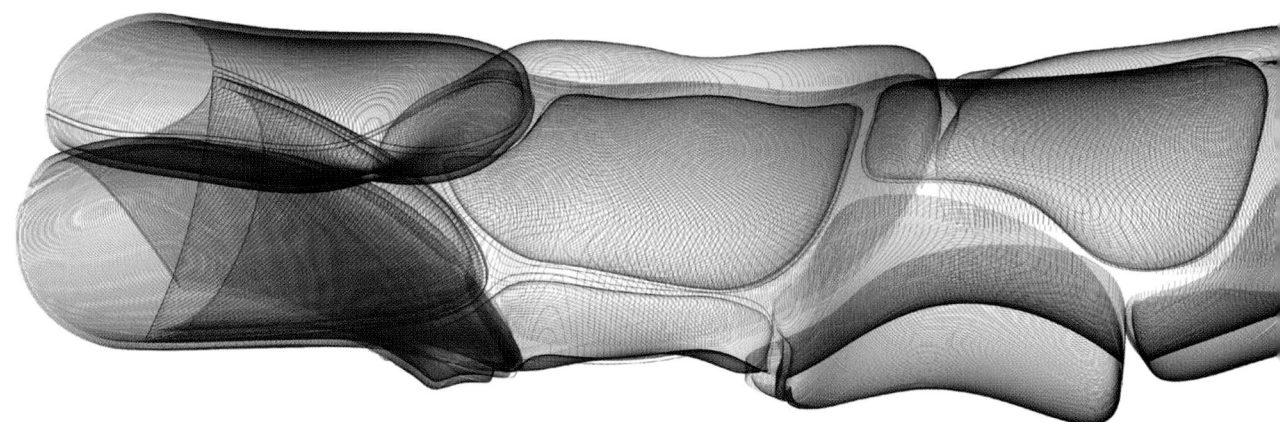

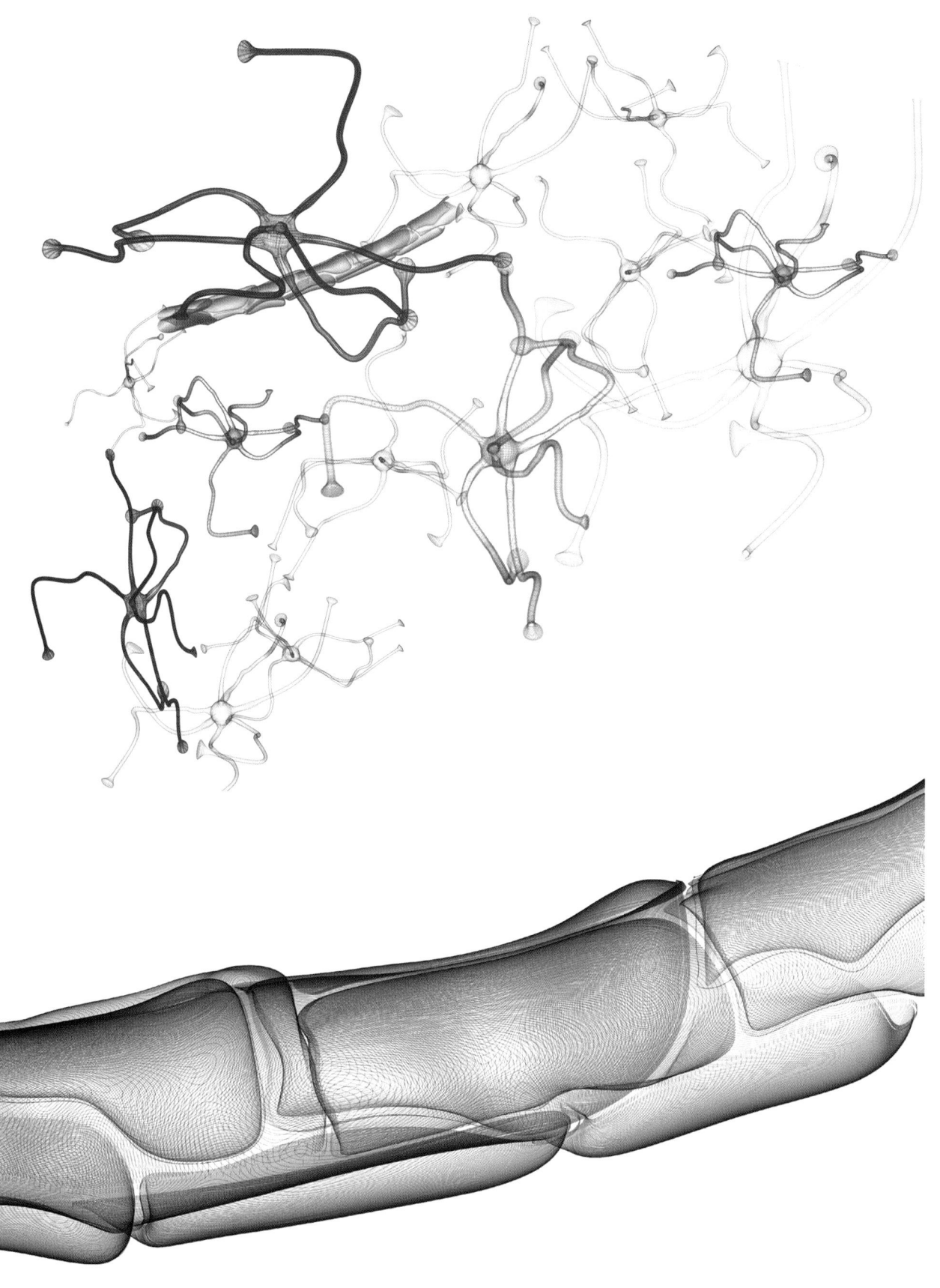

SANDRA MOON

AERENCHYMA TISSUE

This is a study of the aerenchyma tissue inside the stem of a bulrush plant. Aerenchyma is responsible for producing air spaces to allow the exchange of gases.

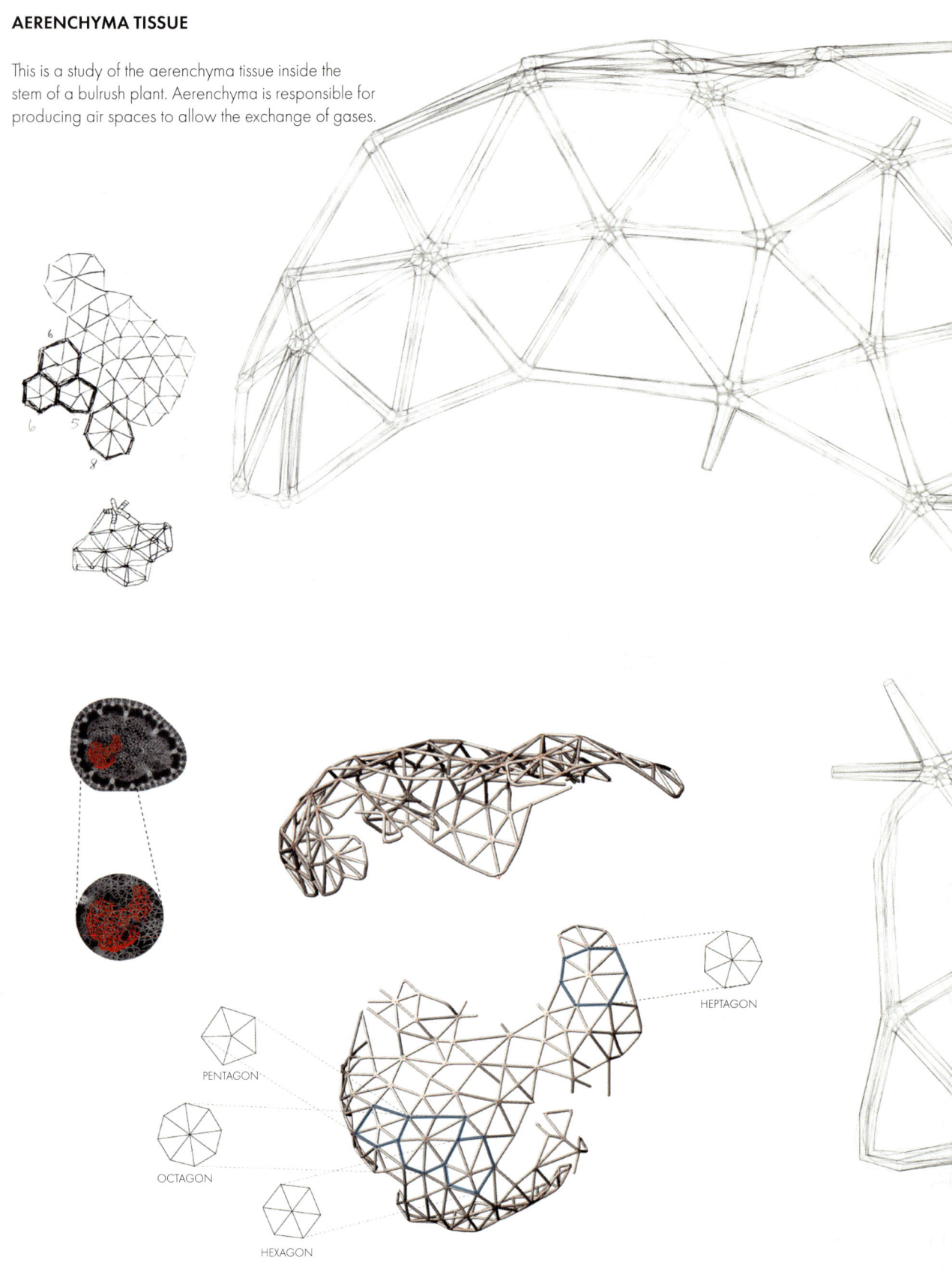

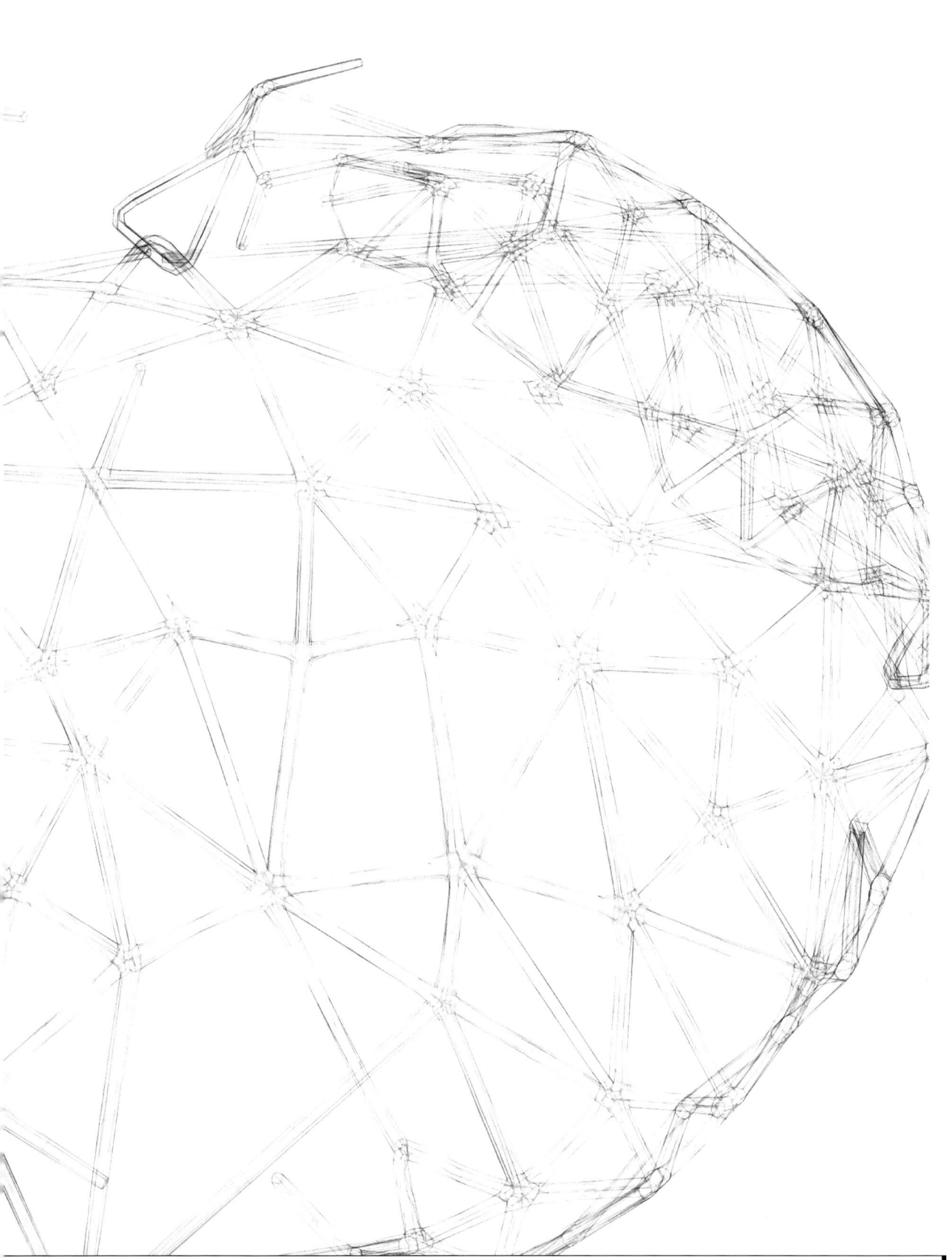

DICTYOSTELIUM DISCOIDEUM

Dictyostelium discoideum is a species of soil dwelling amoeba. Its life cycle consists of free-living unicellular amoebae that feed on bacteria. Under stress conditions, they congregate to form a motile slug that eventually differentiates to form a fruiting body that releases spores.

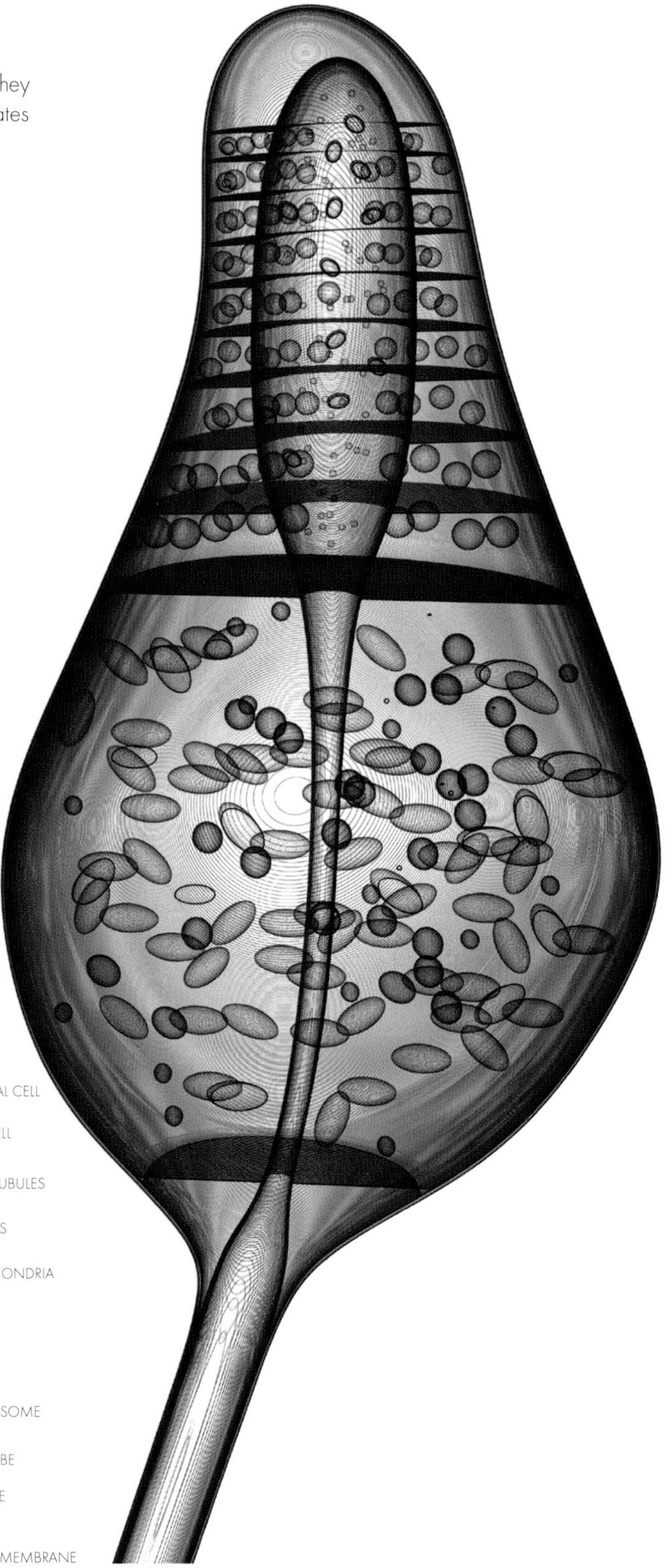

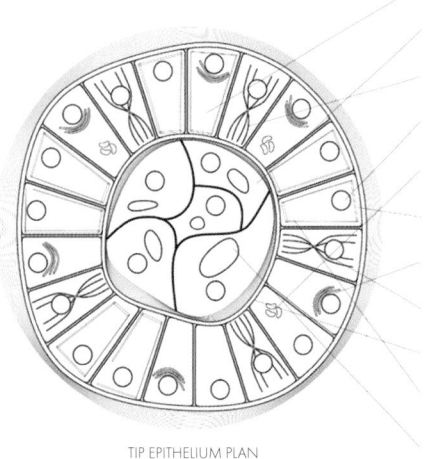

TIP EPITHELIUM PLAN

EPITHELIAL CELL
STALK CELL
MICROTUBULES
NUCLEUS
MITOCHONDRIA
F-ACTIN
GOLGI
CENTROSOME
STALK TUBE
VACUOLE
PLASMA MEMBRANE

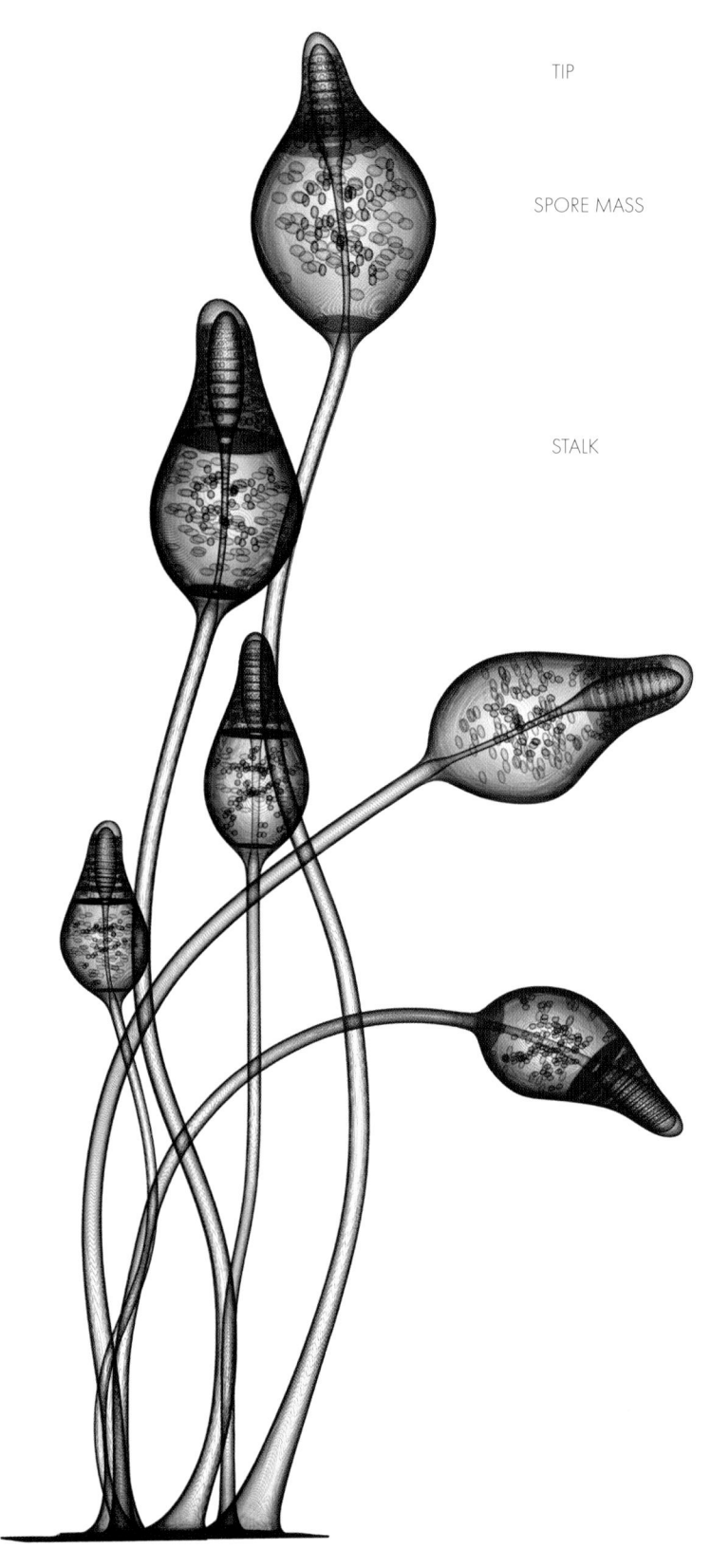

STEREOCILIA OF HAIR CELLS

This drawing of the sensory cilia bundle is of a single hair cell, from the hearing organ in the inner ear. Vibrations made by sound cause the hairs to move back and forth, stimulating and inhibiting the cell. When the cell is stimulated it generates nerve impulses that signal to the brain. In this way, a mechanical sound signal is converted into an electrical signal.

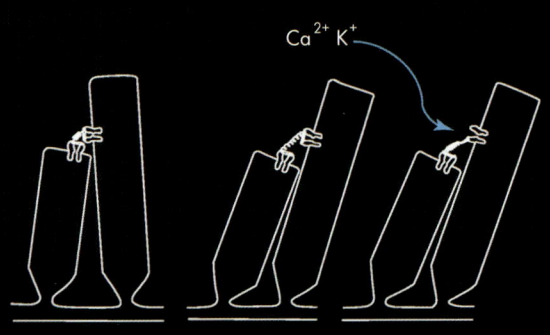

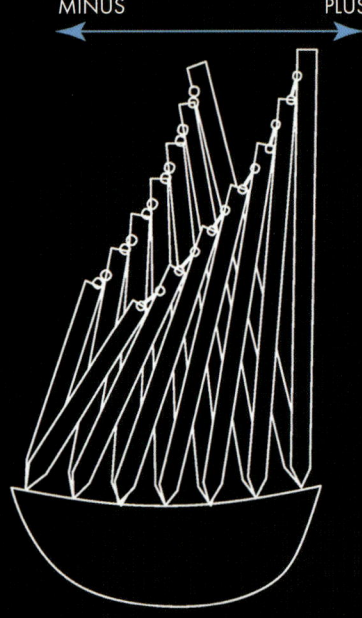

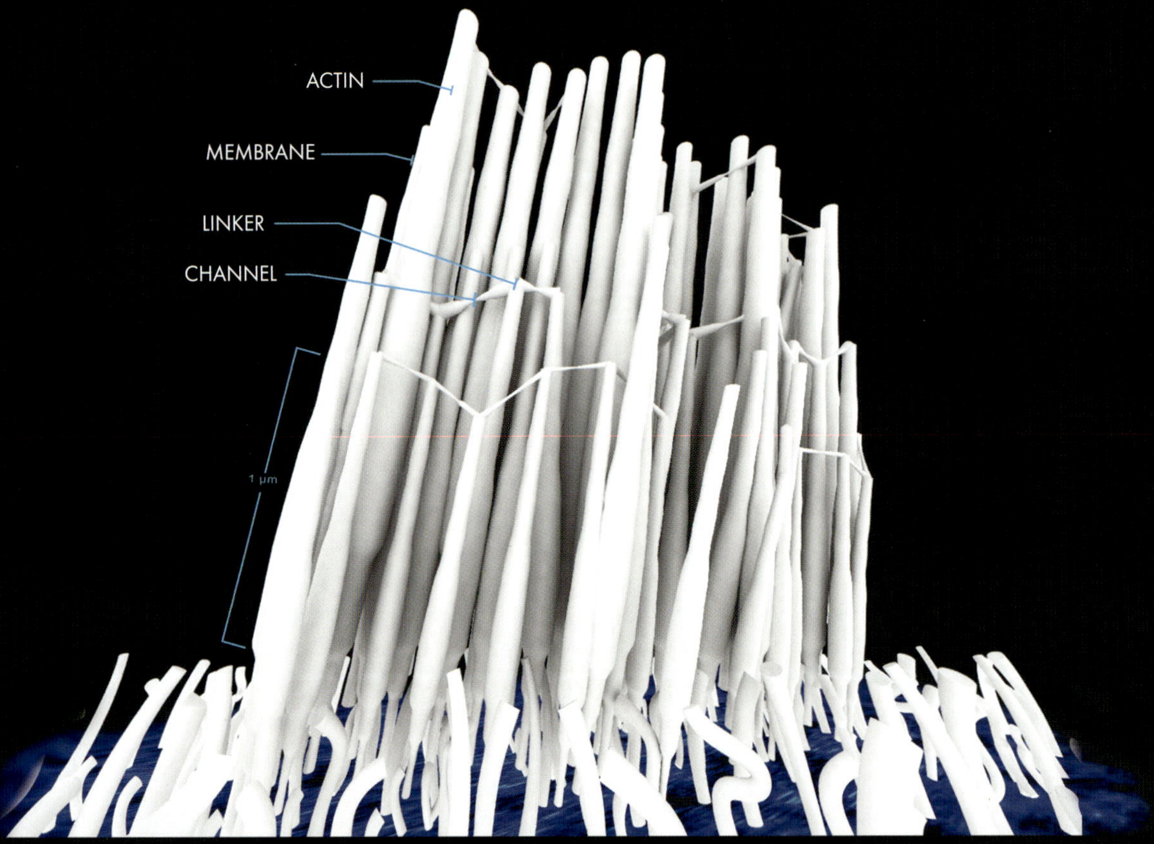

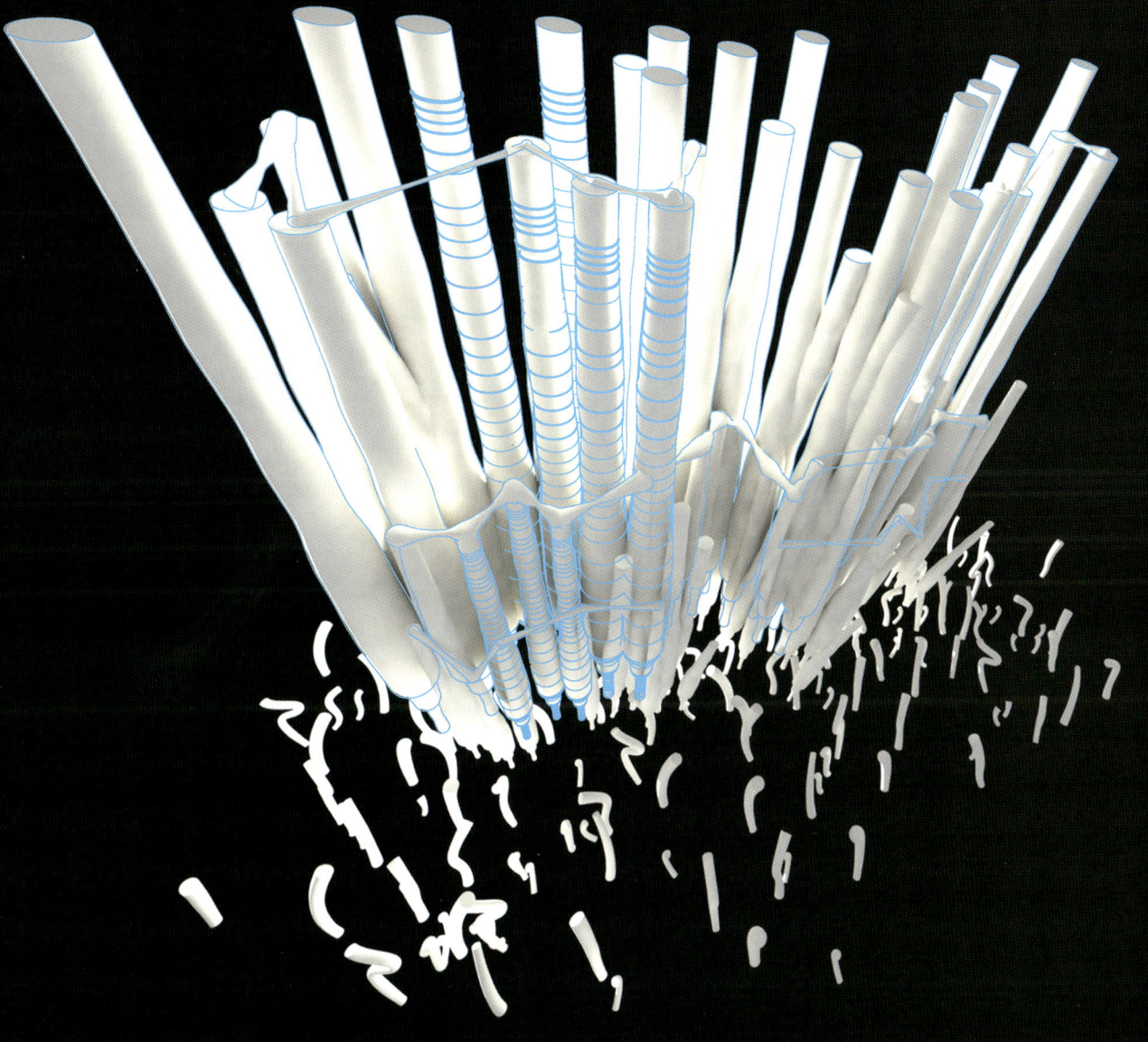

SPINDLE APPARATUS

MITOTIC SPINDLE FORMING

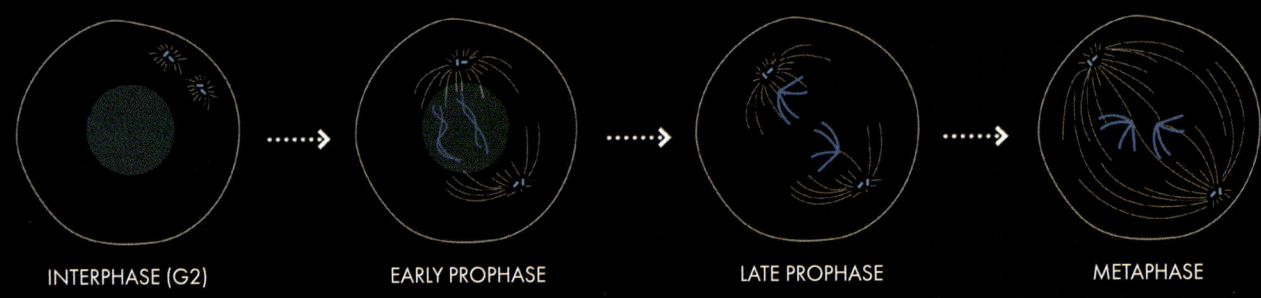

INTERPHASE (G2) → EARLY PROPHASE → LATE PROPHASE → METAPHASE

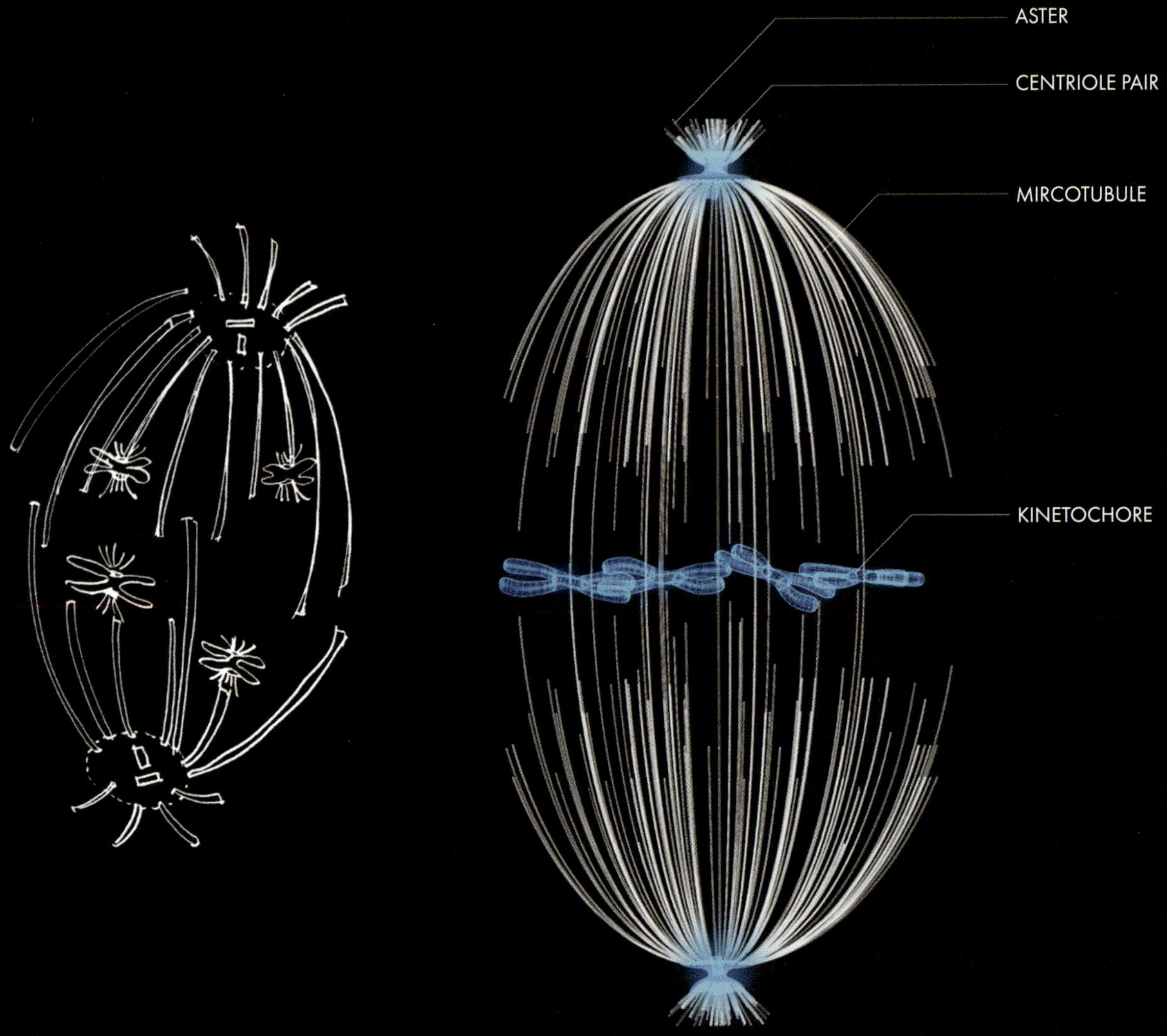

- ASTER
- CENTRIOLE PAIR
- MIRCOTUBULE
- KINETOCHORE

ANAPHASE
TELOPHASE
INTERPHASE (G1)

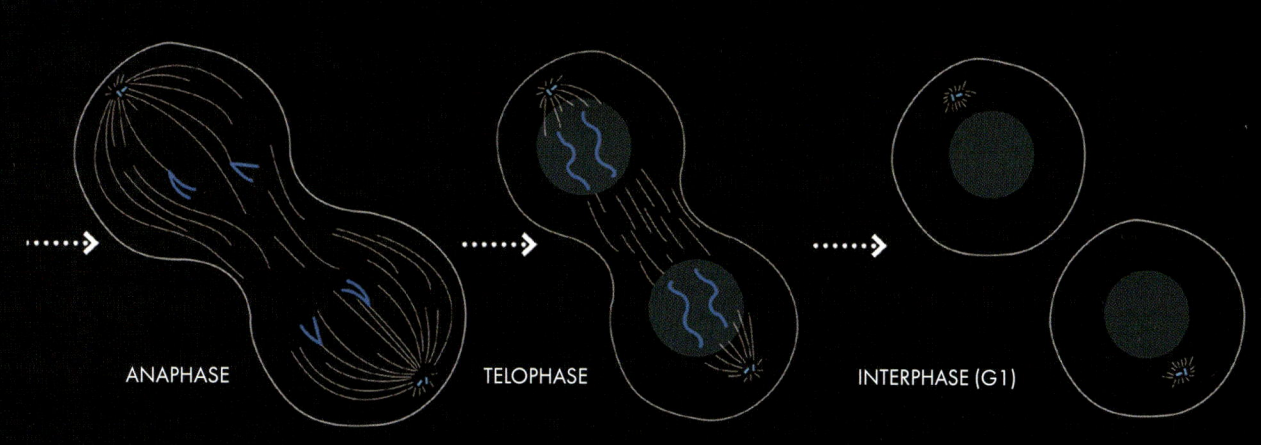

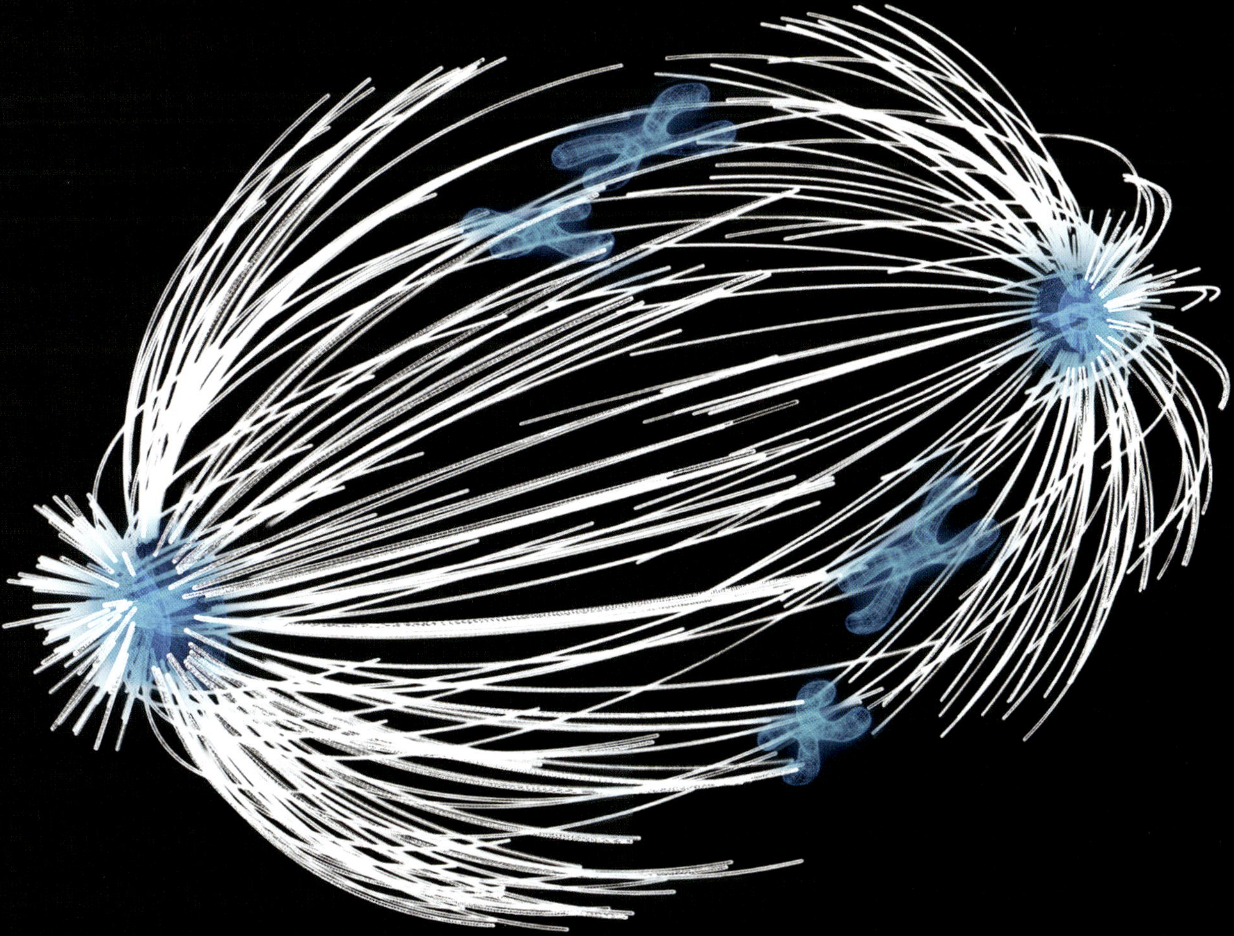

JENNY LIU

PYRAMIDAL CELL

The peculiar tree-like branching structure of pyramidal neurons allows them to receive and integrate multiple inputs. These neurons are commonly found in regions of higher order processing such as the prefrontal cortex. They engage in multiple synaptic interactions that can be excitatory and inhibitory.

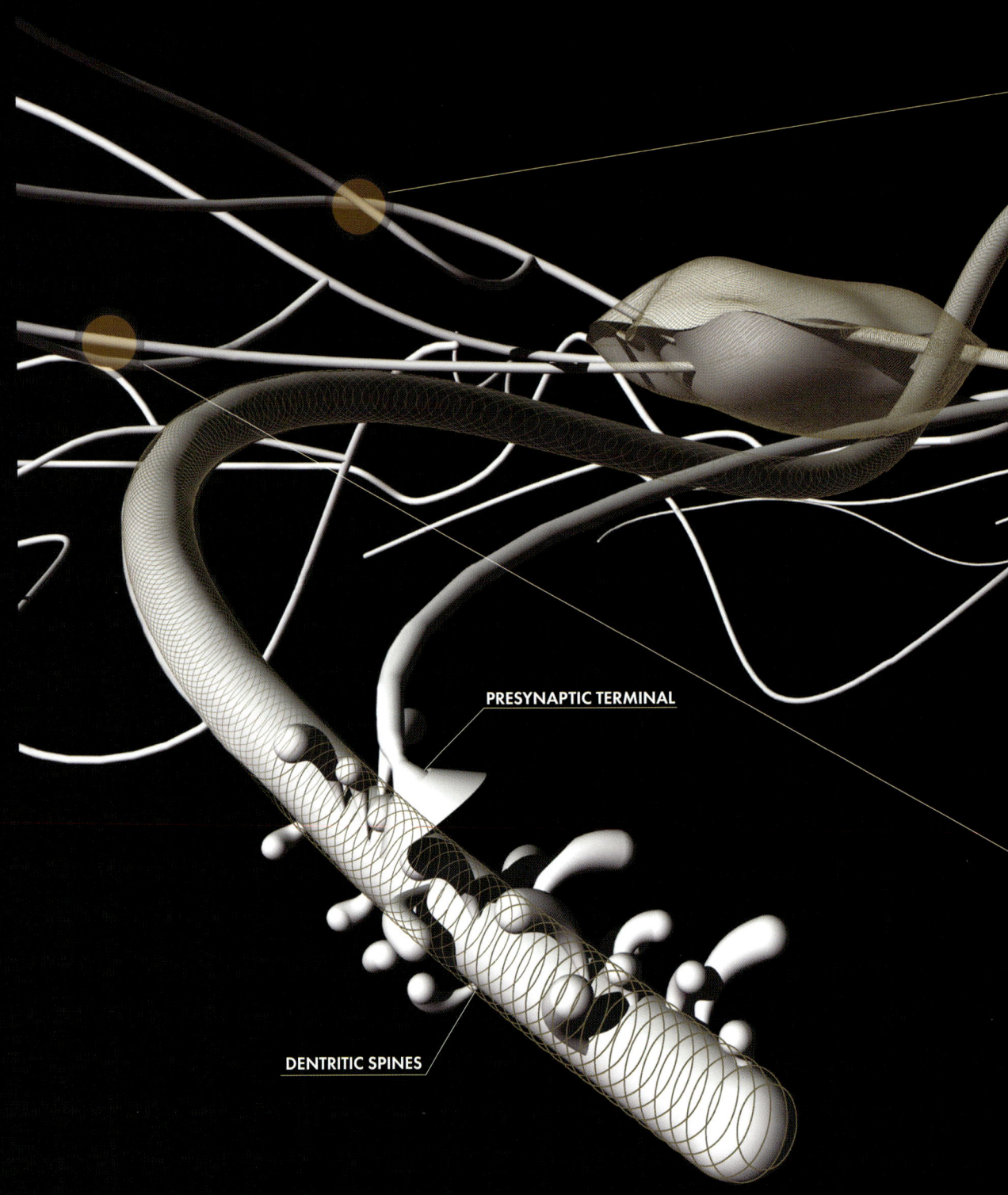

PRESYNAPTIC TERMINAL

DENTRITIC SPINES

BASAL DENDRITE
Input Source: Collaterals & Layer IV Cells
Neurotransmitter: Glutamate
Receptor: N-Methyl-D-Aspartate (NMDA)

APICAL DENDRITE (DISTAL)
Input Source: Cortical & Thalamic Cells
Neurotransmitter: Gamma-Aminobutyric acid (GABA)
Receptor: GABA

APICAL DENDRITE (PROXIMAL)
Input Source: Collaterals & Layer IV Cells
Neurotransmitter: Glutamate
Receptor: N-Methyl-D-Aspartate (NMDA)

AXON
Input Source: Interneurons & Basket Cells
Neurotransmitter: Gamma-Aminobutyric acid (GABA)
Receptor: GABA

NEURAL NETWORKS

A neural network (sometimes called a neural pathway) is a series of interconnected neurons whose activation defines a recognizable linear pathway. The interface through which neurons interact with their neighbors usually consists of several axon terminals connected via synapses to dendrites on other neurons.

ENDING

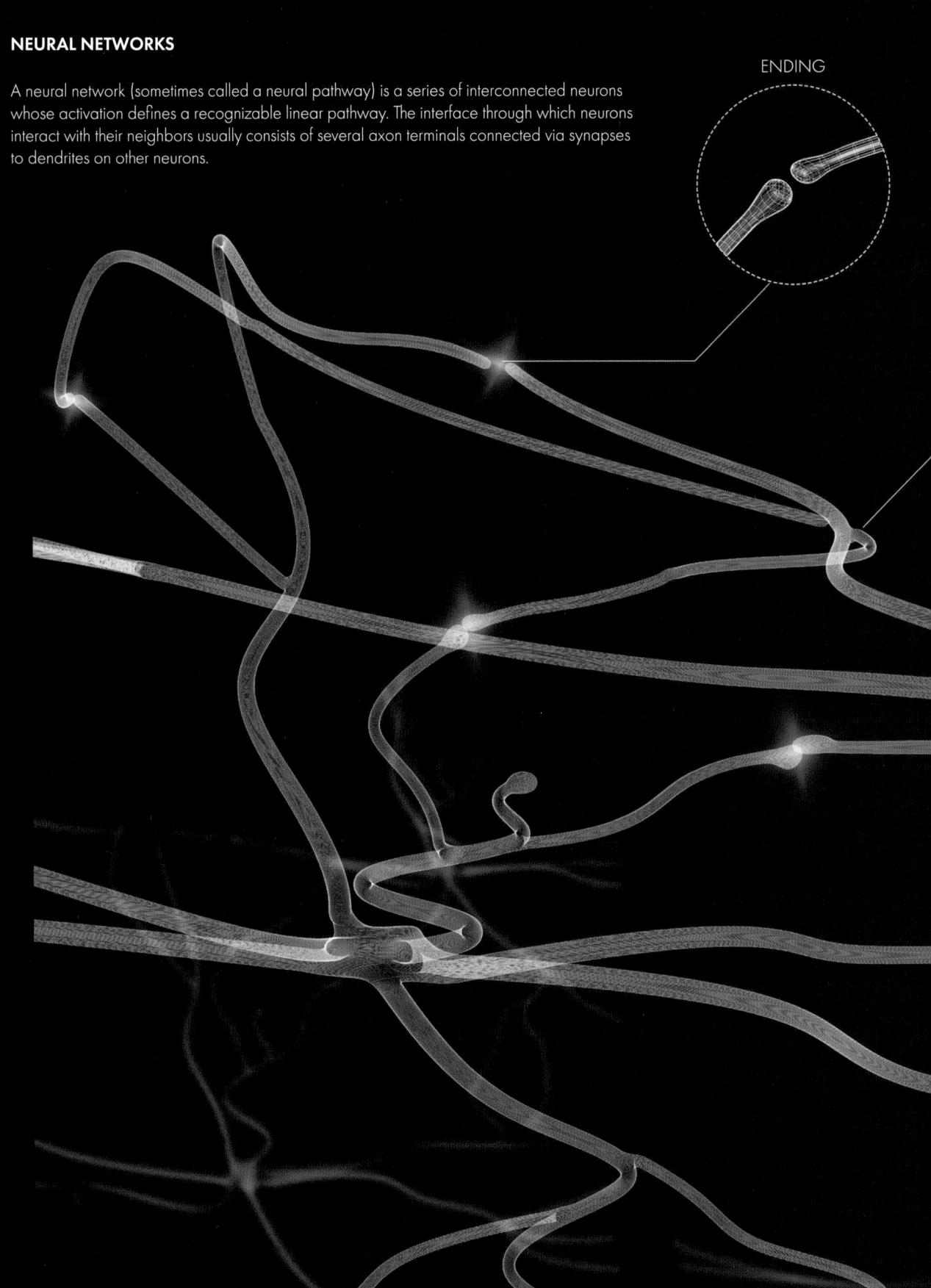

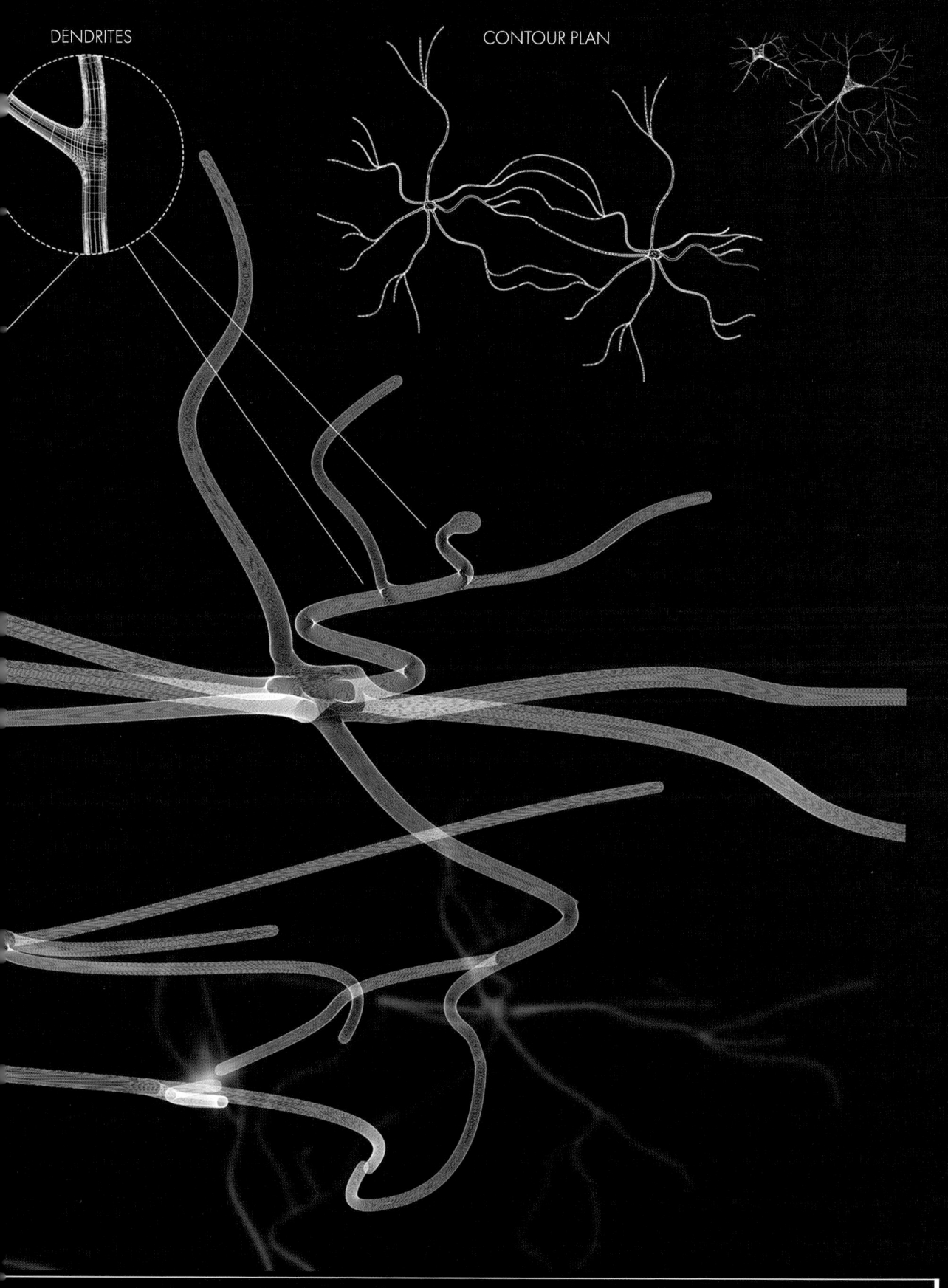

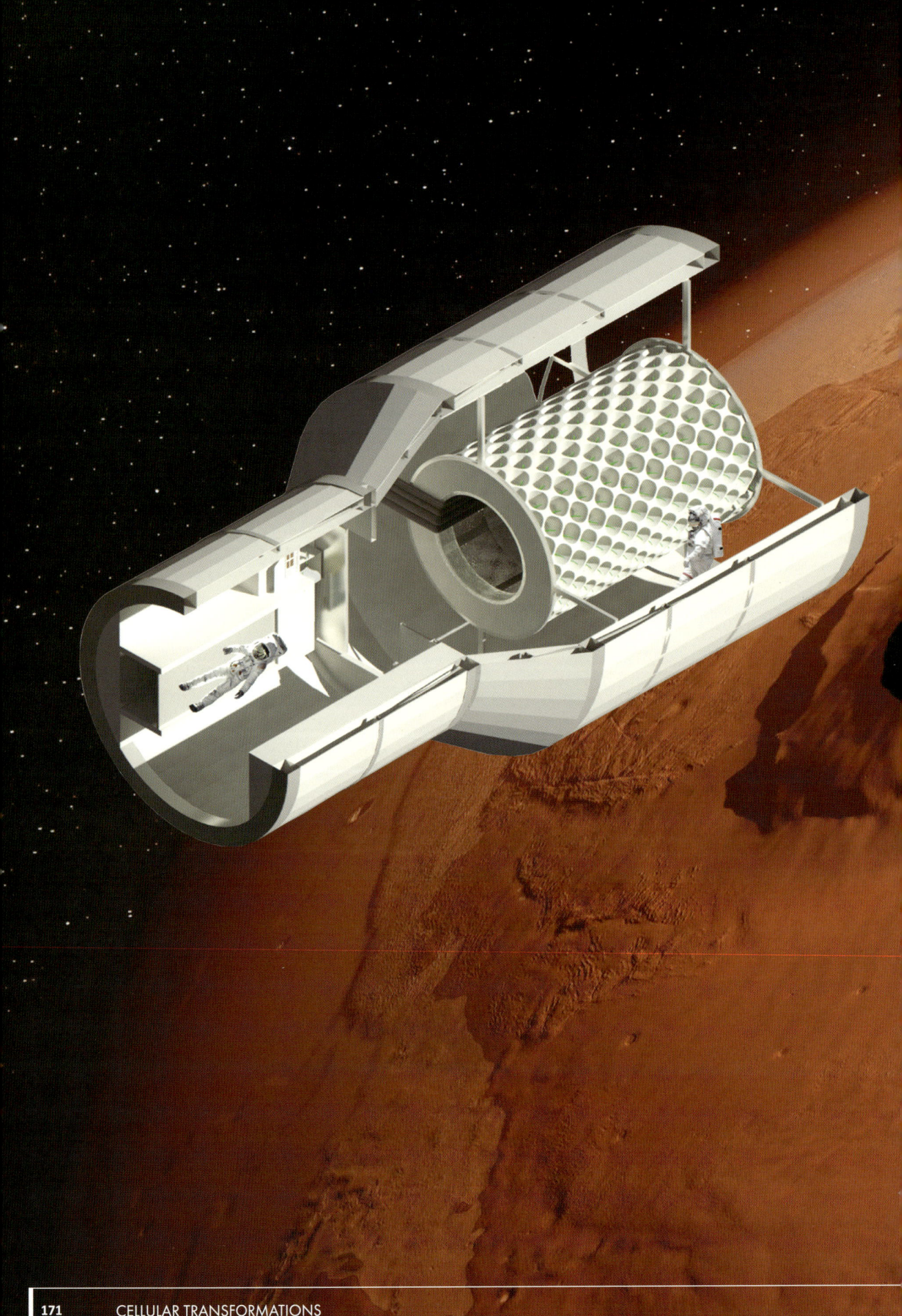

INHABITATION: 2015
MISSION TO MARS RESEARCH

The Mission to Mars research project was the first in which biology and architecture students worked together to develop cross-disciplinary designs. Mars is the next frontier in human space travel. Compared to the Apollo moon missions, the journey to Mars poses significant new challenges due to the much longer travel duration. The journey from Earth to Mars takes between 7 to 9 months one way and a total of 14 to 18 months round trip. The projects proposed new aerospace-engineered habitations that responded to the human physiological and psychological stress of long-term space travel. The projects used plants to provide oxygen, fuel, food, building materials and psychological relief to astronauts on their journey to Mars. Students designed growth pods within space crafts that can grow plants or algae for various purposes. These projects look to the future of environmental and architectural design and especially how the connection between design, technology and science will impact the human race.

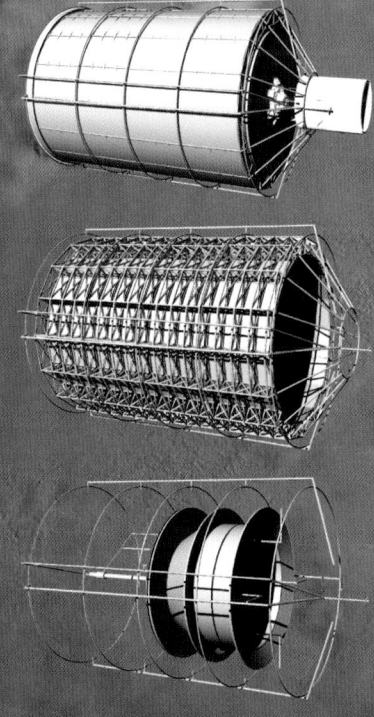
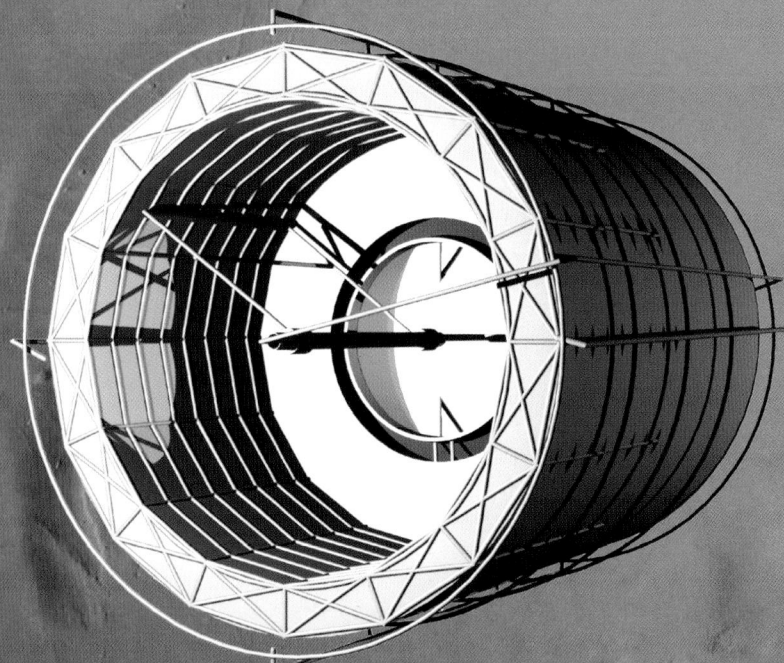

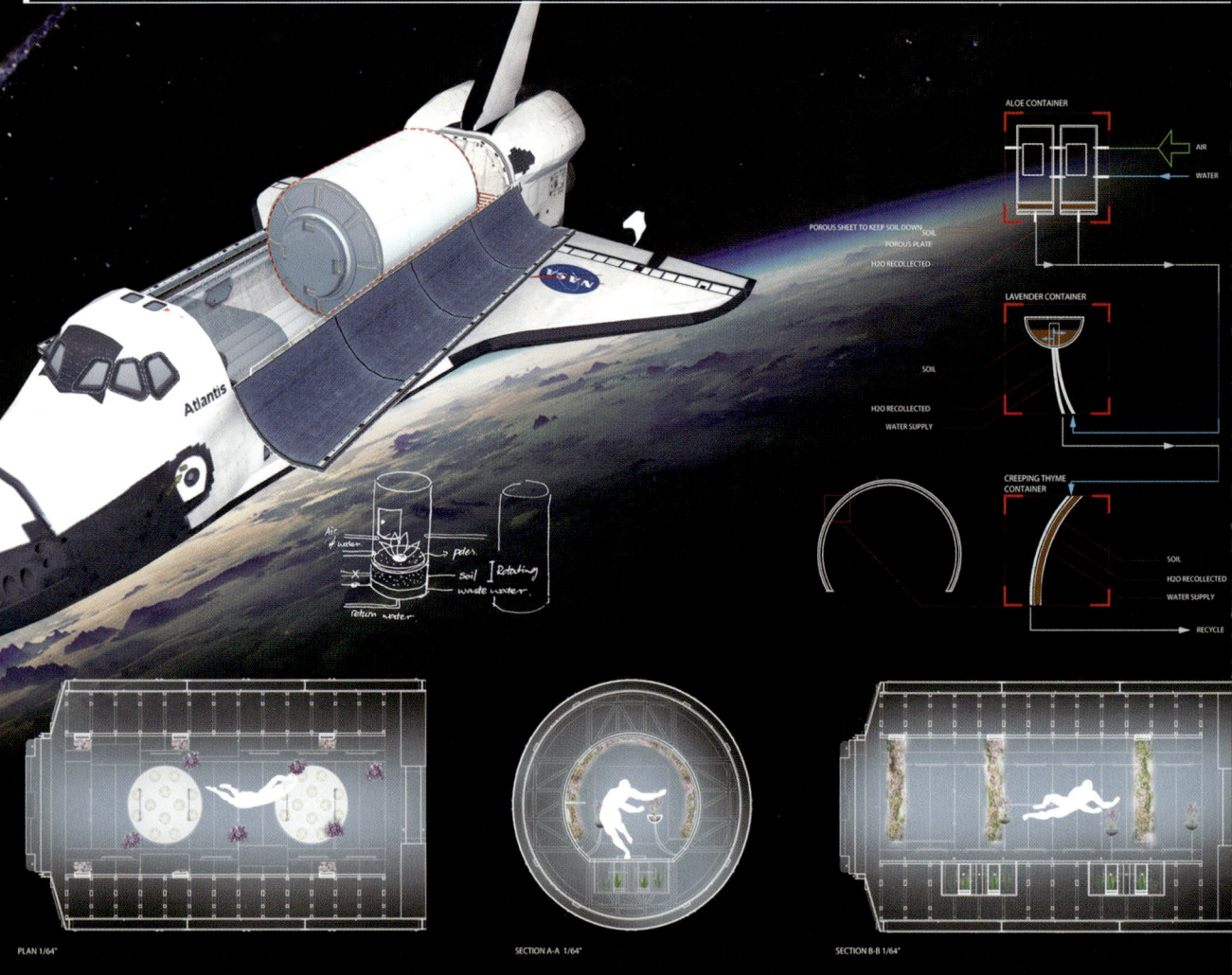

Green Habitations in Space

Space is the canvas of the universe. Its mind boggling vastness holds at least 100 billion galaxies, each populated by countless stars, planets and other celestial objects. While humanity has been pinioned on Earth for most of our time, outer space has ever lured us to explore the great beyond. Humans have been pondering outer space since we looked up at the night sky. Objects in space were attributed divine powers and their regular motions were mapped and studied. Galileo and his telescope allowed us to peer at these objects more closely. But, paradoxically, as space got closer to us through advanced telescopes, its vastness grew. The immensity of space only worked to further ensnare the human imagination as evidenced by countless books, art and movies.

While physical exploration of space is as old as hot air balloons seeking to break Earthly bonds, it is only relatively recently that rockets enabled humans to experience the thrill of being in outer space. We have been to the moon and astronauts now inhabit the International Space Station for long durations. But space is a hostile environment. Instead of air, there is vacuum. The ambient temperature of outer space is a frigid -270 °C. There are no barriers to shield us from hazardous radiation. Therefore, to survive in space, we must carry our dwellings like hermit crabs, replete with the basic necessities for human life.

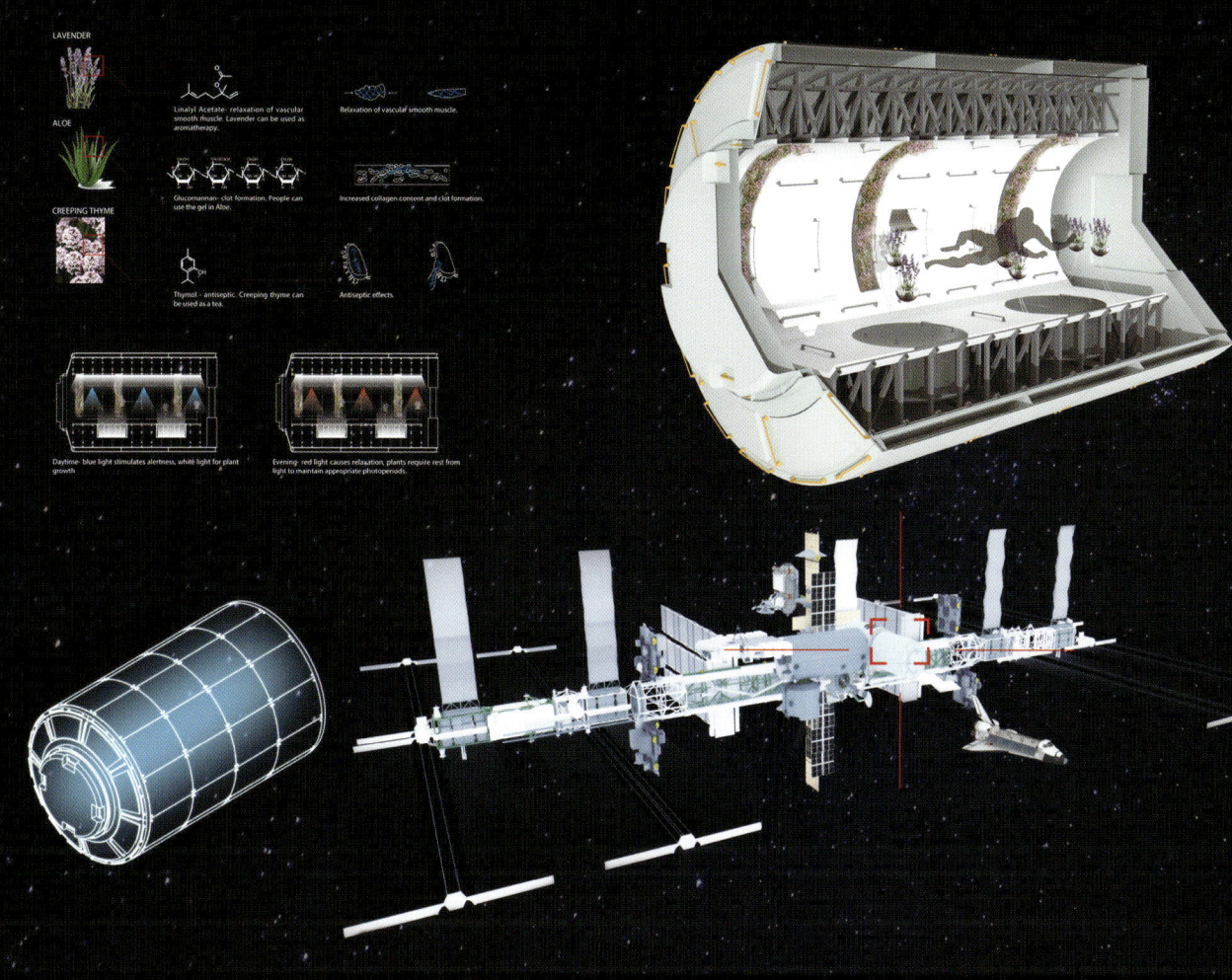

Mars is the next frontier for human space travel. With current launch technology, it will likely take close to 2 years for a round-trip mission to Mars. The long duration of this trip will require the crew to take enough food, water, oxygen, medical supplies, and fuel. In addition, the obligatory 3-4 months stay on Mars dictated by the optimal orbital alignment required for efficient return to Earth will require building materials for habitats on Mars. In addition to posing physical hardships to the crew, long-duration space travel will also challenge their mental health. Our vision is to use plants as an economical and renewable solution to many of these challenges.

Because plants are photosynthetic, they require only water, light, minerals and air to grow and thrive. In return, they yield food, fuel, fiber, medicines and building materials. In addition, their beauty, color and scent provide psychological relief. While plants have been grown in space extensively for research, their use in space travel has been lacking. Here, we propose to design living green spaces to harness the power of plants to provide practical and psychological benefits during the long journey to Mars and beyond.

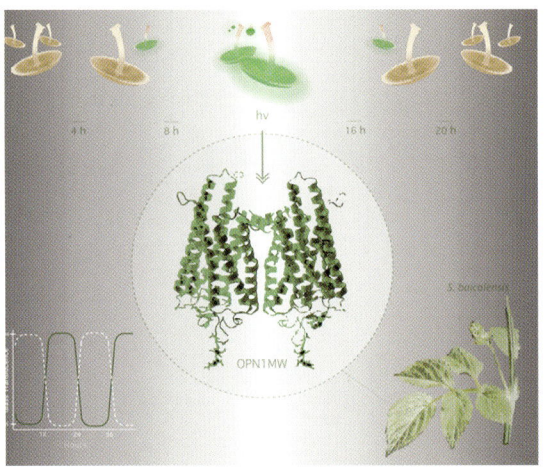
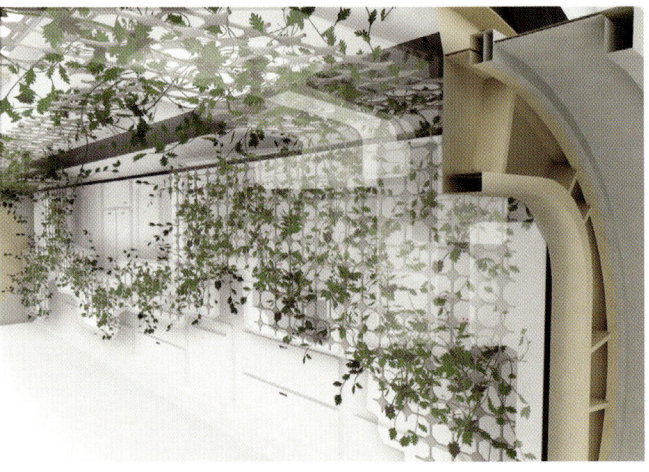
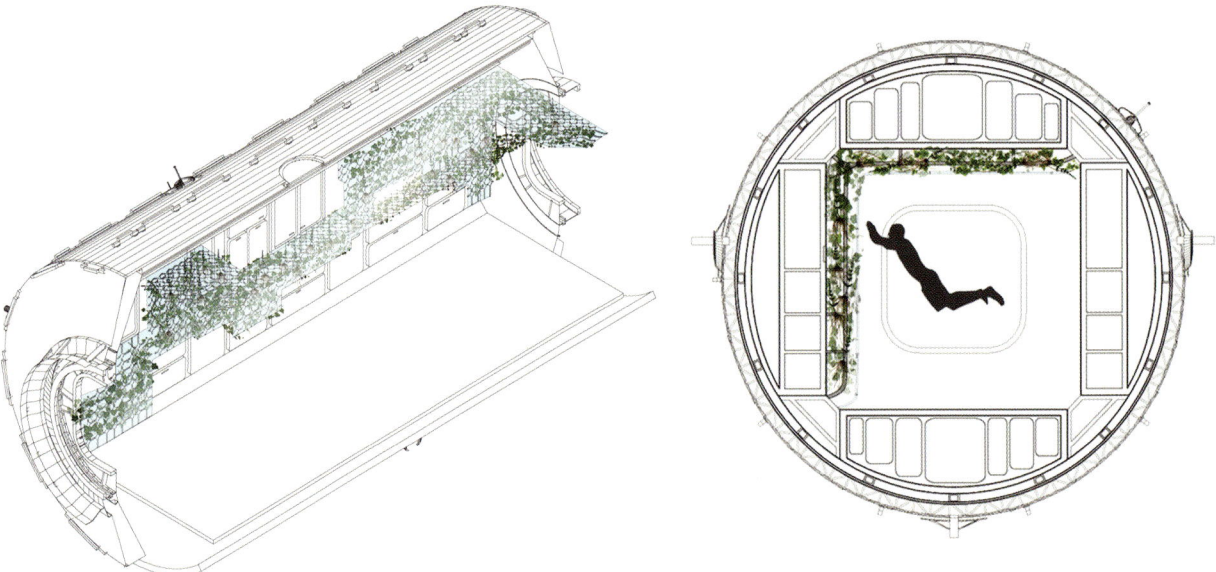

Humans have long exploited the medicinal properties of plants. By judiciously selecting hardy plants that produce useful therapeutic compounds, we can have botanicals in space. During the 9-month journey to Mars or even longer future space travels, imagine entering a pod lush with the vibrant color and soothing aroma of lavender. Besides aromatherapy, lavender produces linalyl acetate that relaxes vascular smooth muscles to promote cardiovascular health. The same pod contains creeping thyme growing along the walls that can be used as a tea and aloe that can be used as a salve to heal wounds and sunburn and consumed to promote digestive health. Similarly, one can design pods to grow herbs such as *Scutellaria baicalensis*, which is an excellent source of melatonin. Due to lack of day-night cycles in space, consuming this herb will benefit the sleep cycle and improve overall crew wellbeing. Thus, incorporating these small garden pods on space ships will provide much-needed physical and mental benefits.

JENNY LIU | SANDRA MOON

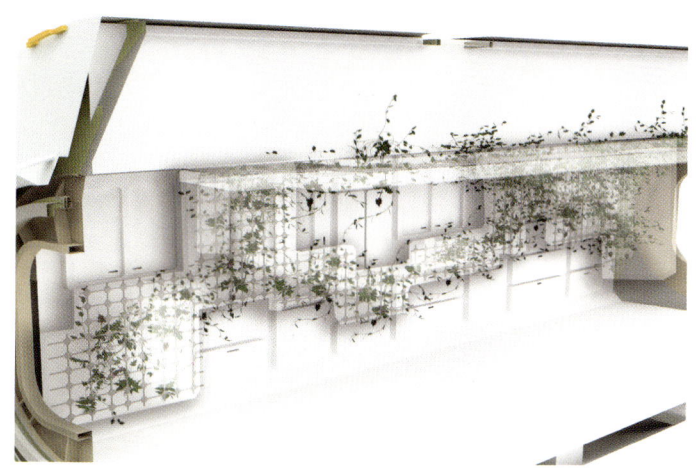
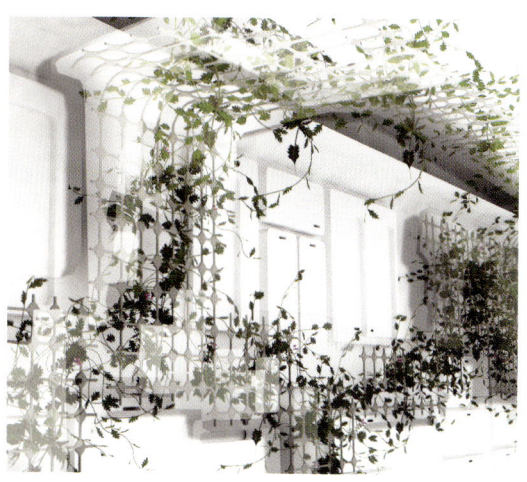

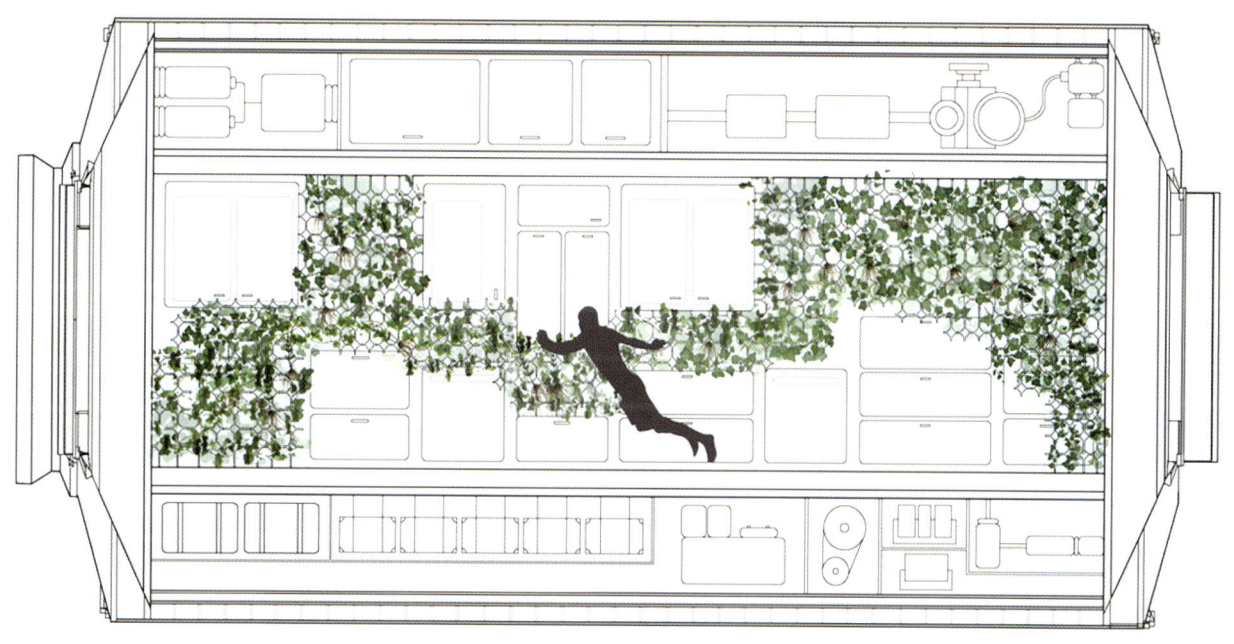

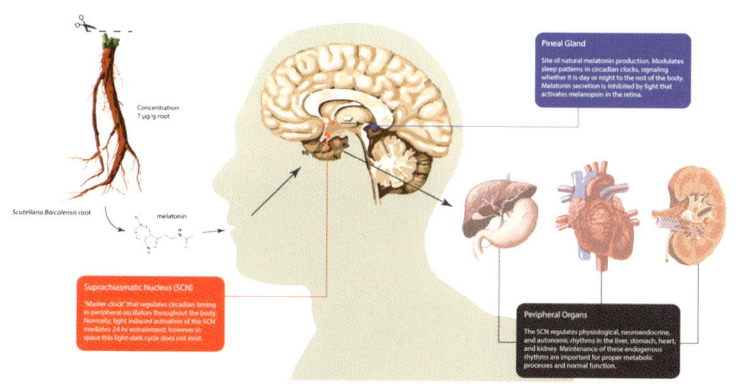
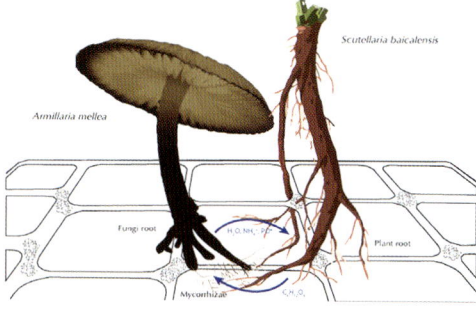

MISSION TO MARS RESEARCH

YUCHEN SHEN | SHAO LIU | ARI GAO

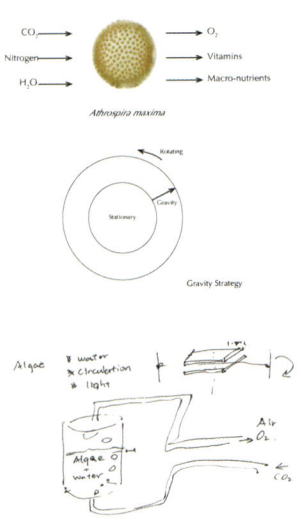

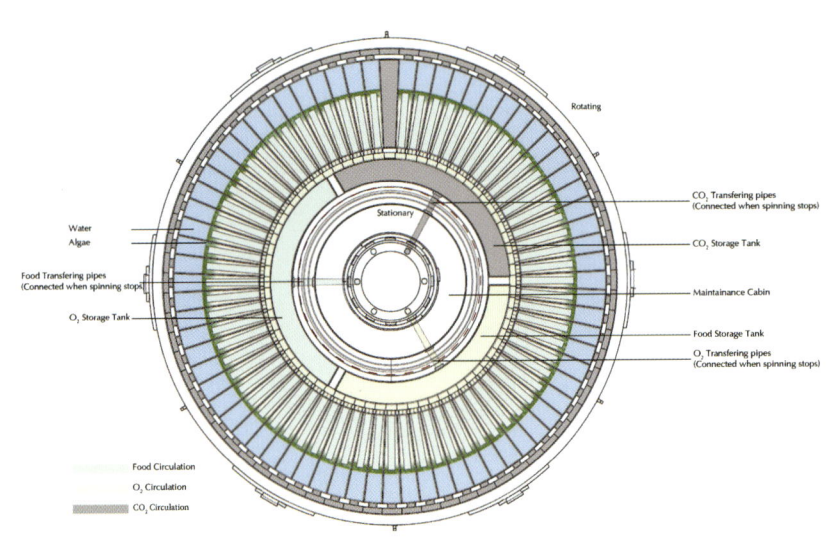

CELLULAR TRANSFORMATIONS

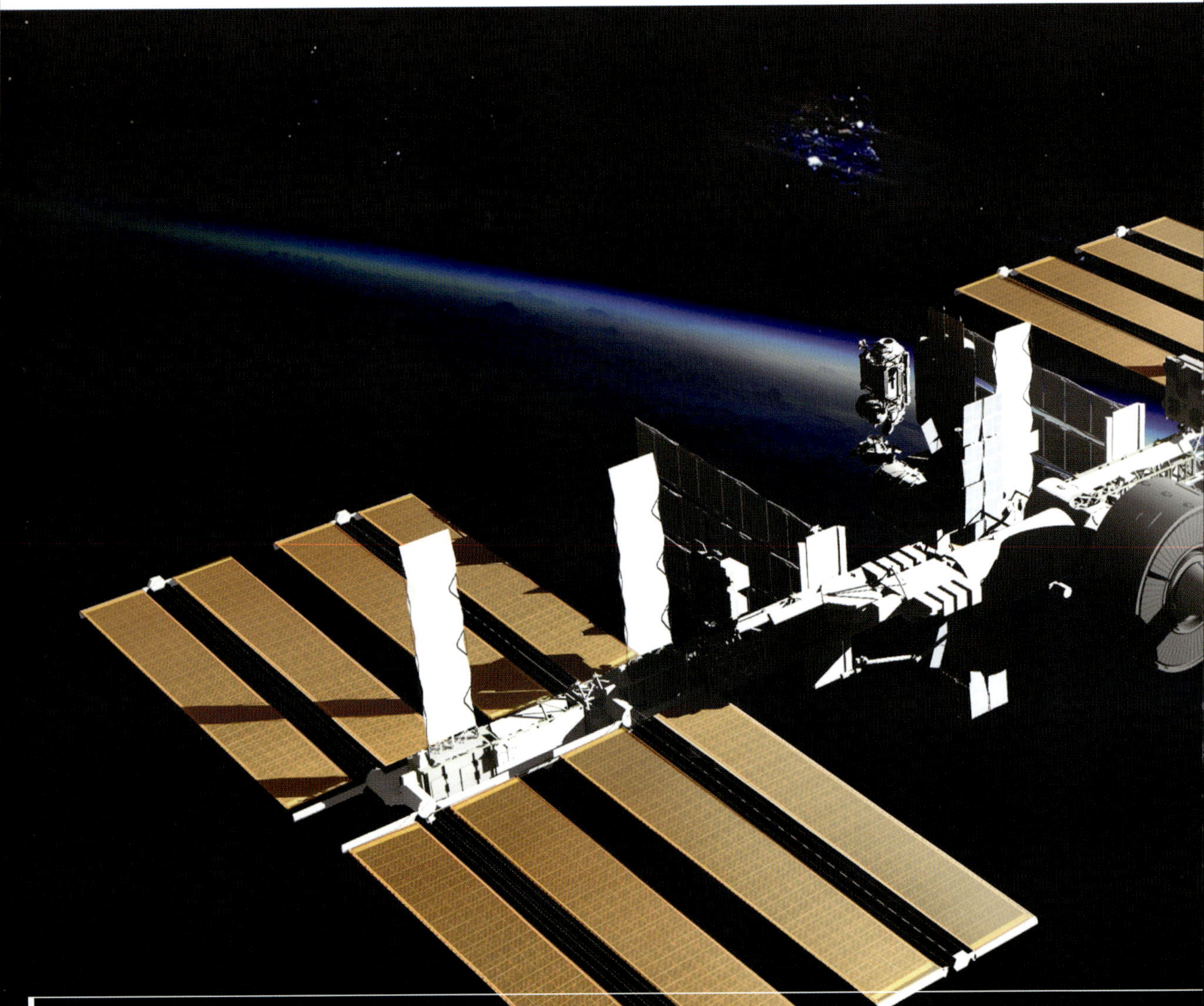

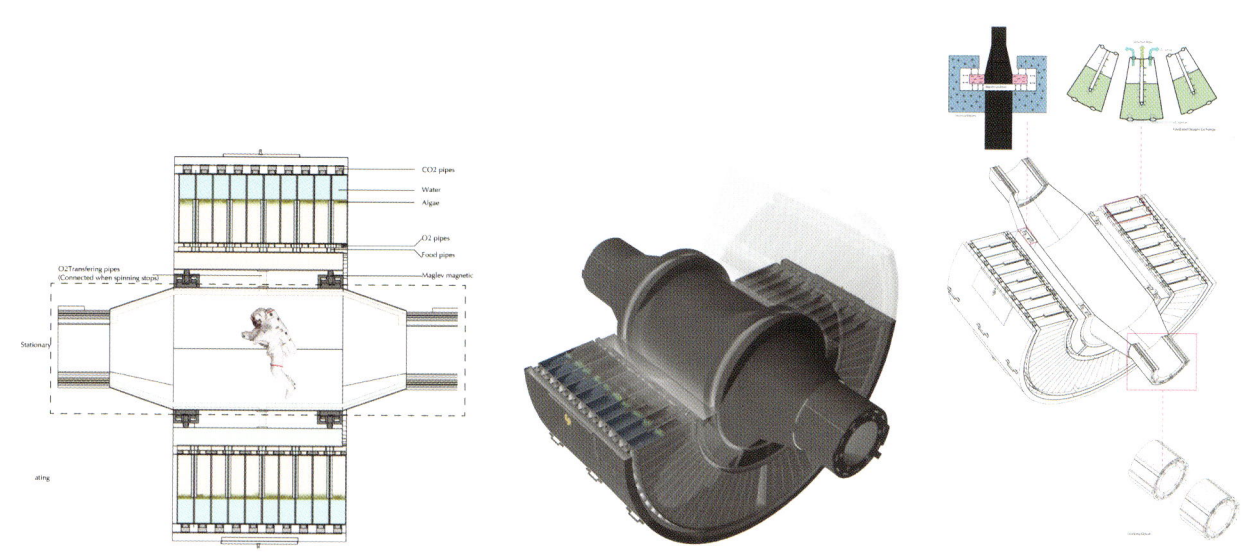

A different approach would be to grow algae in liquid culture. Just like their photosynthetic cousins did on ancient Earth, green algae can be used to oxygenate space ships as well as harvested for consumption. They can even be used to seed large-scale algal ponds on Mars to produce biofuel locally instead of carrying an enormous amount of fuel on board.

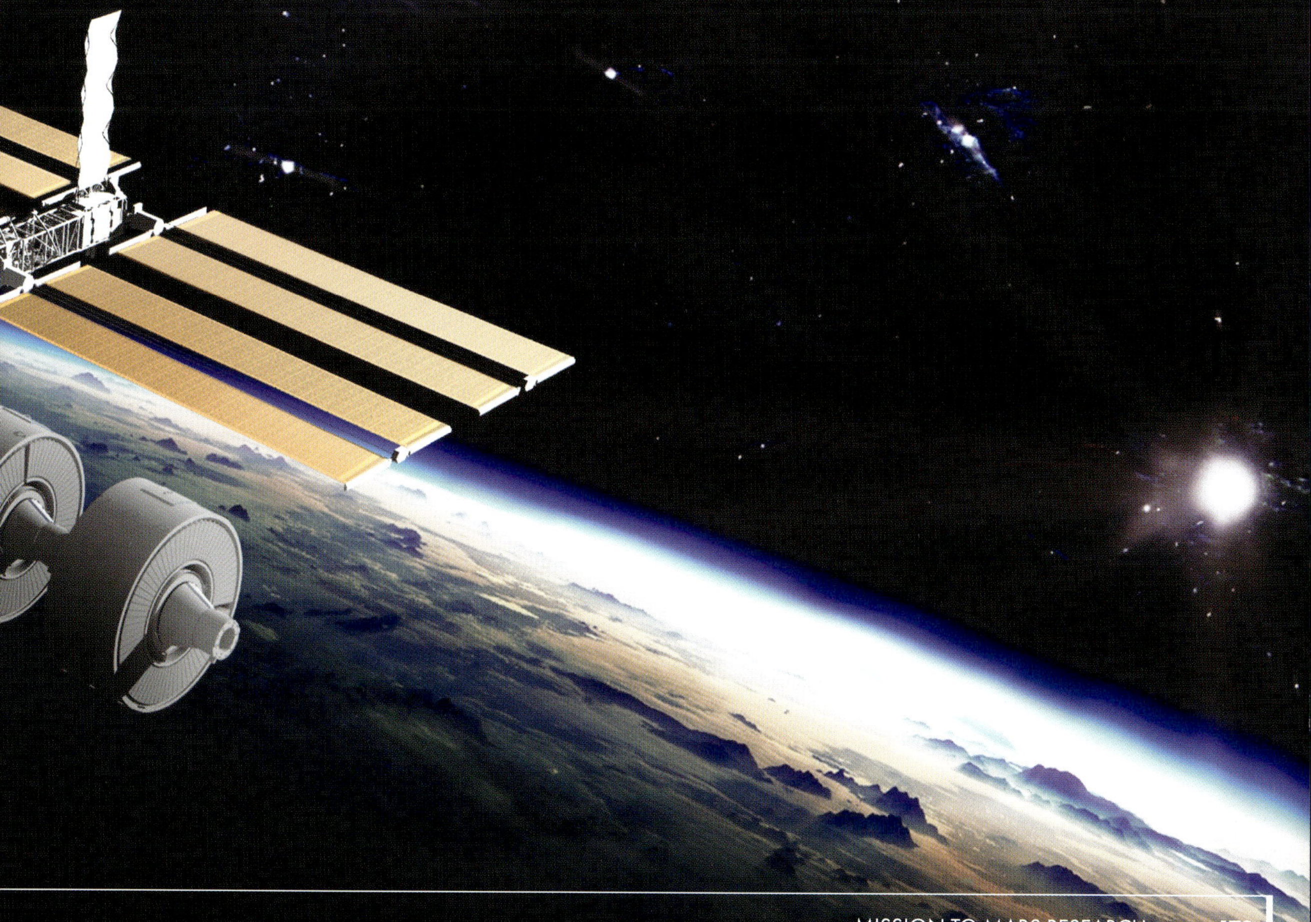

The botanical gardens and algal ponds will be grown in space ships by using liquid and solid waste from crews to water and fertilize the plants. Instead of CO_2 scrubbers, the CO_2 exhaled by the crew will be pumped into the growth chambers or algal containers for photosynthesis. Rotation will be used to simulate gravity for directional plant growth. These green spaces will significantly reduce the amount of food, oxygen and medicine that would have to be carried to sustain a crew for a long journey.

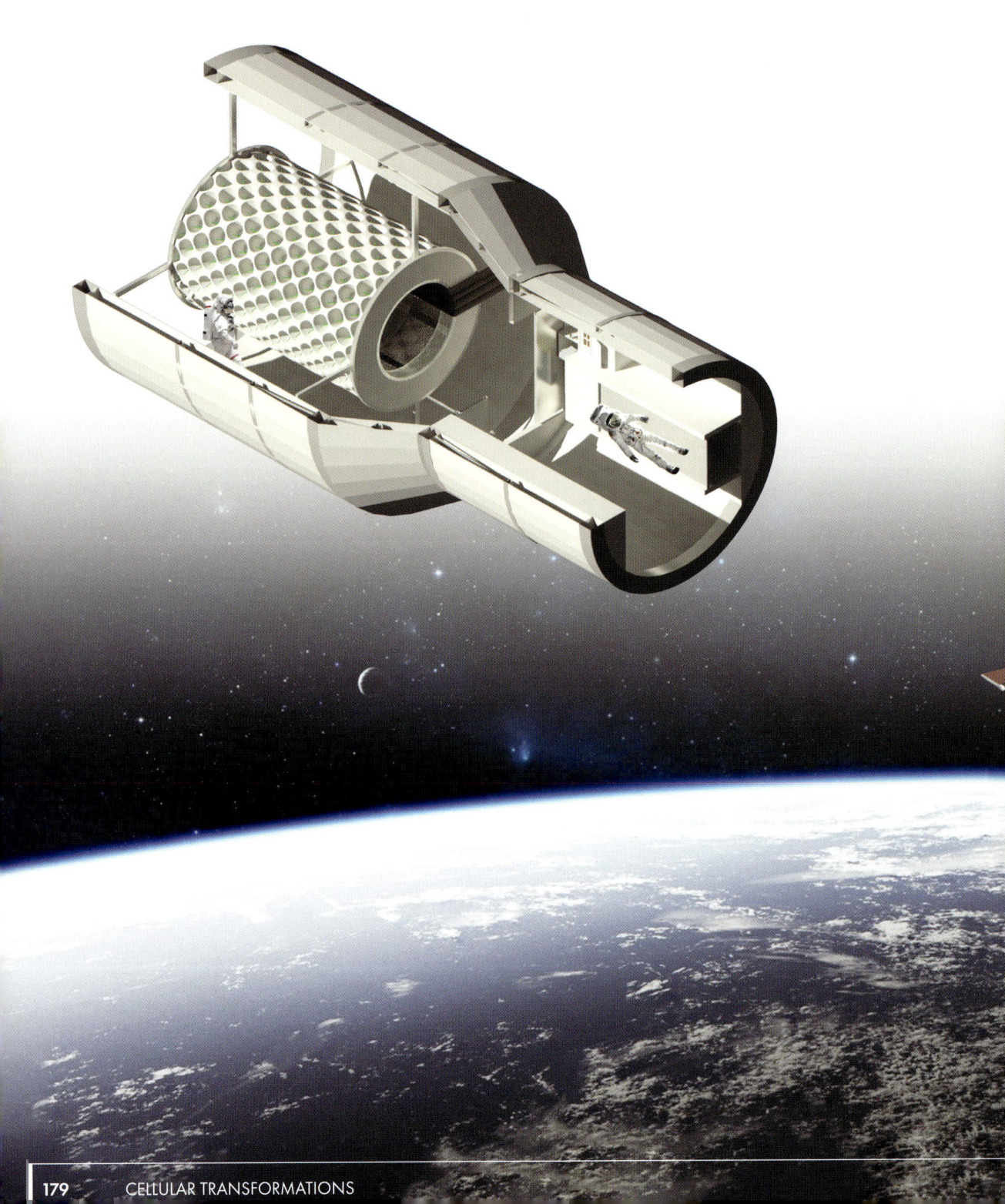

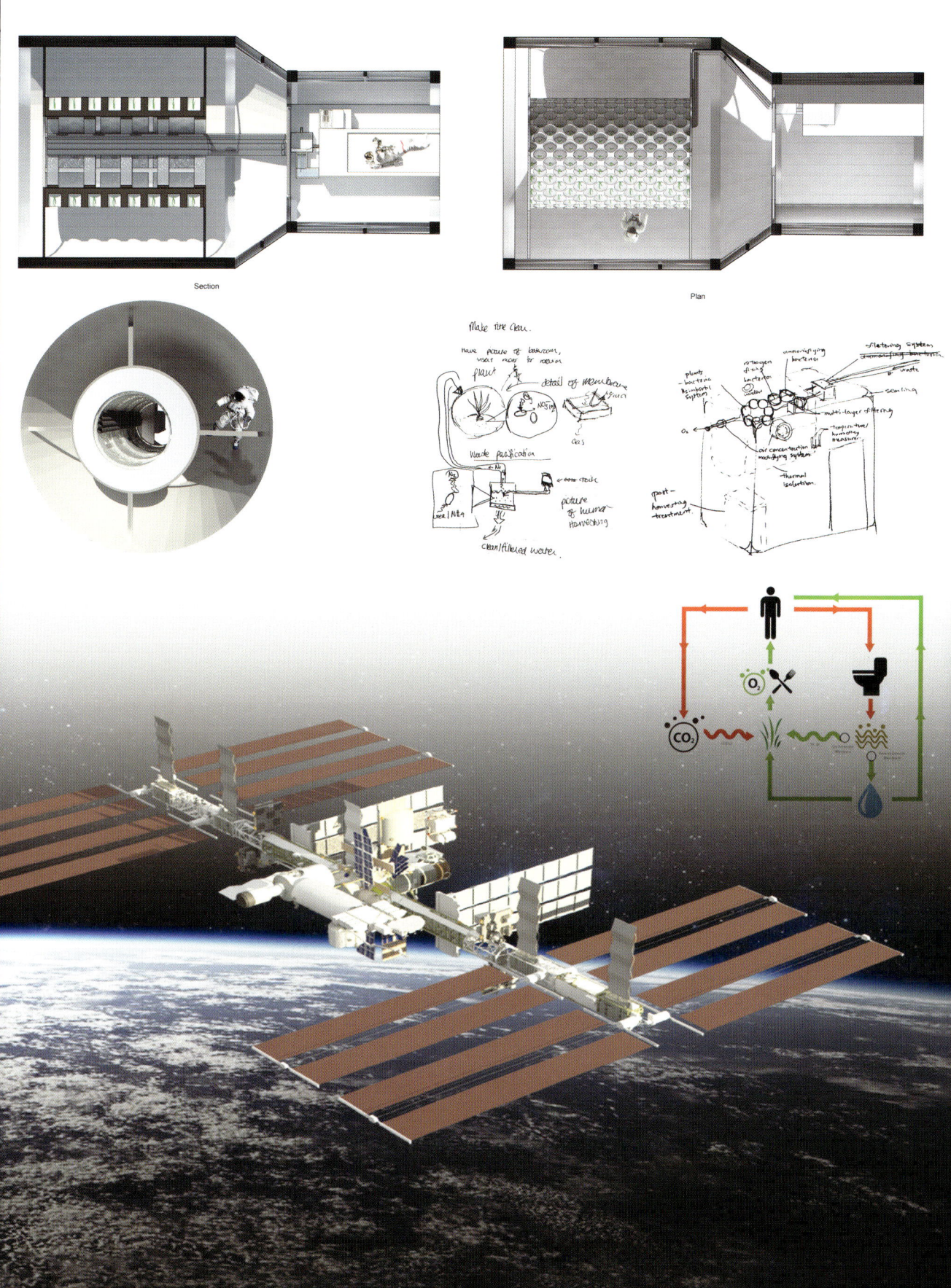

MISSION TO MARS RESEARCH

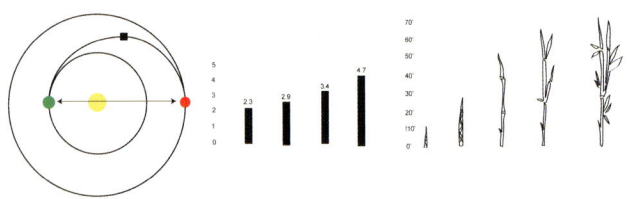

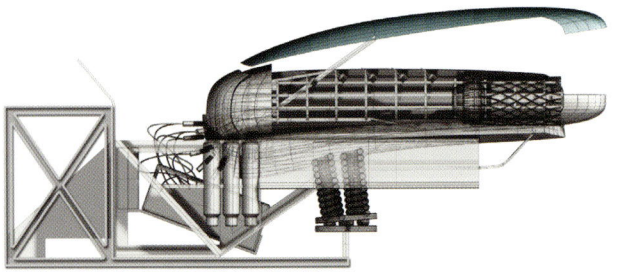

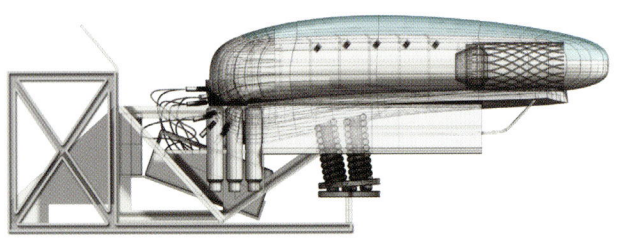

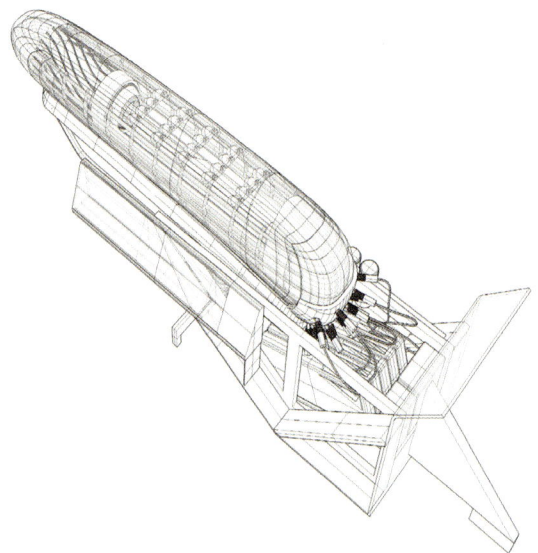

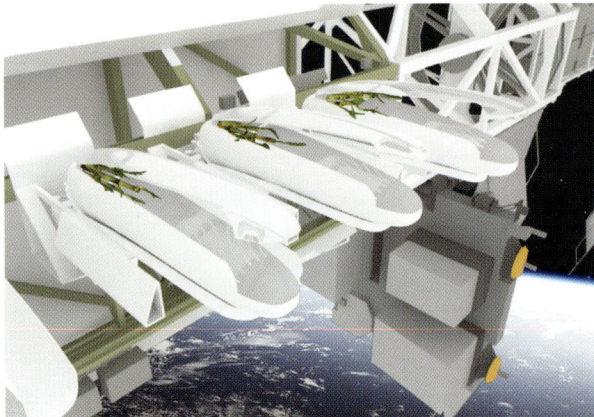

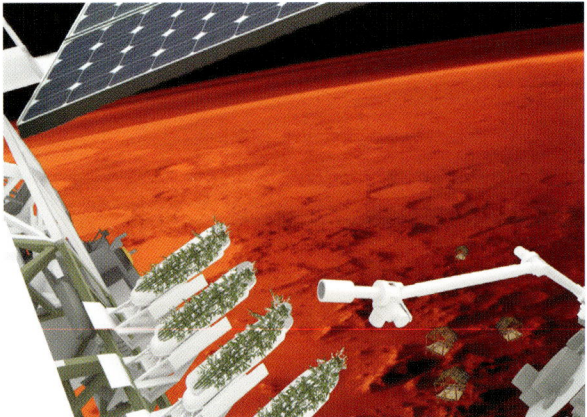

Finally, upon arrival to Mars, the crew will need building materials to construct living, research and growth spaces. Here, bamboo will come to the rescue. Bamboo is one of the fastest growing land plants and is an excellent building material. Bamboo saplings planted at the start of the journey would reach maturity over the 9 months that it would take to reach Mars. The mature bamboo can then be robotically harvested and used for construction purposes. For the trip home, the bamboo growth pods would be jettisoned to reduce weight and save on fuel.

Plants satisfy much of our Earthly needs. Here we show how they can help us meet our space exploration needs as well. We believe that the awesome power of plants is the key to bring our desire to visit and put down roots on other worlds to fruition.

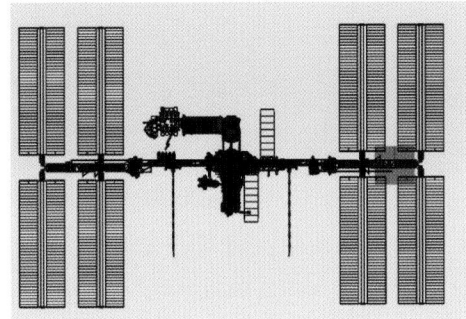
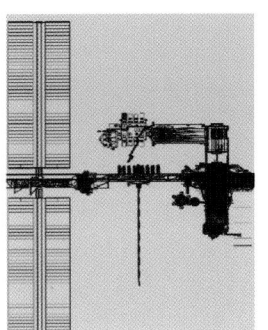
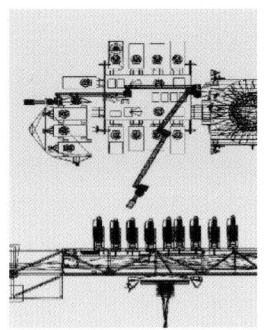
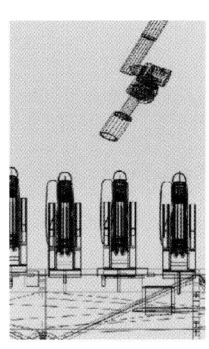

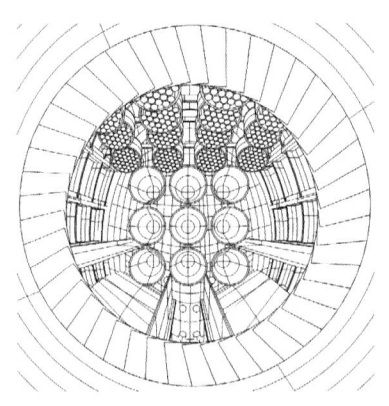
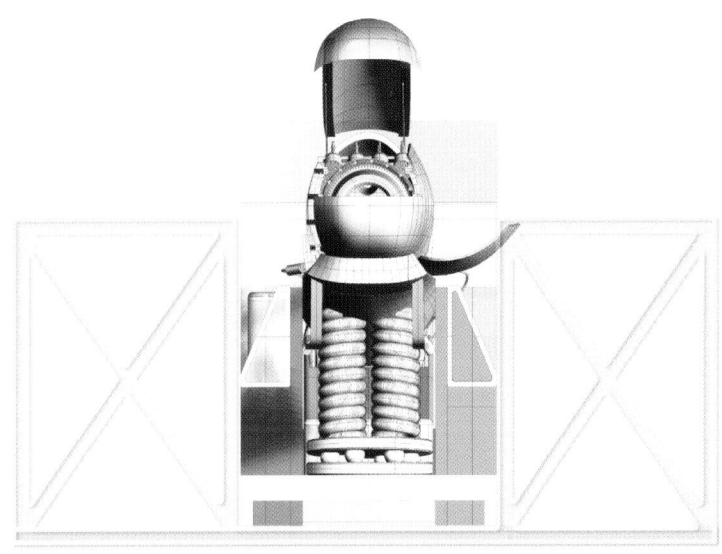

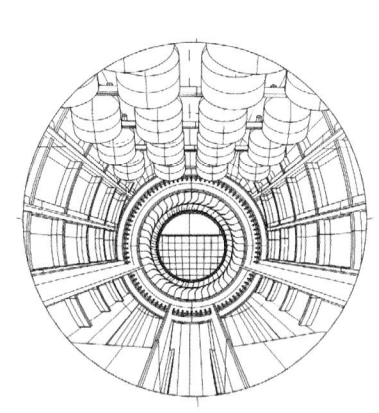
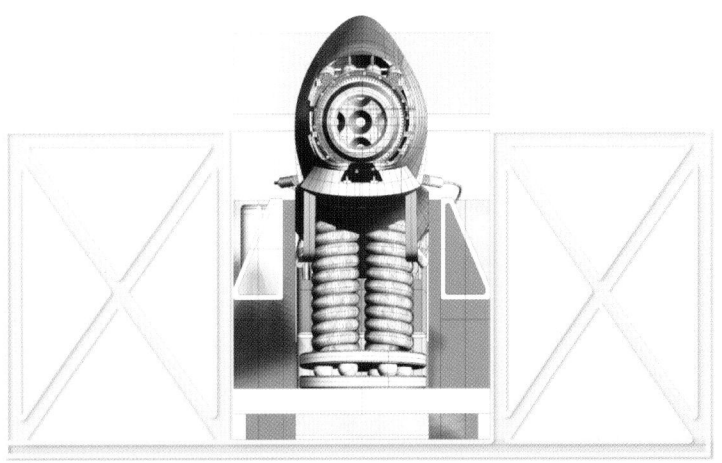

MISSION TO MARS RESEARCH

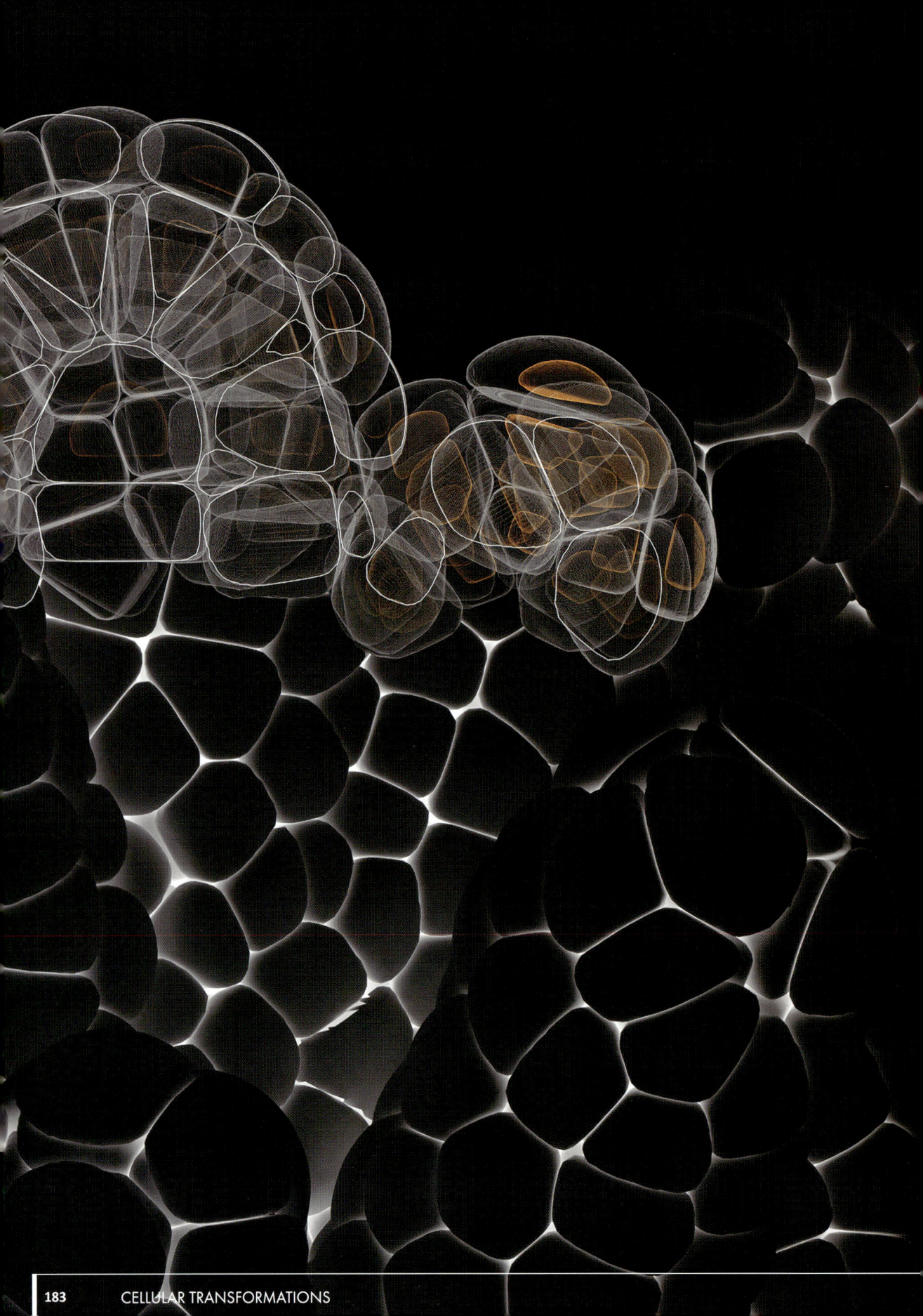

CELLULAR TRANSFORMATIONS

TRANSFORMATION: 2018
ADVANCED CELL ANALYSIS 03

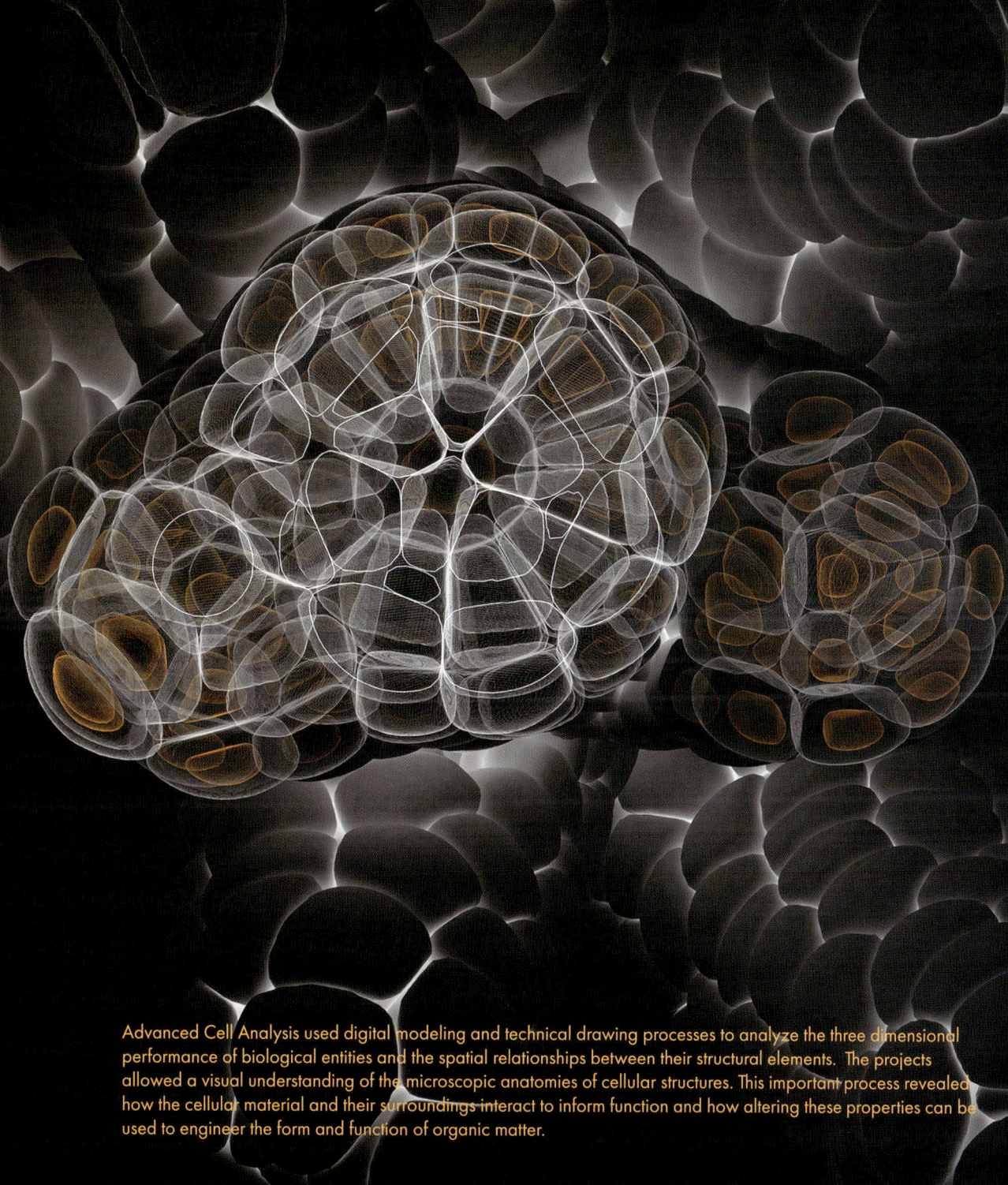

Advanced Cell Analysis used digital modeling and technical drawing processes to analyze the three dimensional performance of biological entities and the spatial relationships between their structural elements. The projects allowed a visual understanding of the microscopic anatomies of cellular structures. This important process revealed how the cellular material and their surroundings interact to inform function and how altering these properties can be used to engineer the form and function of organic matter.

Synaptic Cleft

The synaptic cleft is the small junction of space between two neurons that interact with each other. When one neuron sends information to the next, it produces an electrochemical stimulus called an action potential. The action potential travels down the length of the neuron until it reaches the synaptic cleft and triggers the release of vesicles filled with neurotransmitters. Synapses are the vital unit that wire information through neurons all over the body, allowing us to interact with the environment, and enable us to produce conscious thoughts and memories.

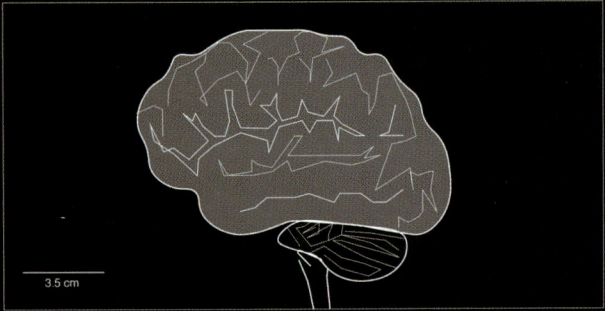

brain

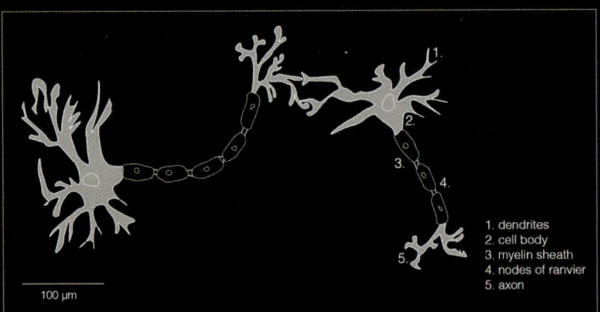

1. dendrites
2. cell body
3. myelin sheath
4. nodes of ranvier
5. axon

neuron

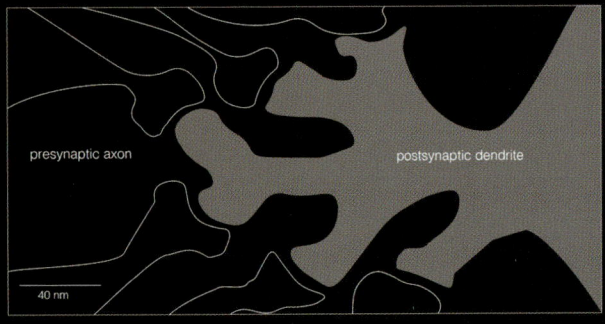

connections

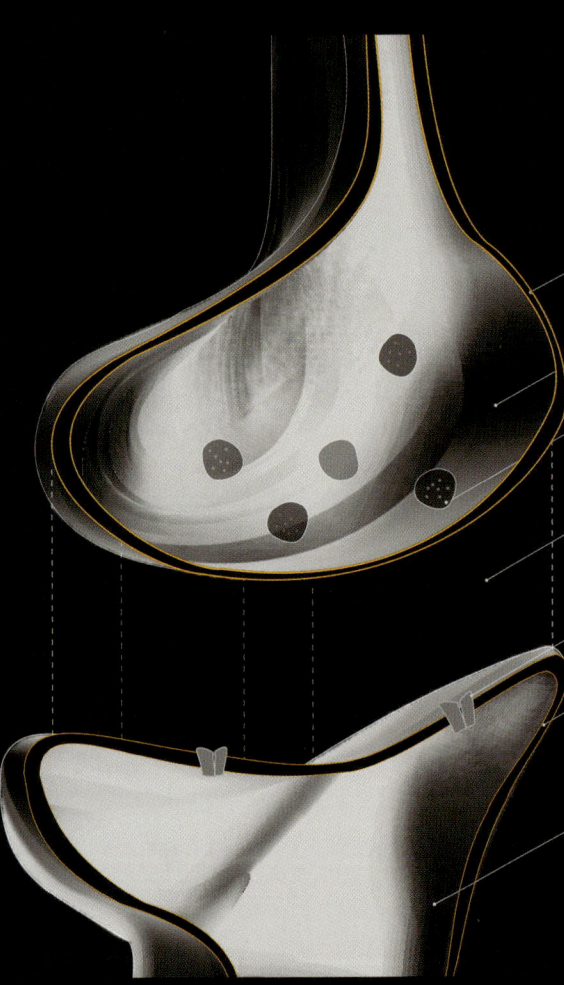

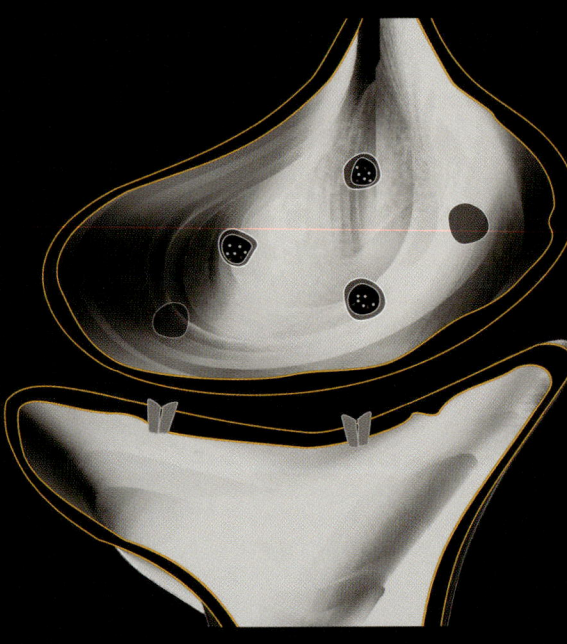

01 pre-action potential

pre-synaptic membrane

cytoplasmic space

vesicle

cleft gap

receptor

post-synaptic membrane

cytoplasmic space

signal transduction process

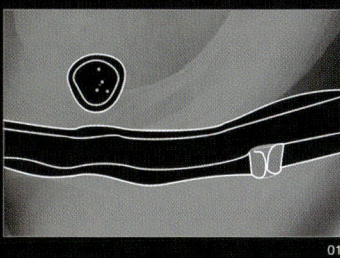

01

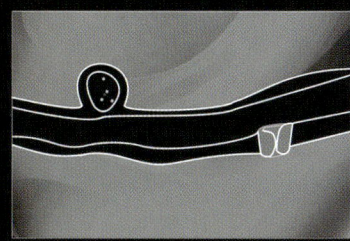

02

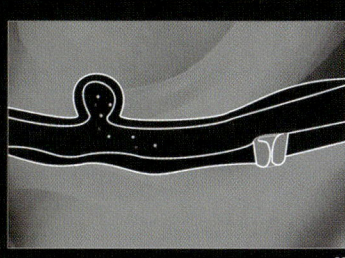

03

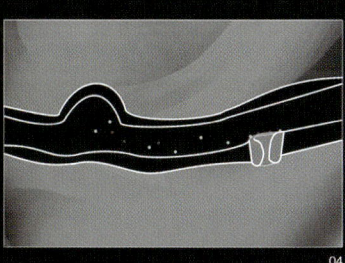

04

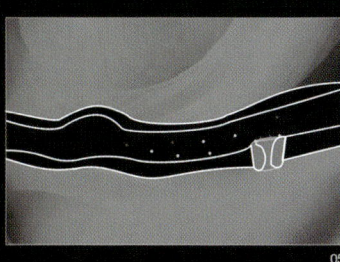

05

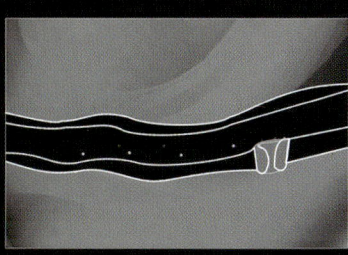

06

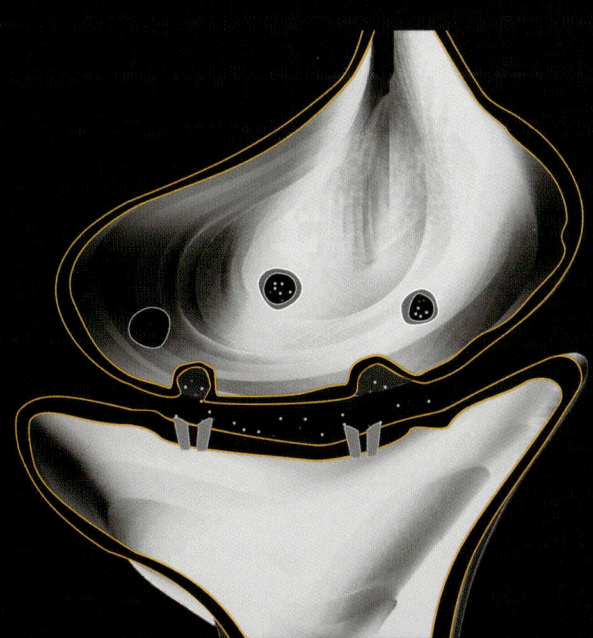

02   post-action potential

Bacterial Flagellum

A flagellum is an appendage that protrudes from some bacterial cells. It serves as a means of movement by propelling the cell forward in the medium it is in. It comprises of three main parts: the basal body, the hook, and filament. The filament and hook are made up of singular repeating protein units with additional proteins to cap or serve as conjunction points. The basal body generates rotational movement powered by the proton motive force of protons moving across the stators of the basal body machinery. The hook connects the filament and the basal body and is fixed in a right angle orientation. As such, when the motor in the basal body rotates, the filament coils around generating a propulsive force. The rotations are very fast, often amounting to 200 to 1000 rpm which can equate to roughly 60 cell lengths per second.

BACTERIAL COLONY

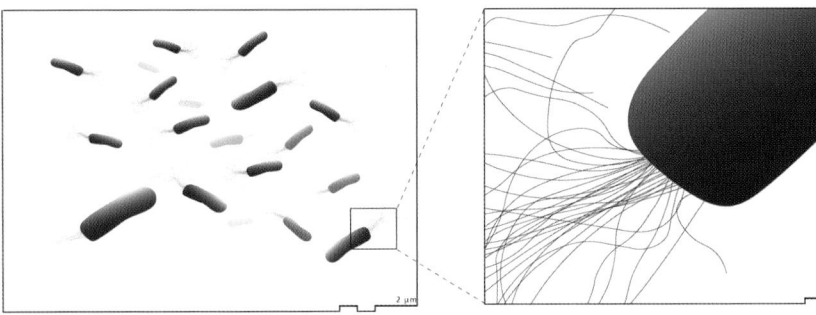

SECTION THROUGH CELL MEMBRANE

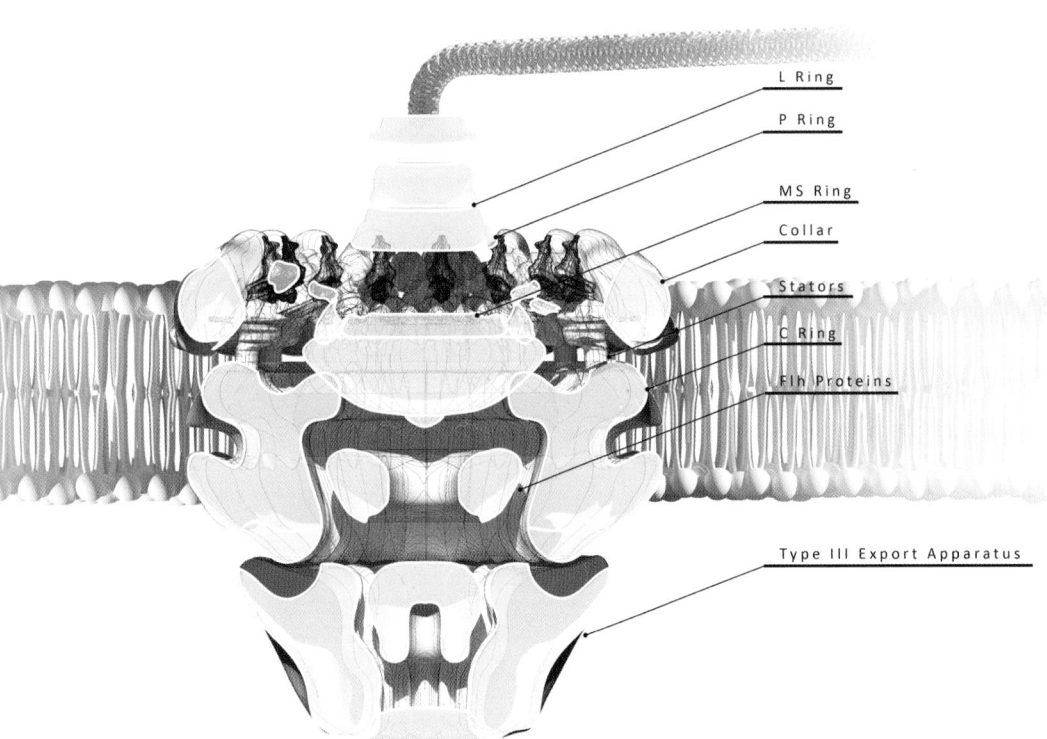

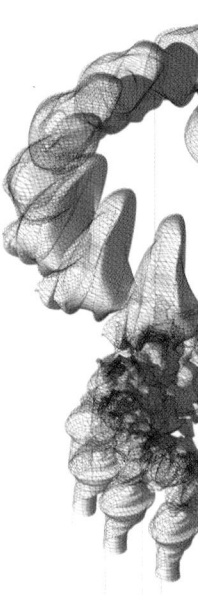

ANDREA TRINKLE | SIAN ZHANG

Hook and Filament
The visible components of the flagellar apparatus and propels the motion of the bacterial cell

L Ring
Anchors the flagella in the liposaccharides in the bacterial cell wall

P Ring
Anchors the flagella in the peptidoglycan in the bacterial cell wall

Collar
Surrounds the MS ring and is loosely associated with the flagellar motor apparatus

Stators
Stationary proteins that act as channels for protons to enter or ext, powering the spinning rotor machinery and serving as a point for the rotor to rotate against

MS Ring
Anchors the apparatus in the cytoplasmic membrane and forms part of the spinning rotor of the basal body

C Ring
Part of the spinning rotor and helps to control the direction and speed of the flagellar rotation

Type III Export Apparatus
Comprised of Fli and Flh proteins to make up an ATPase ring and export gate. This apparatus is involved in flagella assembly. It utilizes ATP and proton gradients to export the proteins that make up the flagella

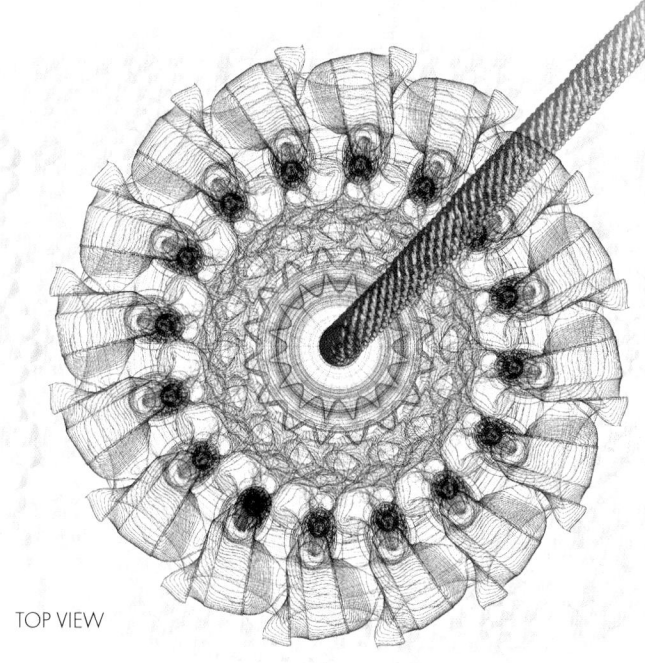

TOP VIEW

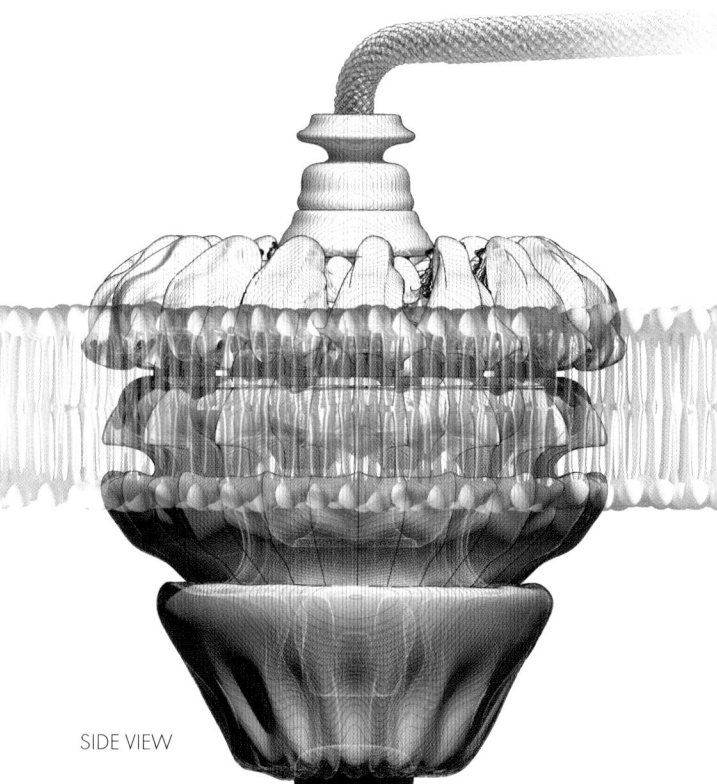

SIDE VIEW

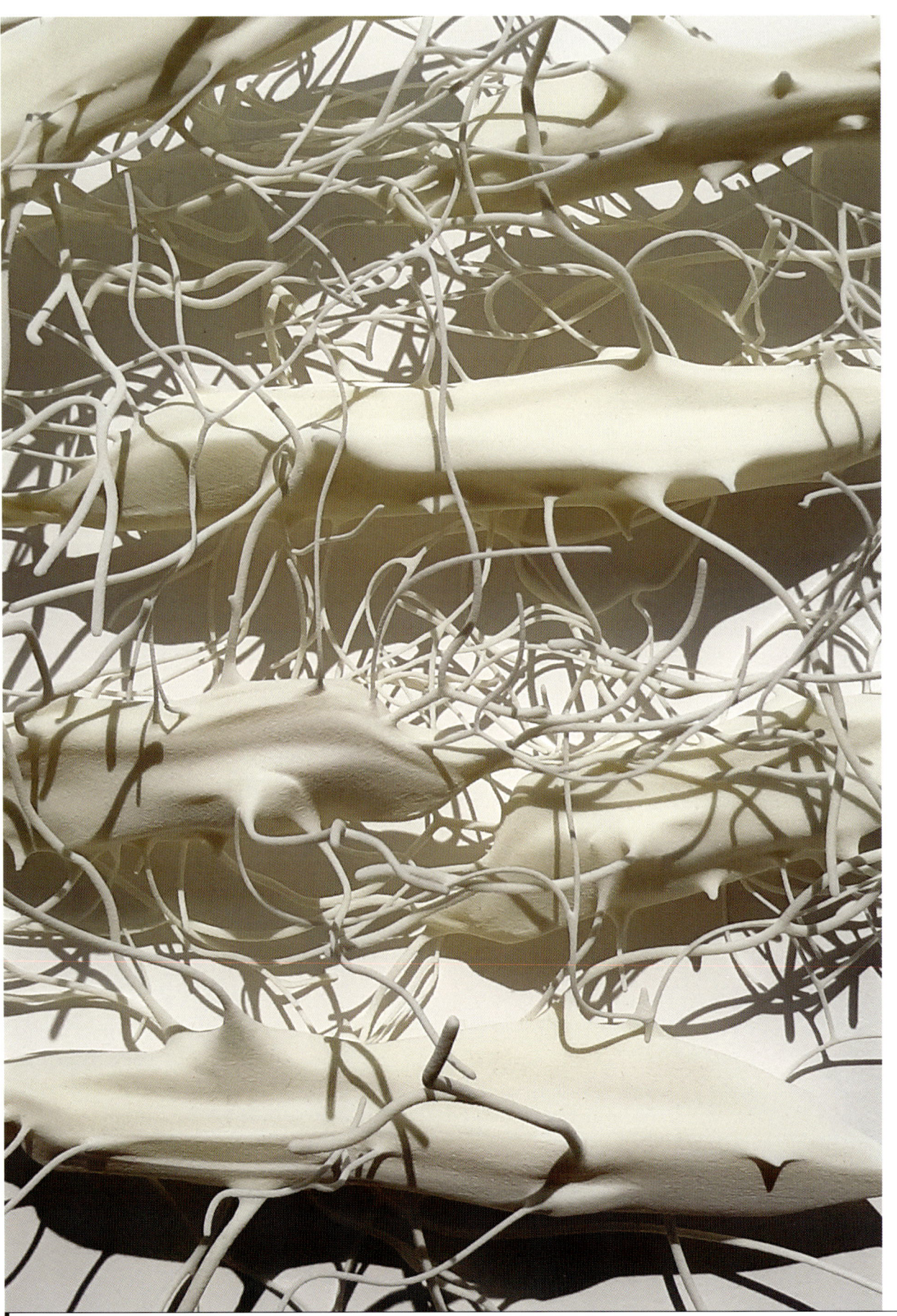

REPLICATION: 2017-2020
3D PRINTED CELLS

The 3D Printed Cells project was a collaboration between biology and architecture students to develop highly detailed digital models of intricate cellular structures and activities that were outputted as high-resolution 3D printed models. Advances in microscopy and fluorescent-protein technology offer unprecedented views of molecular space–time dynamics in living cells. However, digital modeling of the spatially complex and dynamic cellular systems has been lacking. Modeling and analysis of the three dimensional performances of biological structures and the spatial relationships between the structural elements allows deeper investigations into the inner workings of cells. Modeling and outputting in the physical dimension remains an important emerging area of cellular research.

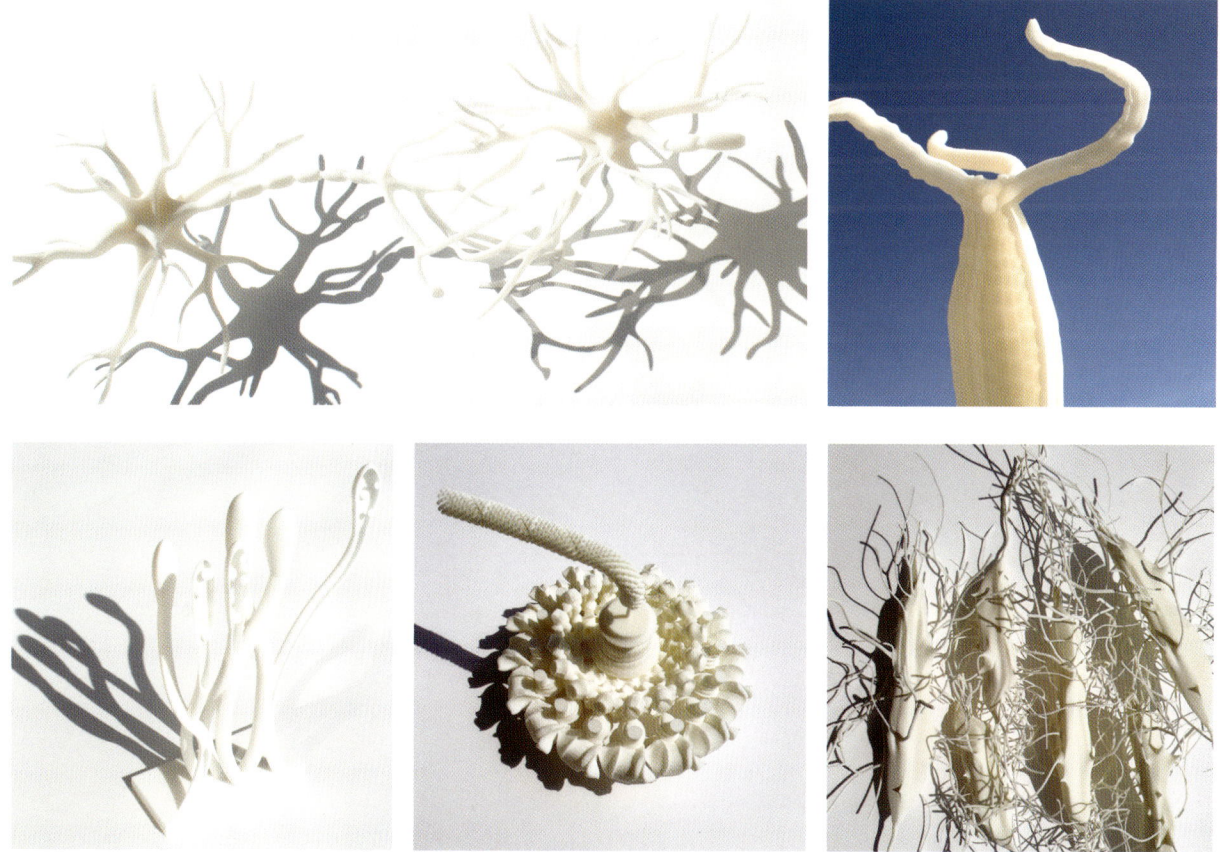

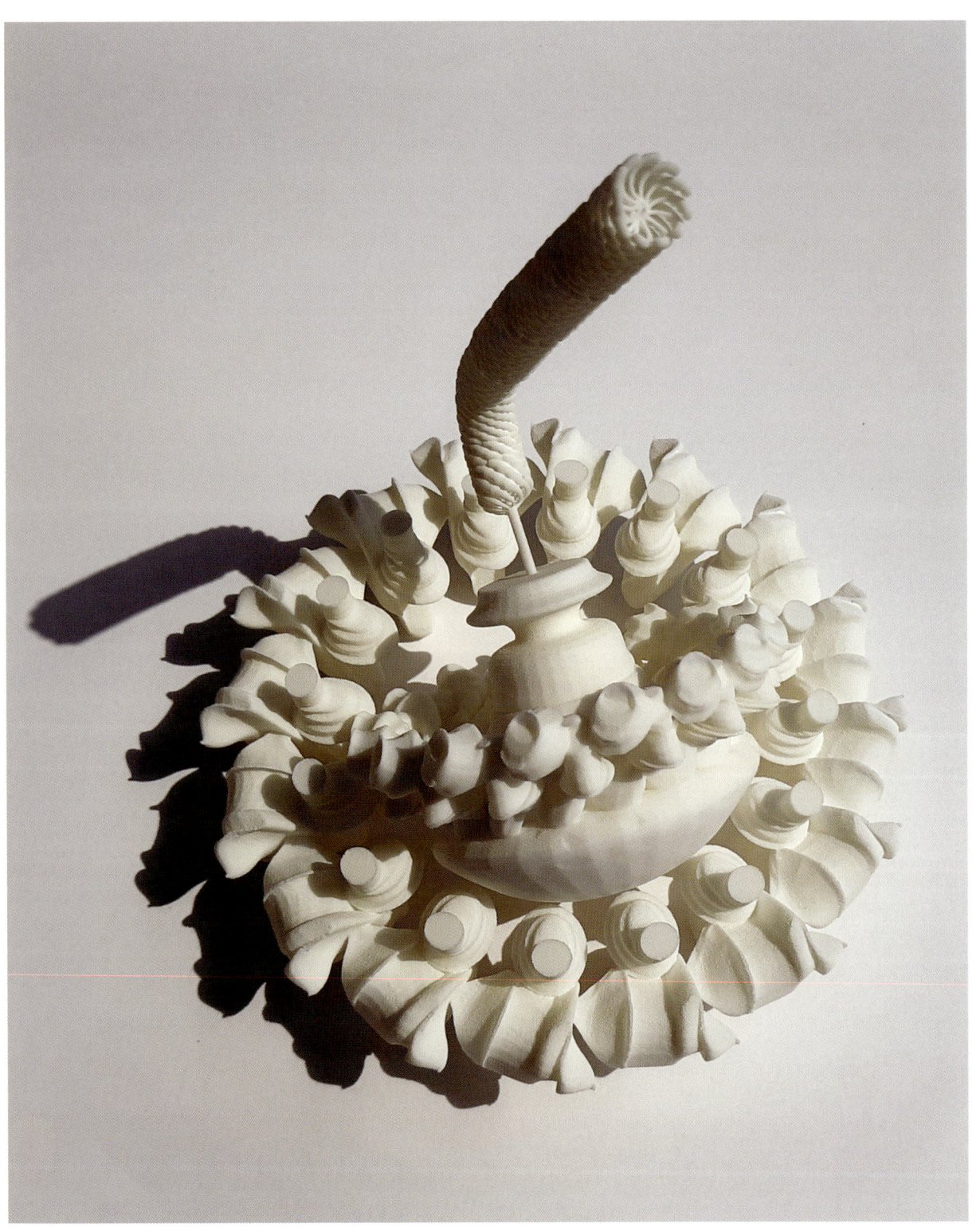

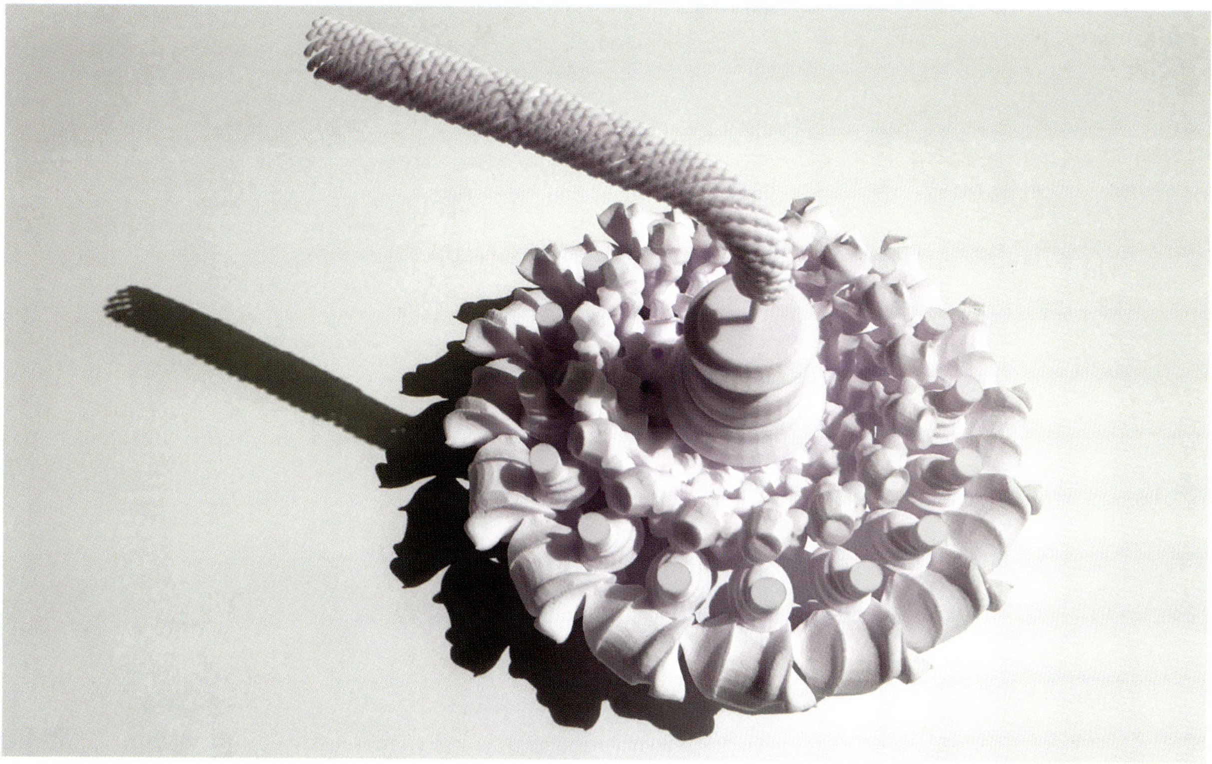

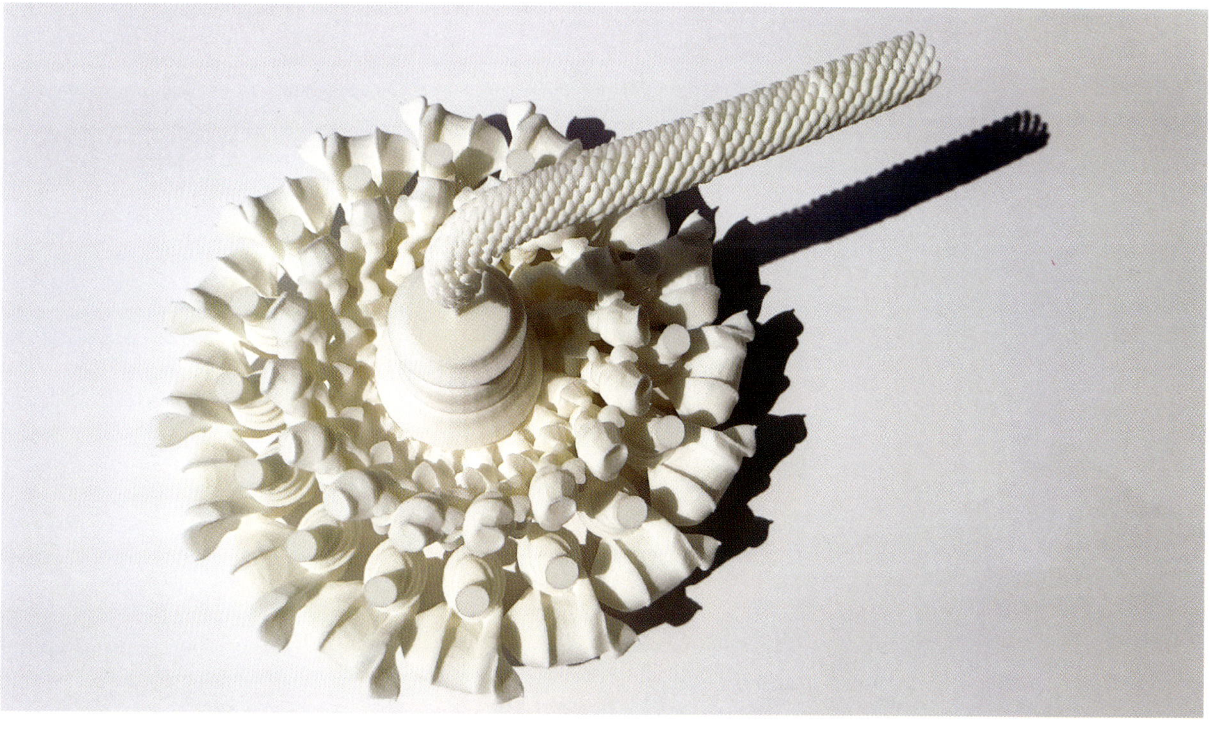

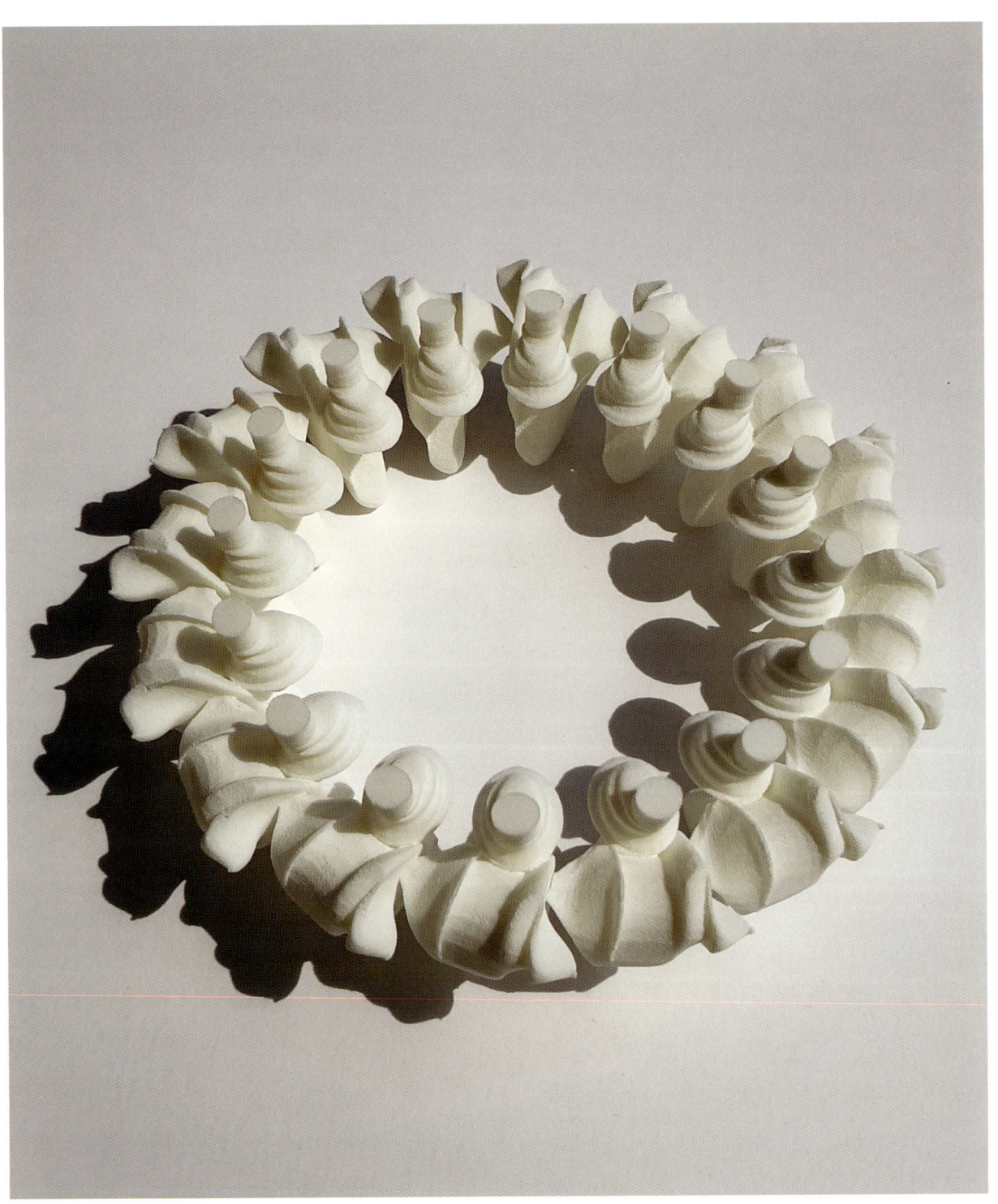

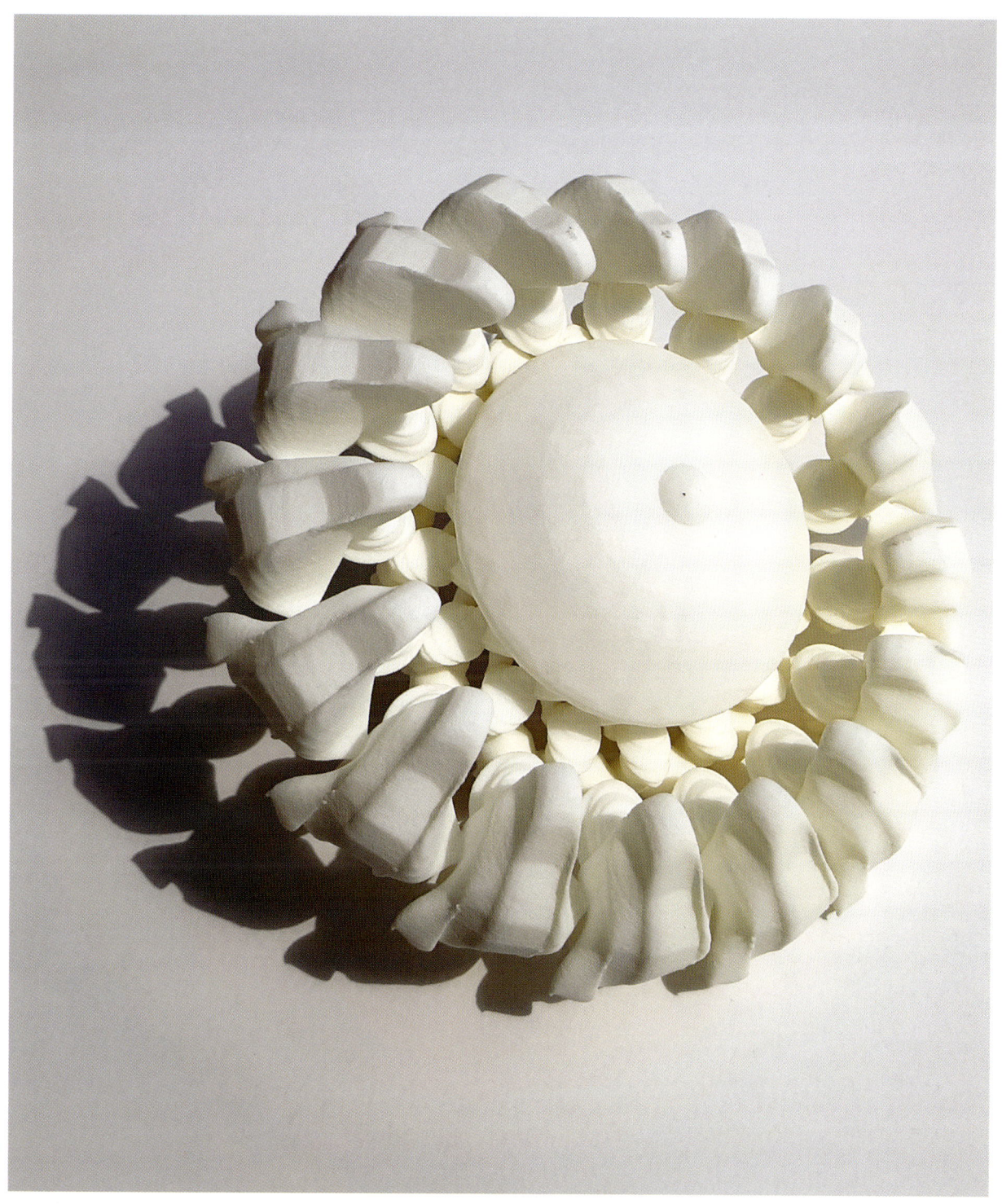

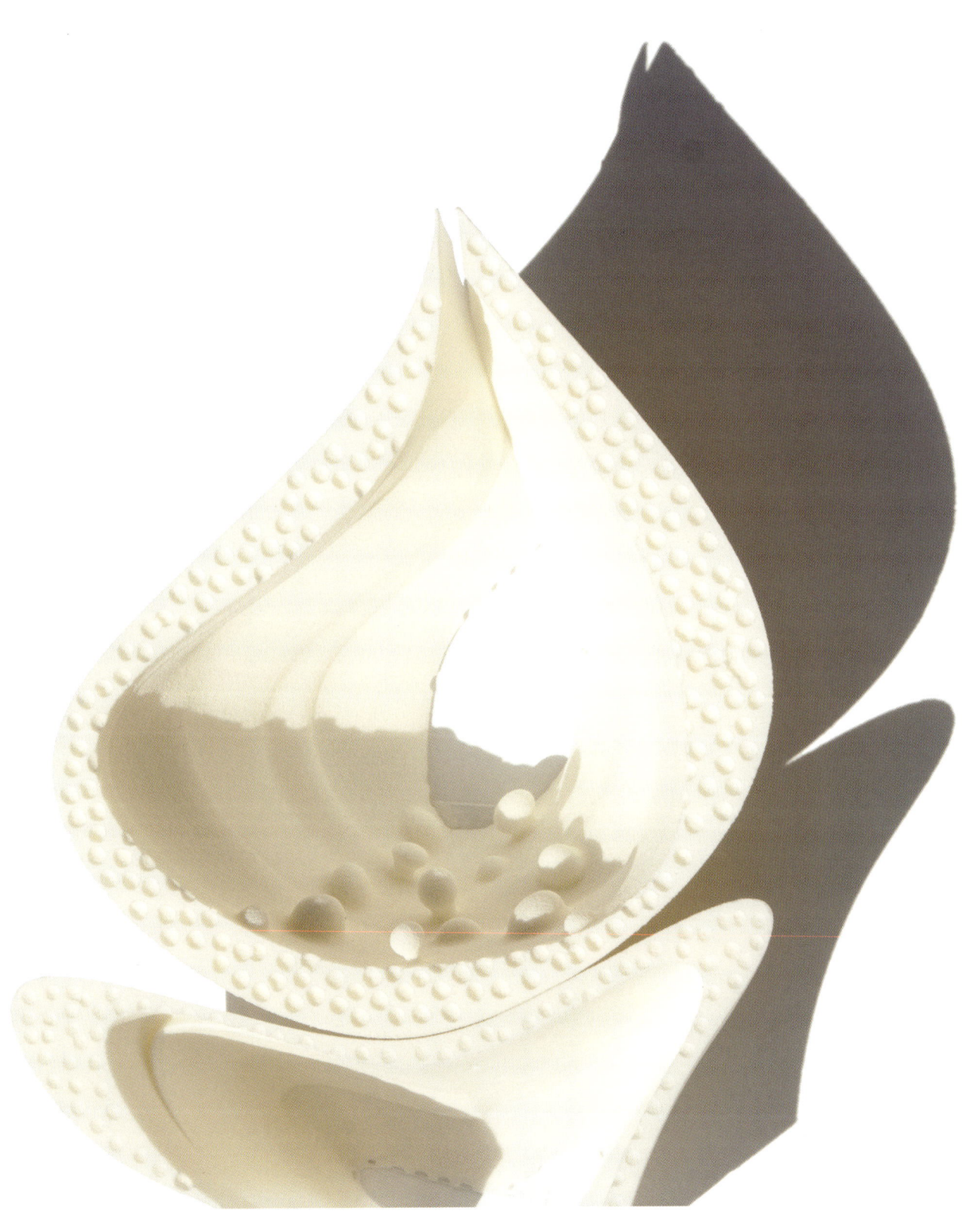

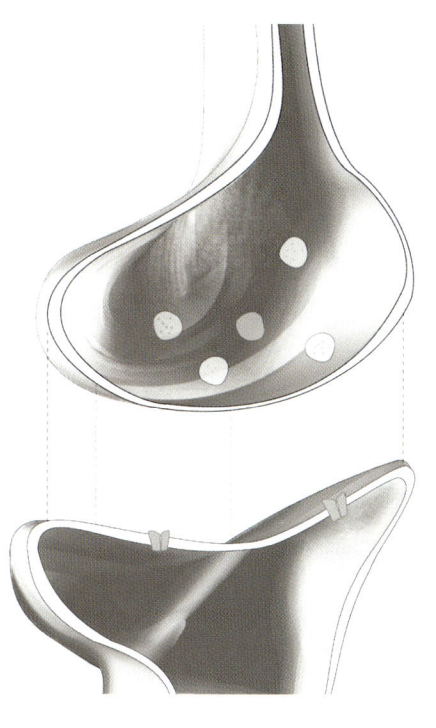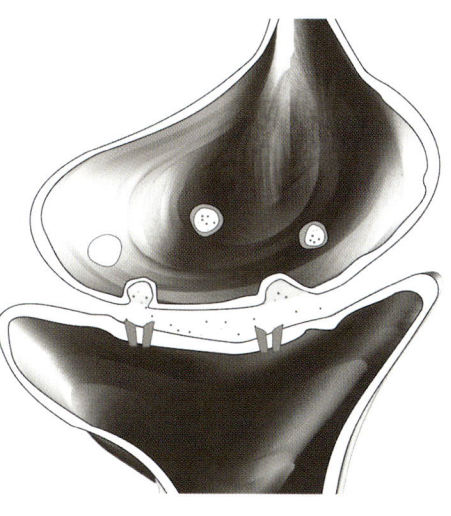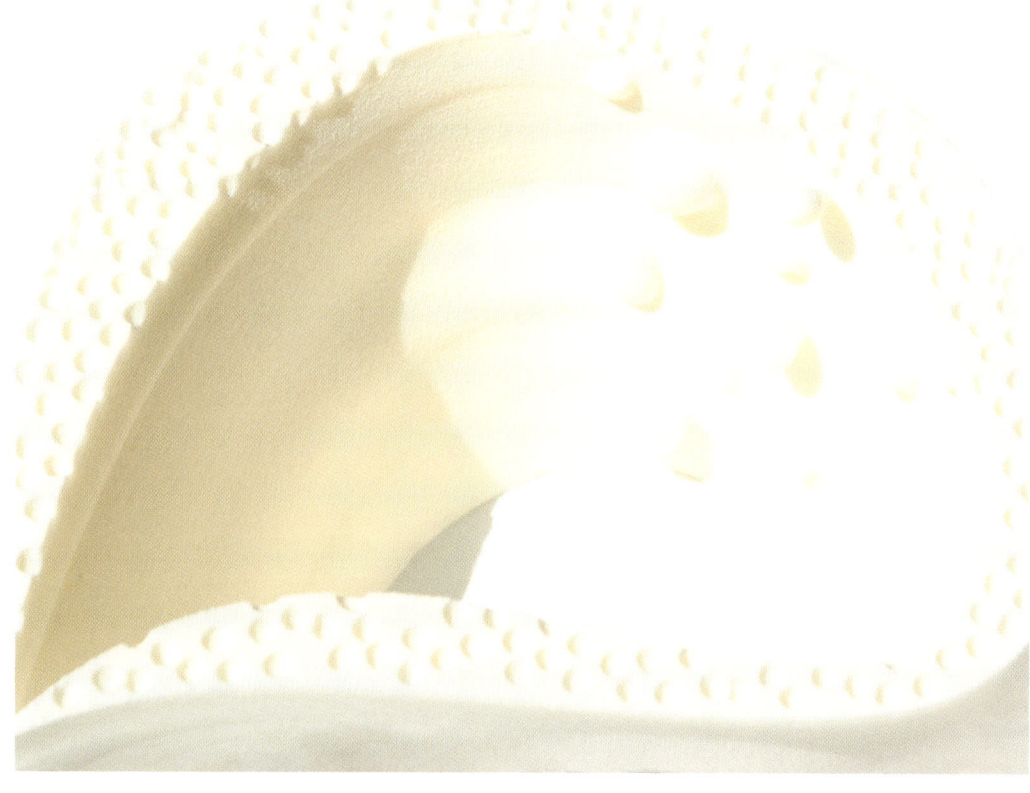

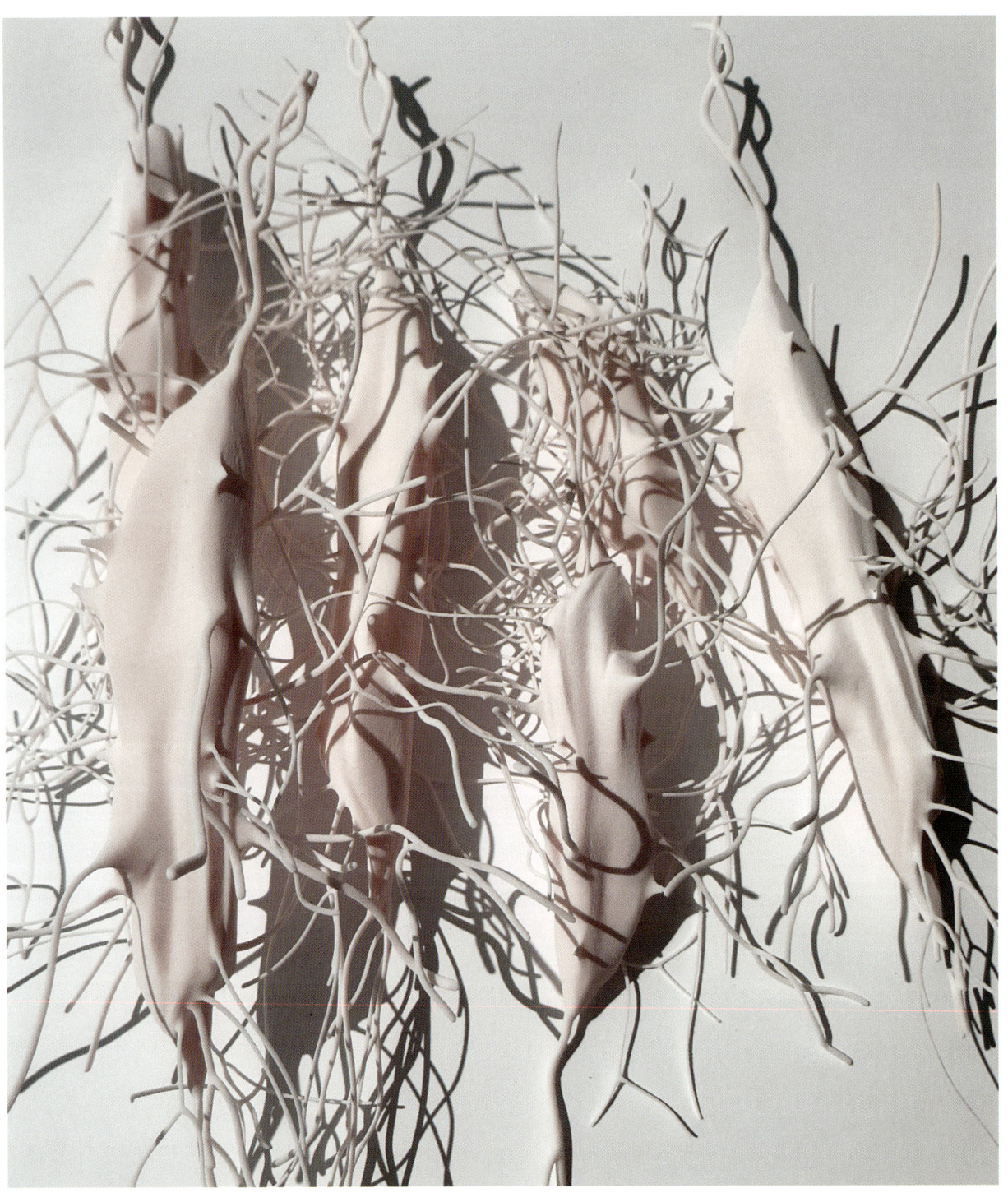

Structure Of An Osteon

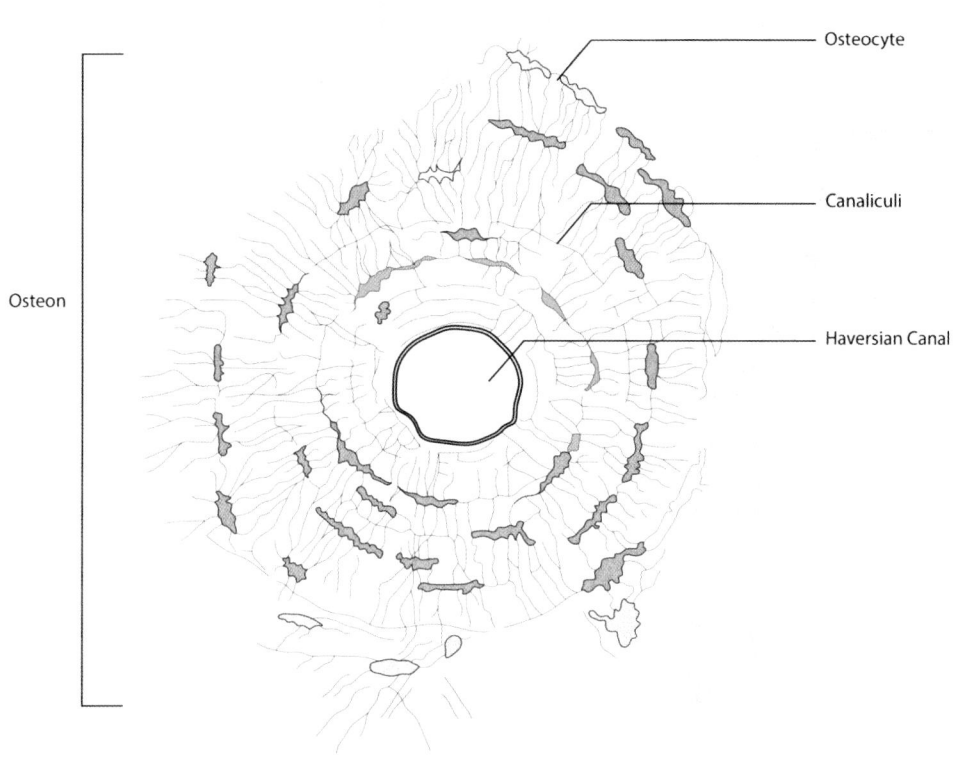

Growth Of An Osteon

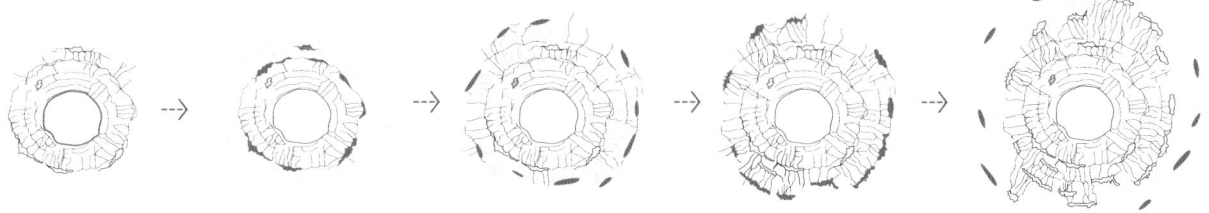

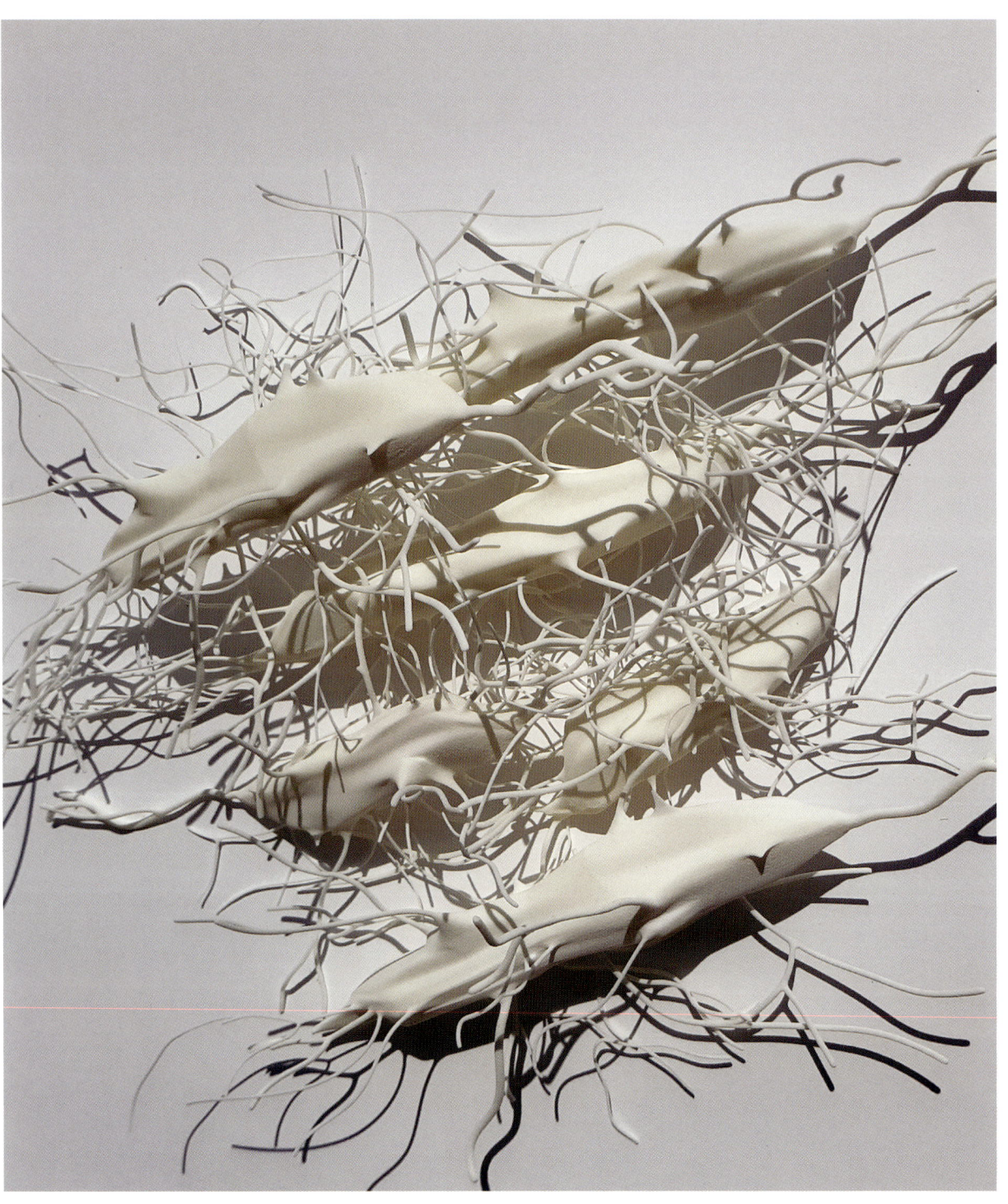

Section Of An Osteocyte

Osteocyte

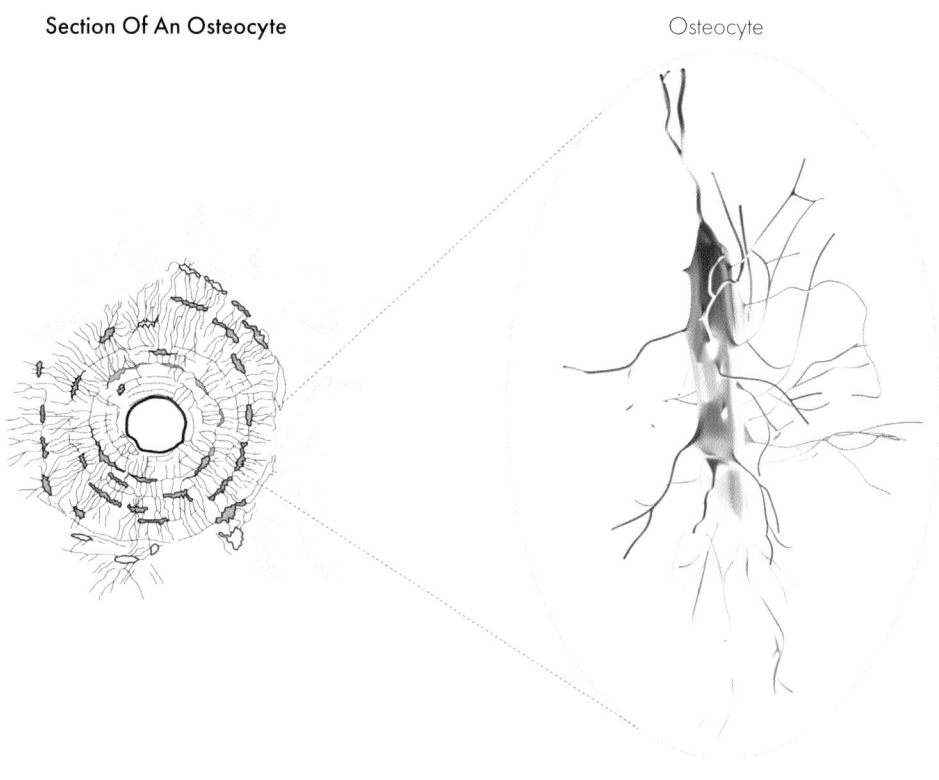

Osteocyte Cell

Osteogenic Cell

Osteoblast

Osteocyte

Osteocyte

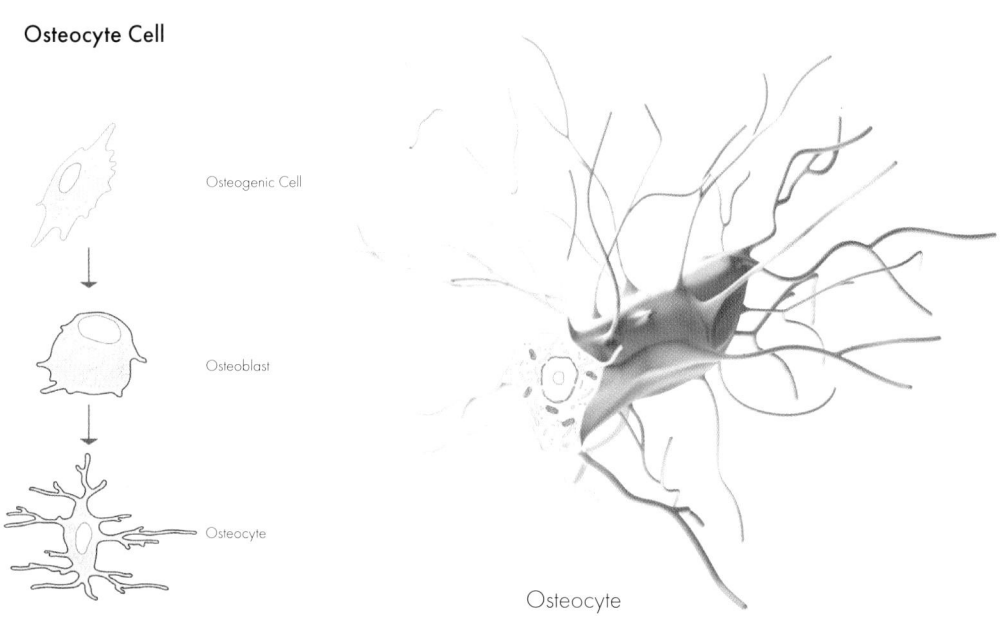

PEZIZA FUNGI

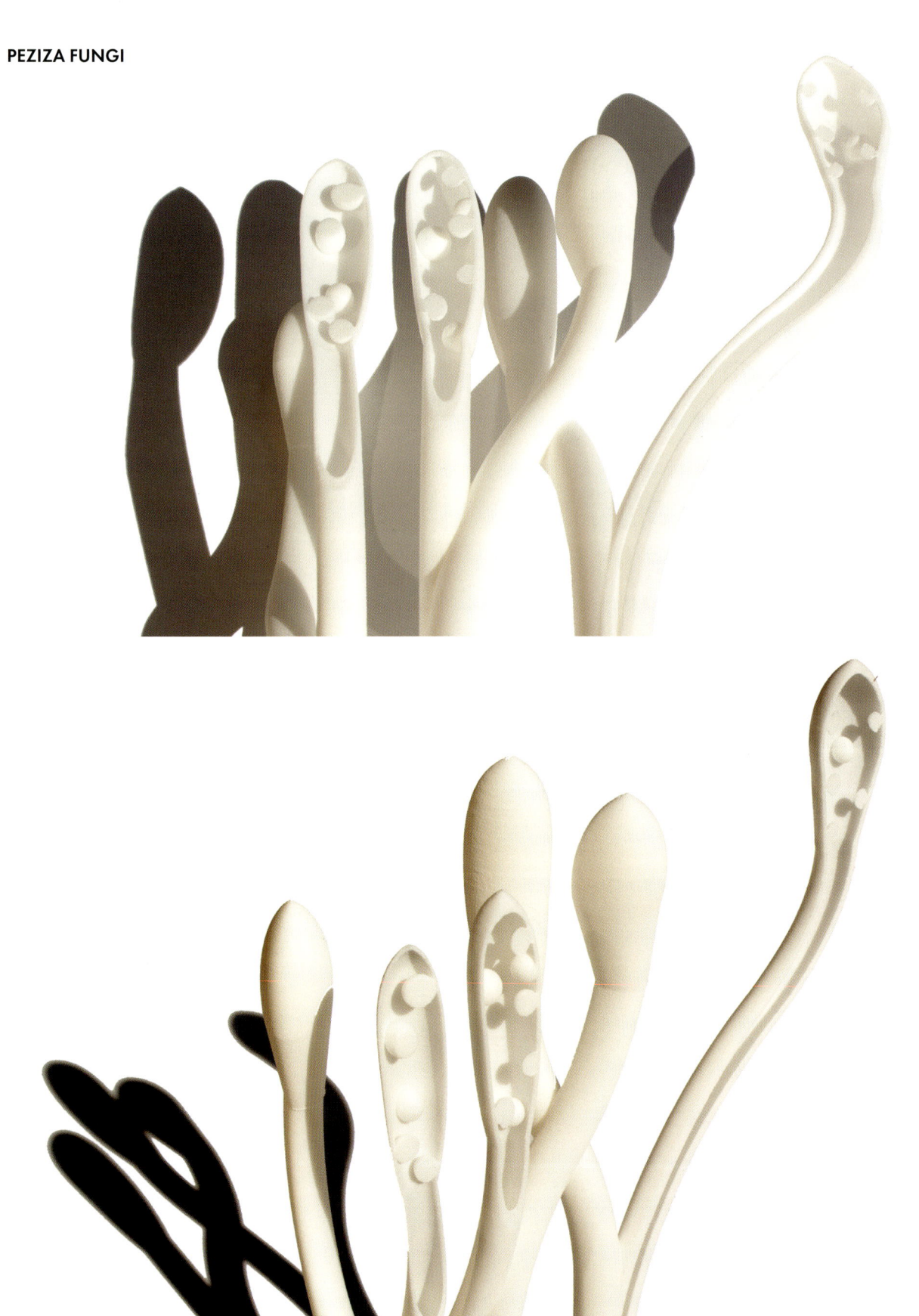

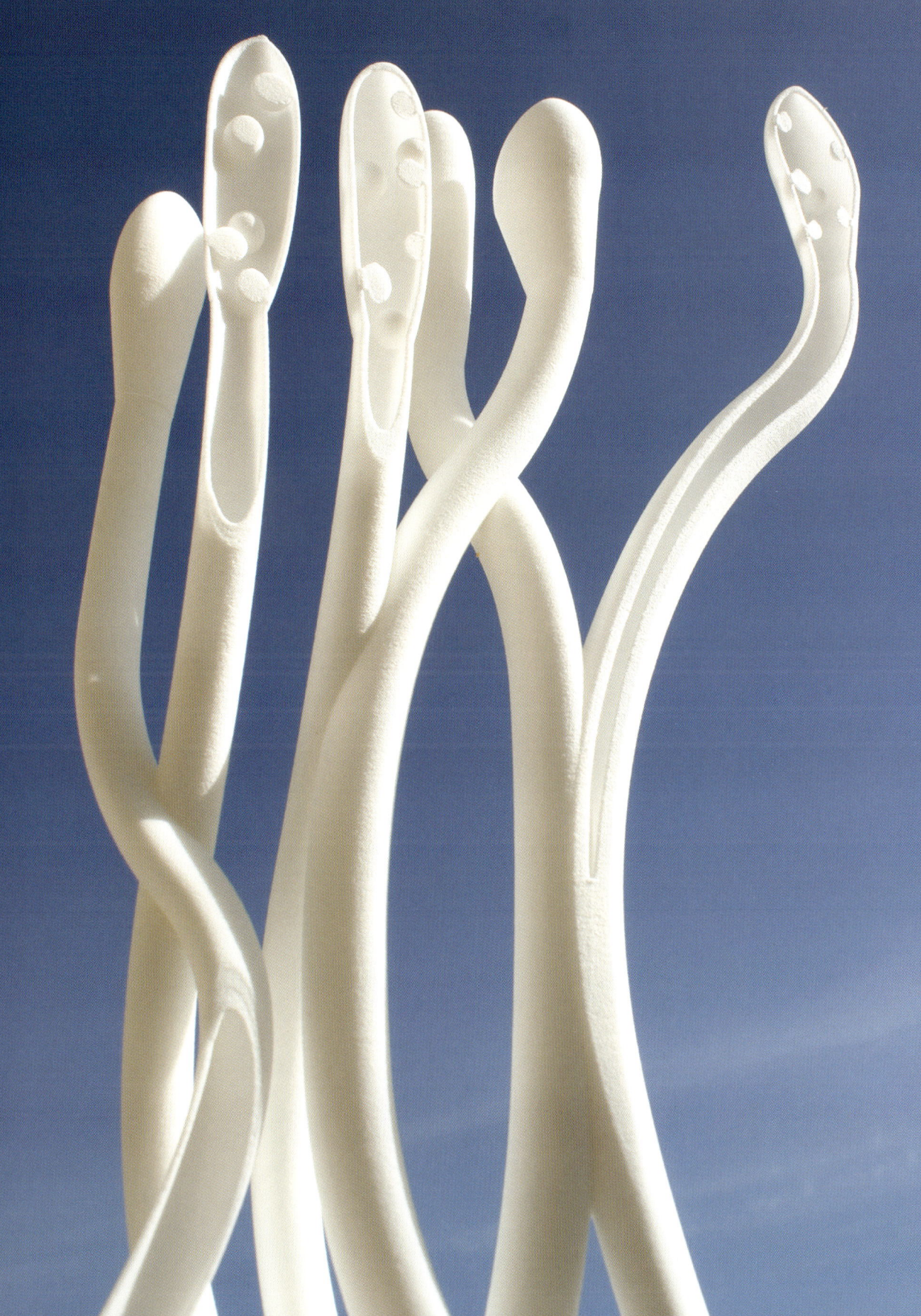

NERVE CELL COMMUNICATION

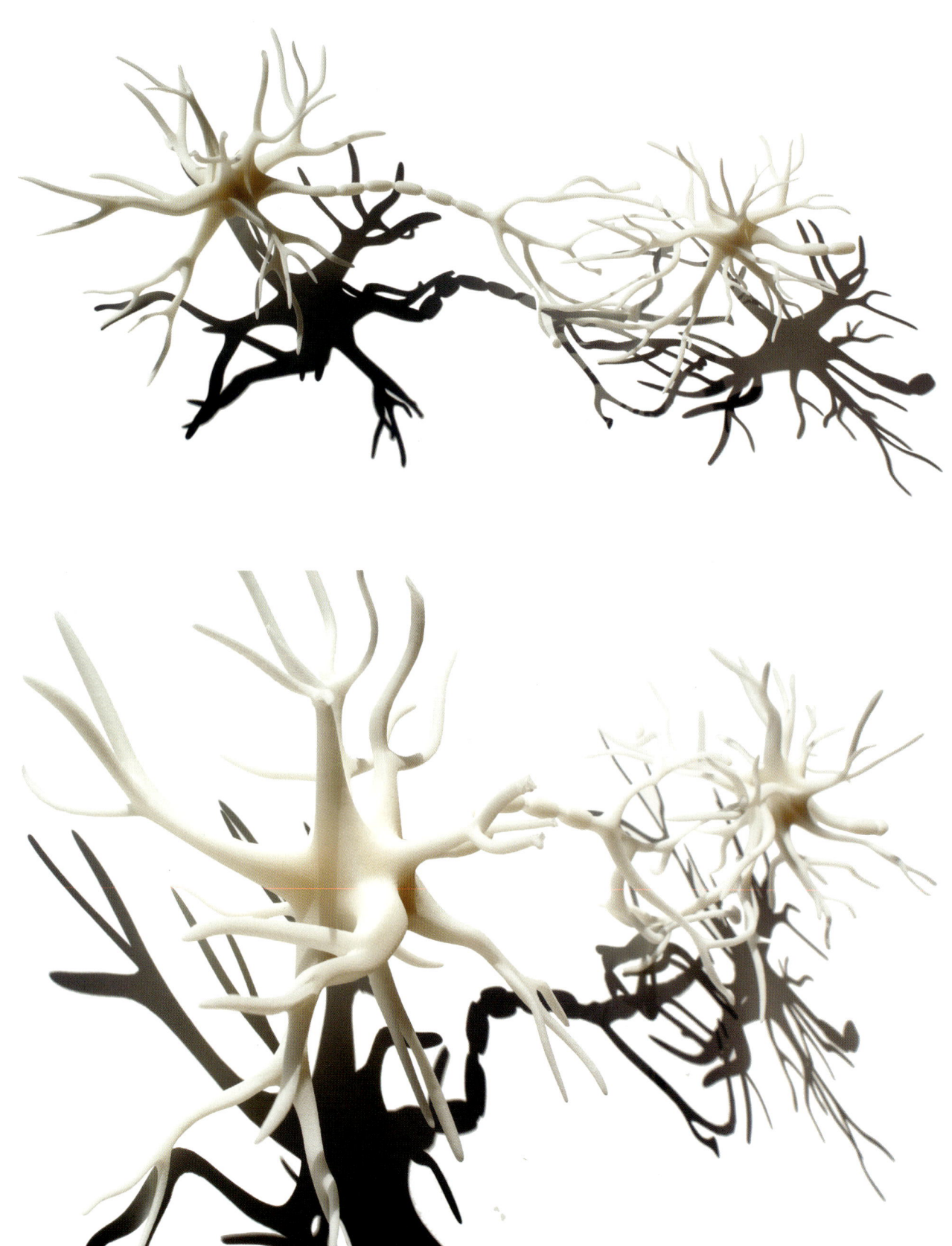

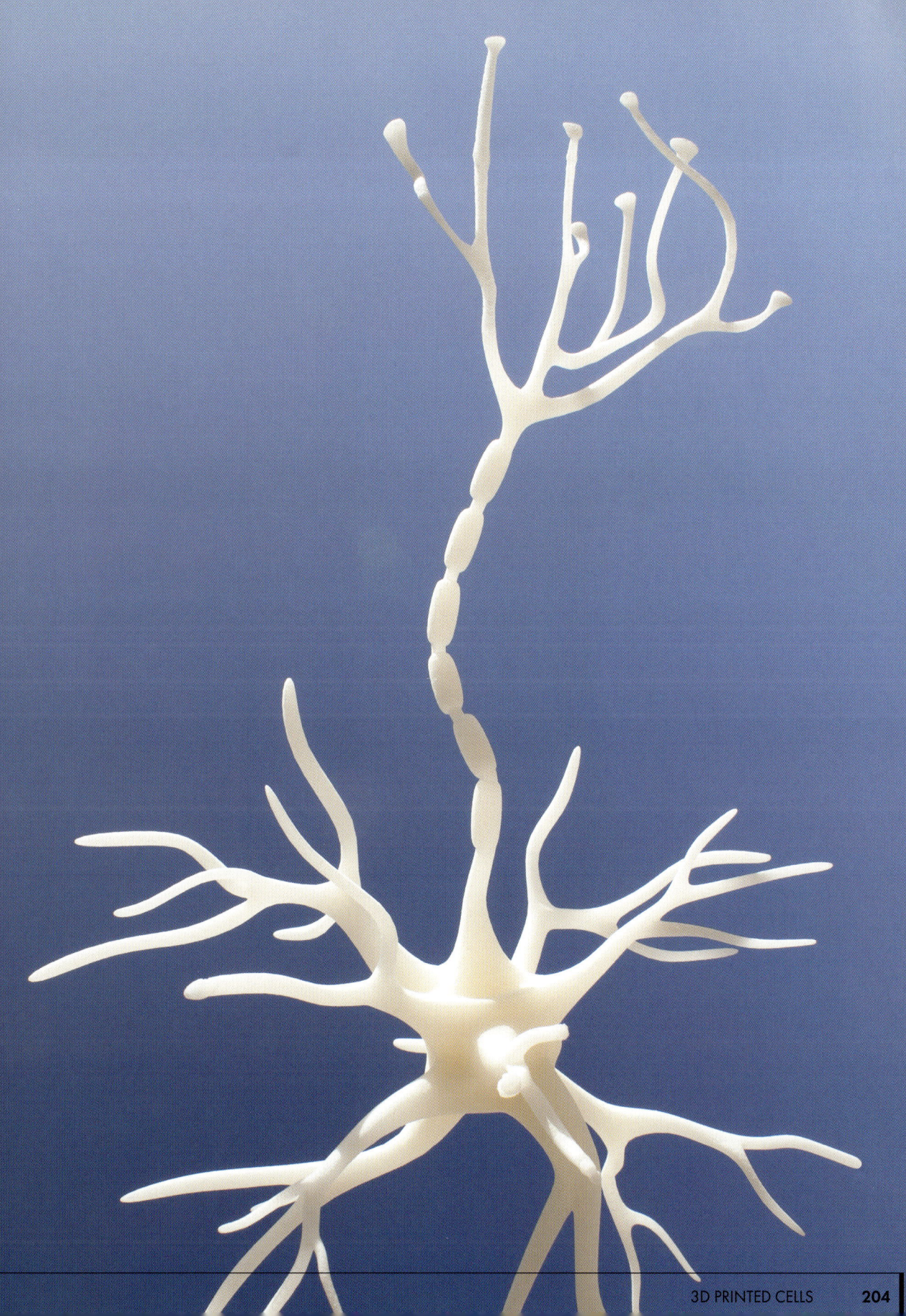

PATRICK MURRAY | YUHAO JI | GUANYU KE

HYDRA

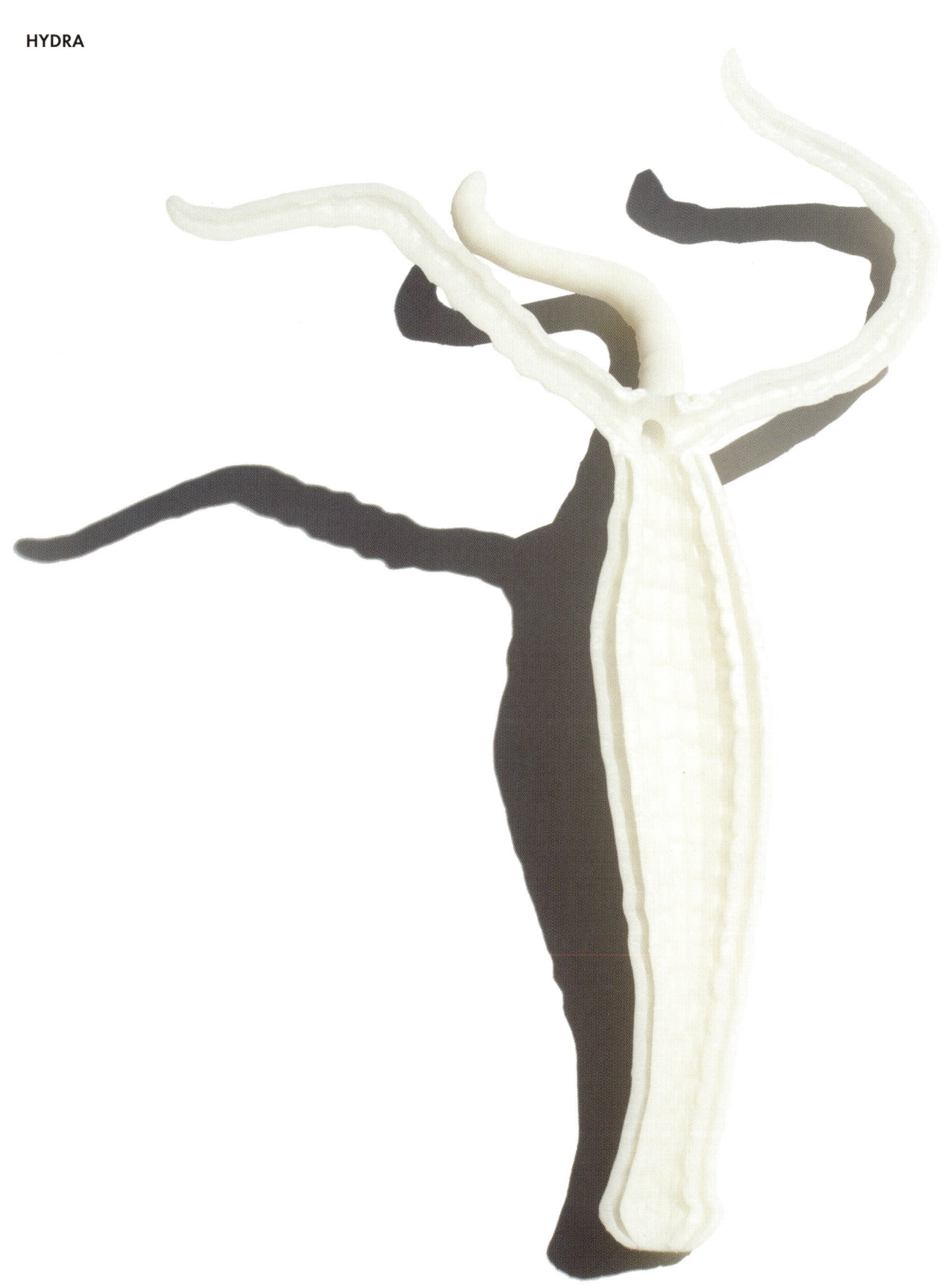

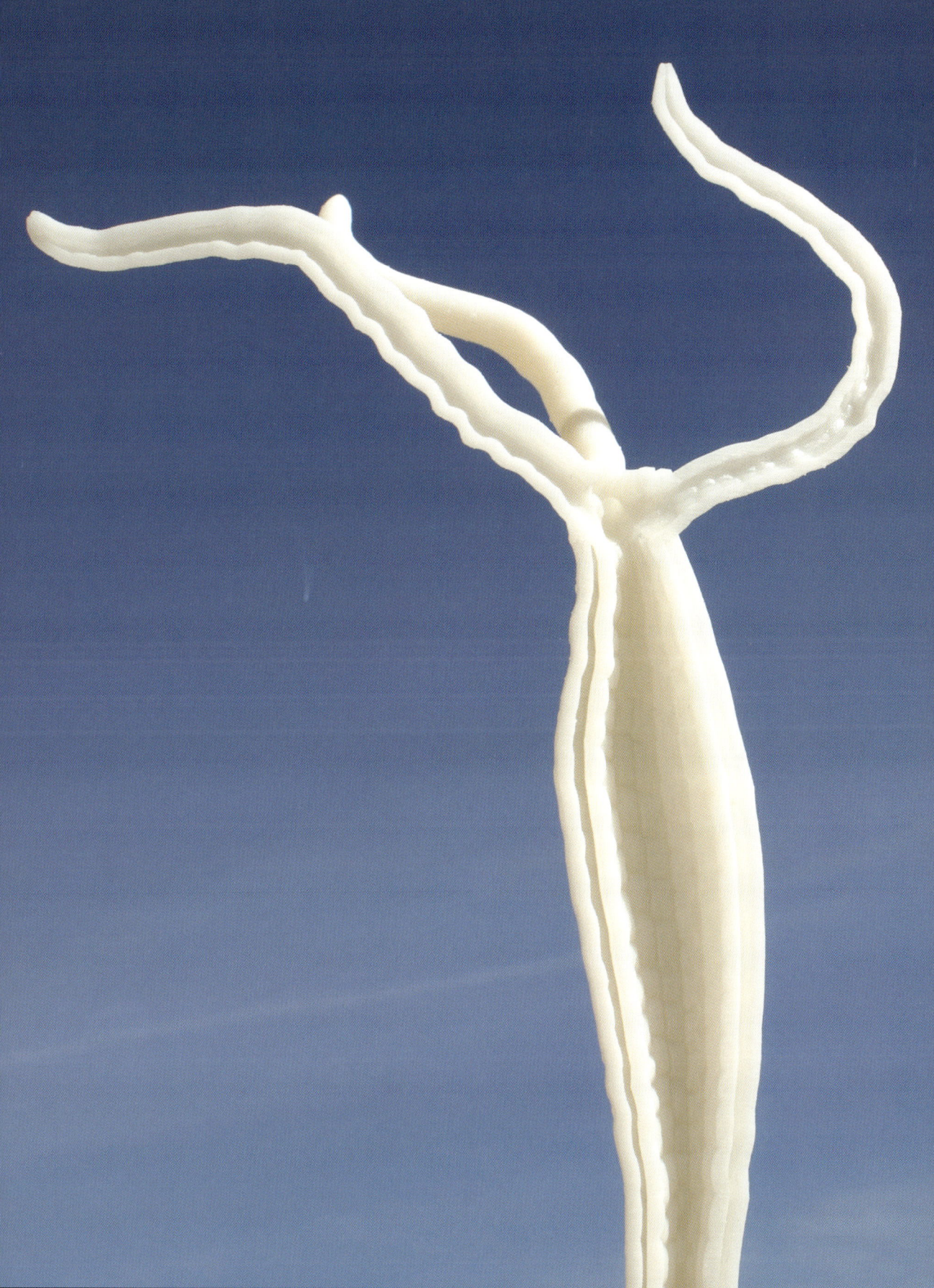

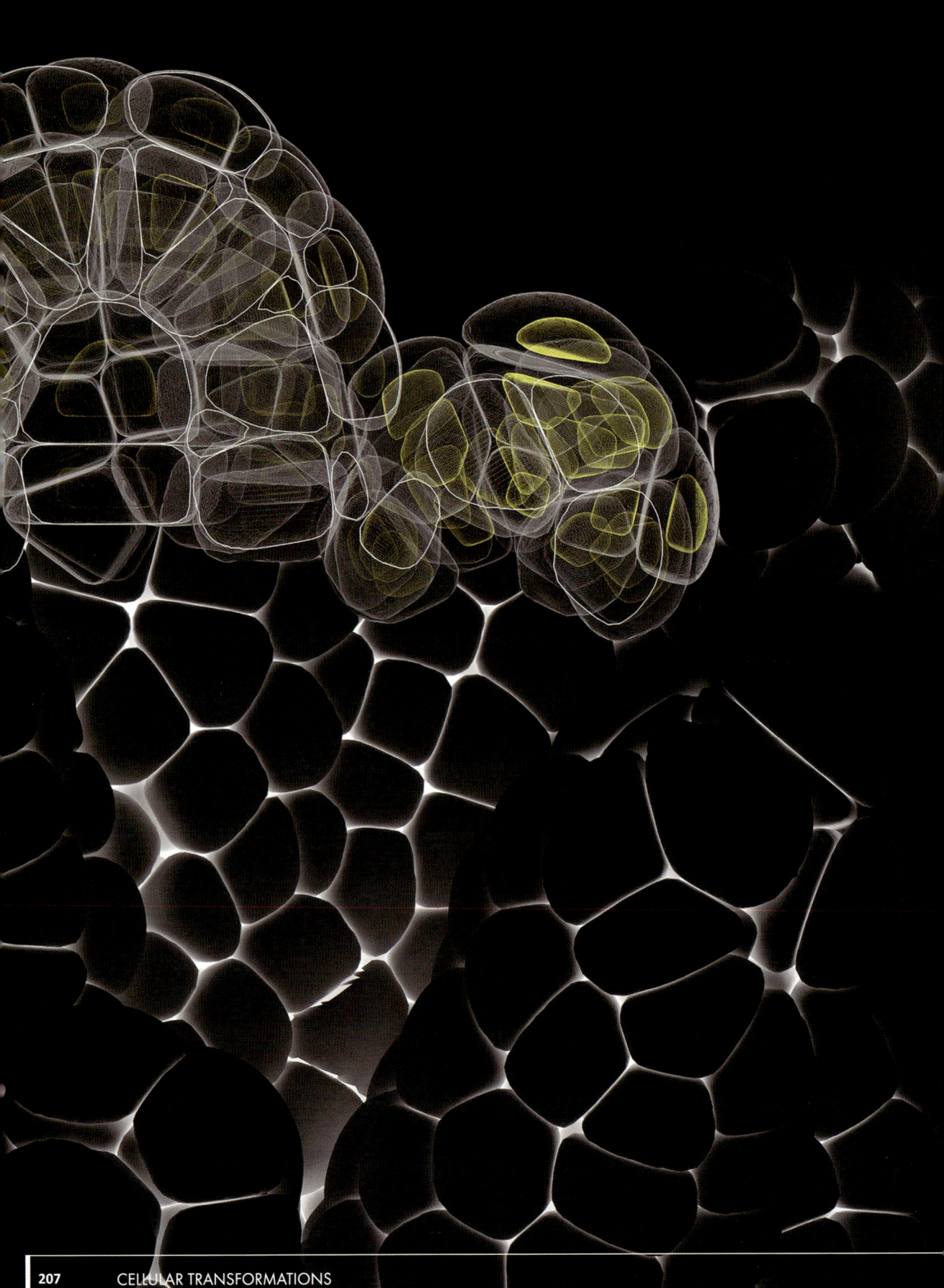

TRANSFORMATION: 2020
ADVANCED CELL ANALYSIS 04

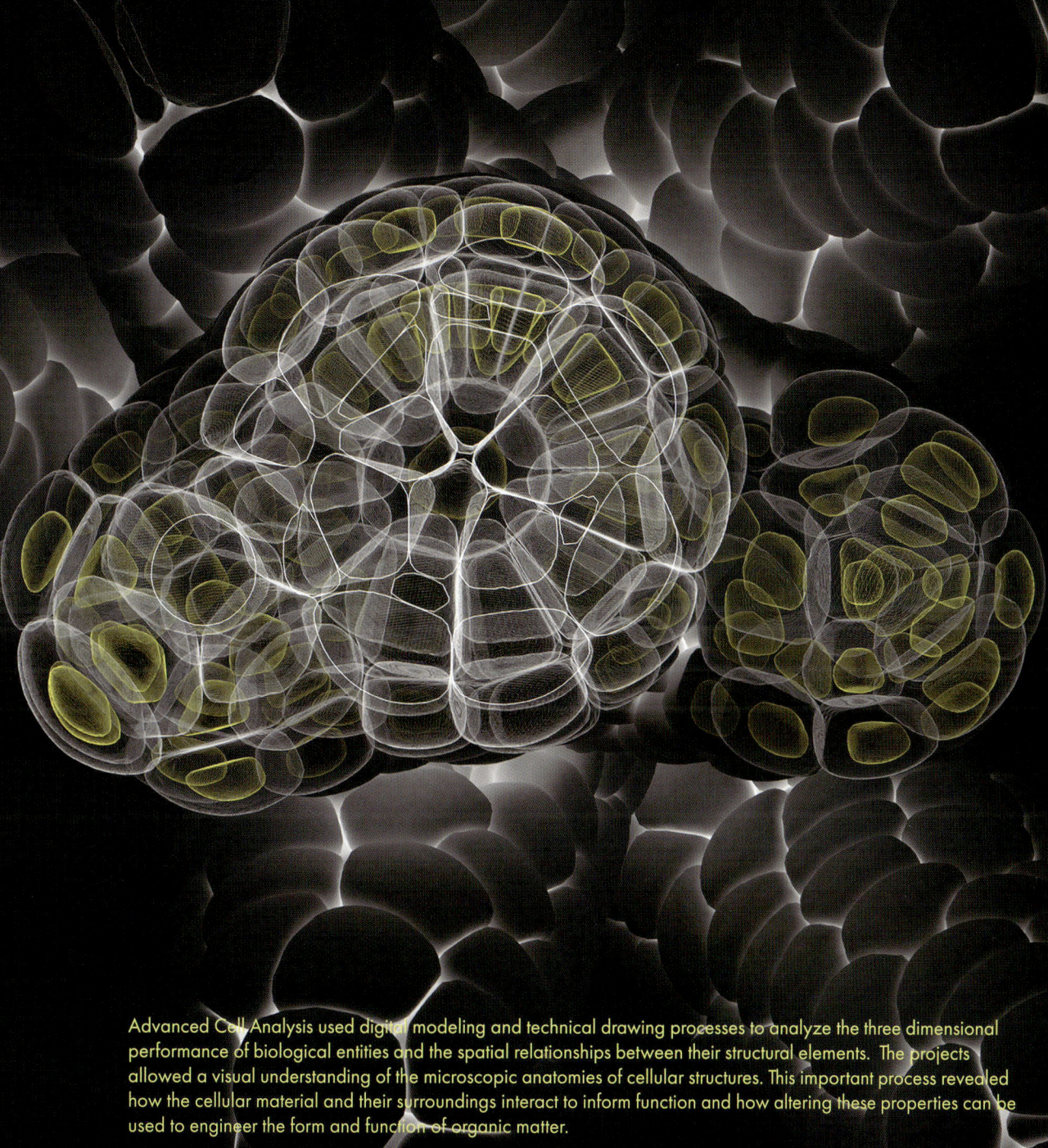

Advanced Cell Analysis used digital modeling and technical drawing processes to analyze the three dimensional performance of biological entities and the spatial relationships between their structural elements. The projects allowed a visual understanding of the microscopic anatomies of cellular structures. This important process revealed how the cellular material and their surroundings interact to inform function and how altering these properties can be used to engineer the form and function of organic matter.

Zhuoxian Deng | Xinfei Tao

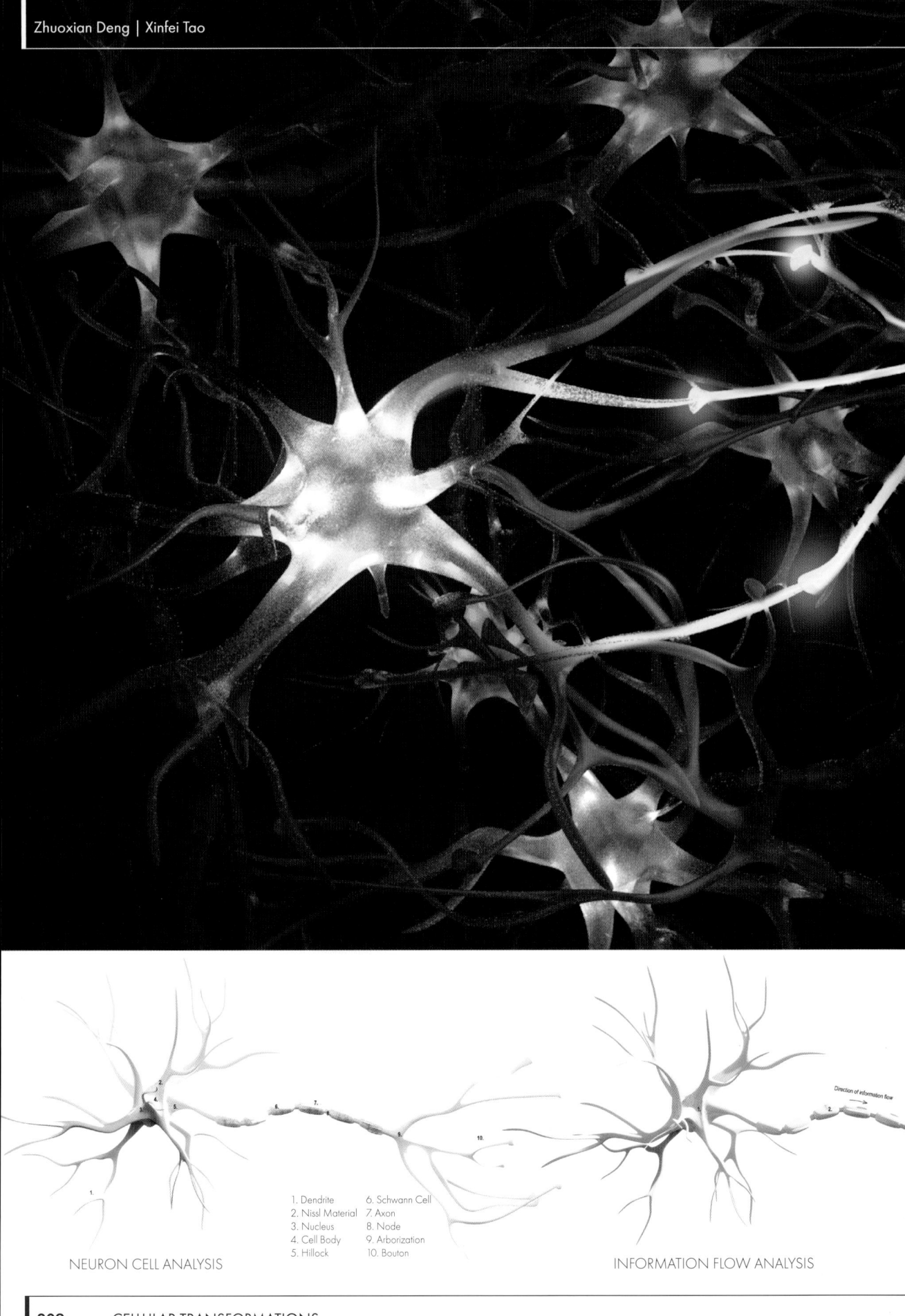

1. Dendrite
2. Nissl Material
3. Nucleus
4. Cell Body
5. Hillock
6. Schwann Cell
7. Axon
8. Node
9. Arborization
10. Bouton

NEURON CELL ANALYSIS

INFORMATION FLOW ANALYSIS

Zhuoxian Deng | Xinfei Tao

INFORMATION FLOW IN THE CENTRAL NERVOUS SYSTEM

A study of how information is transferred from one neuron to another in the mammalian central nervous system. This study includes examination of the shape and interactions between neurons and how their connectivity leads to networks. Here, the dynamic pattern of information flow in neural networks is rendered.

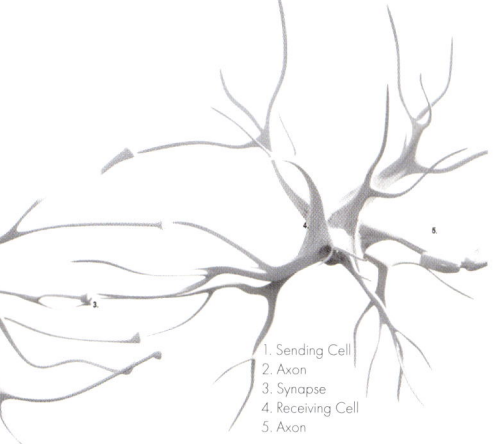

1. Sending Cell
2. Axon
3. Synapse
4. Receiving Cell
5. Axon

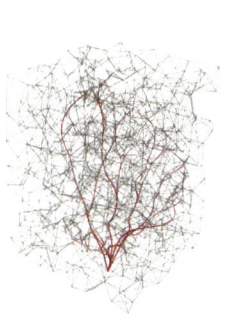 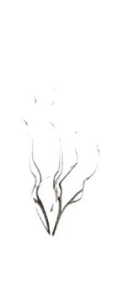 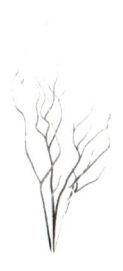 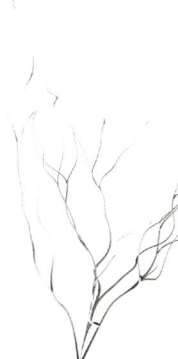

MAPPING NEURON CONNECTION PATH

ADVANCED CELL ANALYSIS 04

ETHAN CHIANG | ZHENGRAN XU

PEZIZA

Peziza grow on decaying wood and organic matter and reproduce by producing ascospores. This rendering mainly shows the fungus' spore containers (asci) each with eight ascospores. The background is part of peziza structure including hyphae and mating type. As the spores mature, fluid builds up behind them; when the pressure gets too much, the tops of the asci open and the spores are flung out into the air.

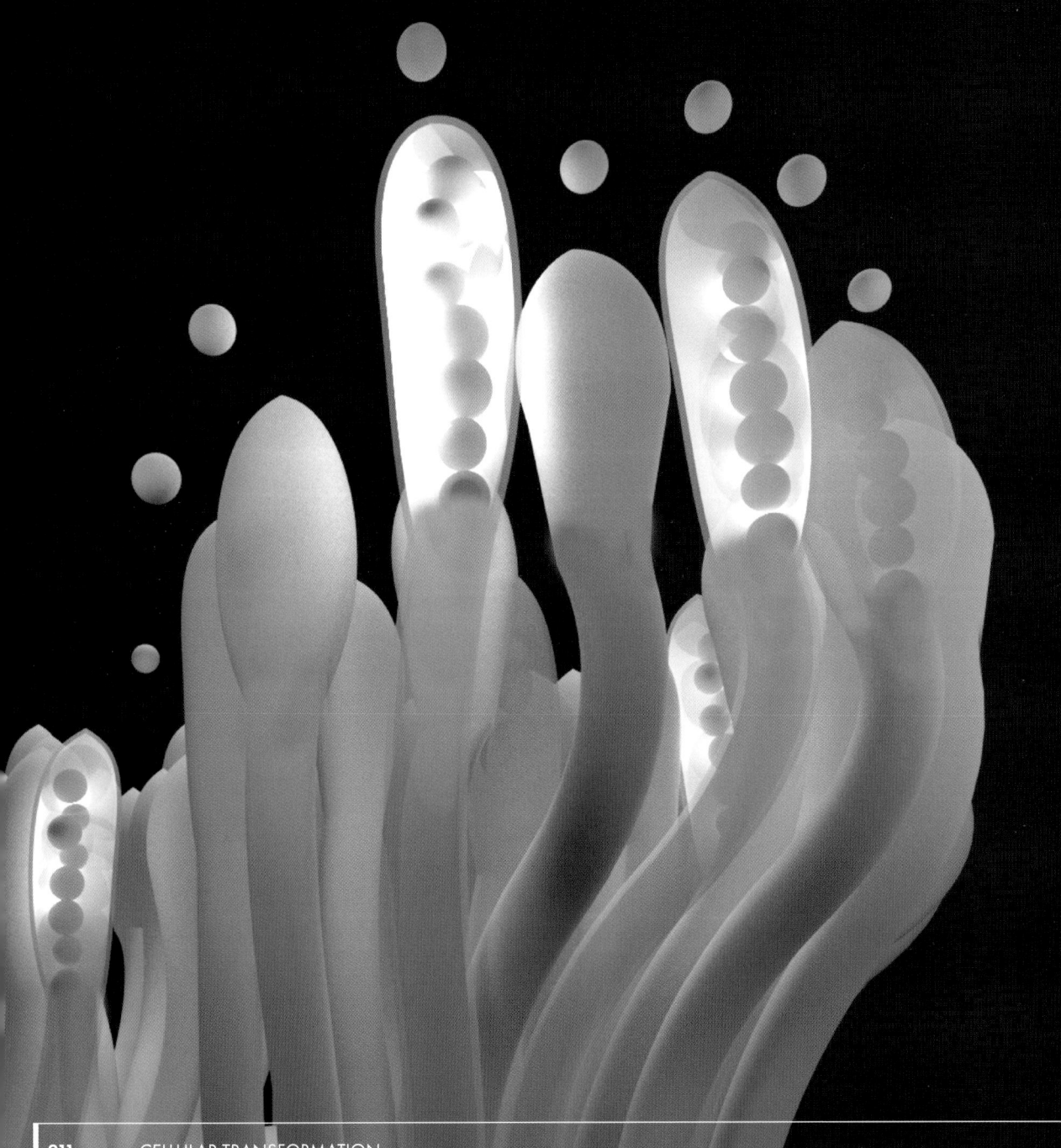

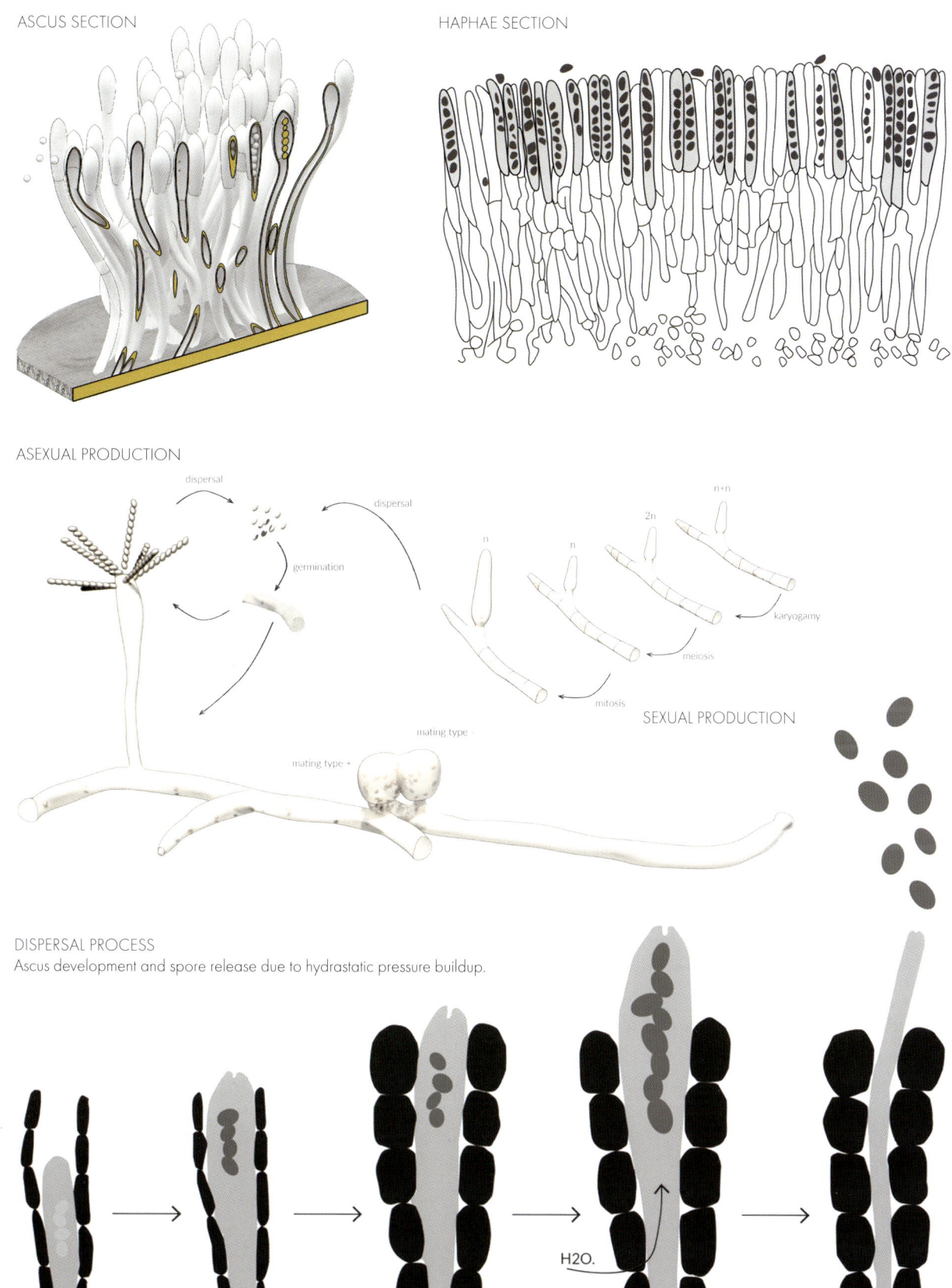

PATRICK MURRAY | YUHAO JI | GUANYU KE

REGENERATION PROPERTIES OF THE HYDRA

The hydra goes through an asexual reproduction process of budding under ideal circumstances. In regeneration, broken hydra tissue can regenerate into a new hydra by reorganizing itself and designating a new mouth area. In addition, hydra cells use pheromones to communicate with each other and know their location in the cell sequence system and transform accordingly through the process known as pheromone transmission.

REGENERATION

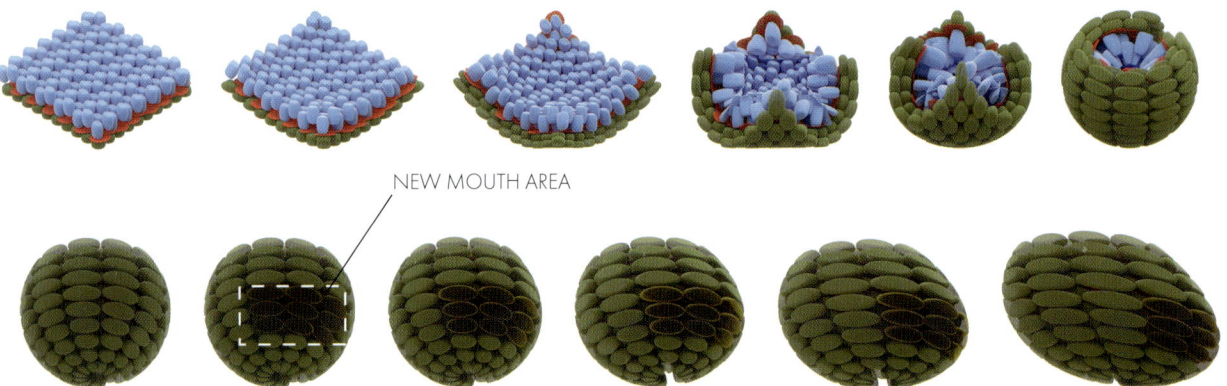

Elongation directed by concentration gradient of hormones secreted by new mouth core (dark green)

PHEROMONE TRANSMISSION

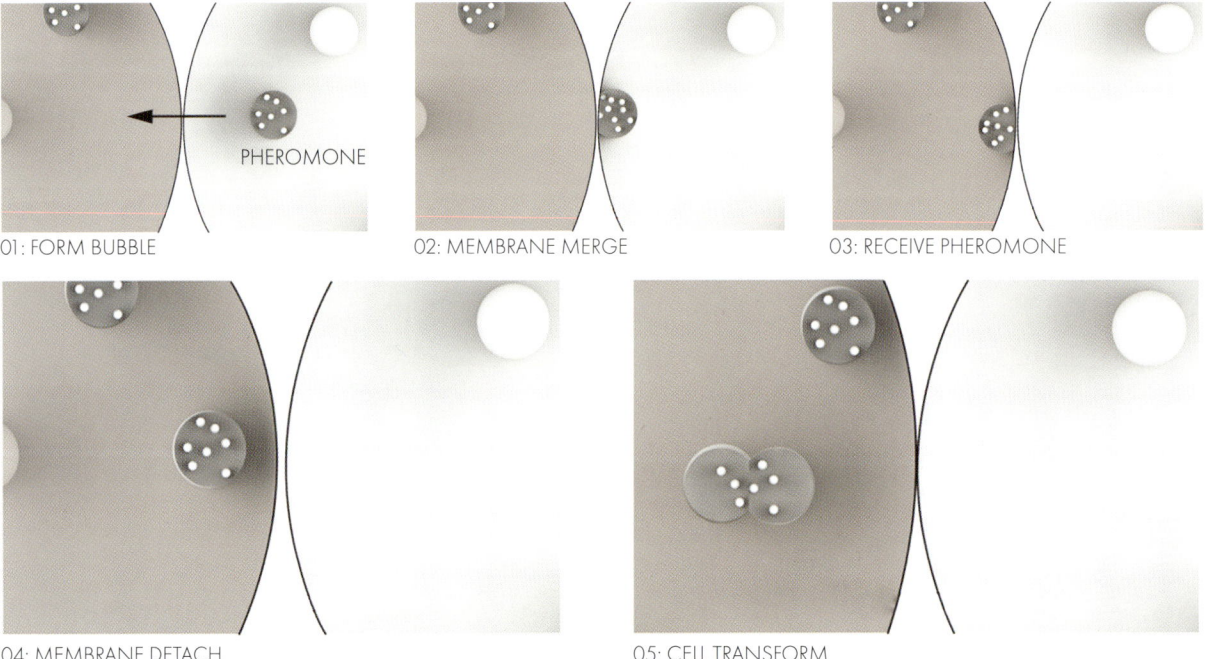

01: FORM BUBBLE   02: MEMBRANE MERGE   03: RECEIVE PHEROMONE

04: MEMBRANE DETACH   05: CELL TRANSFORM

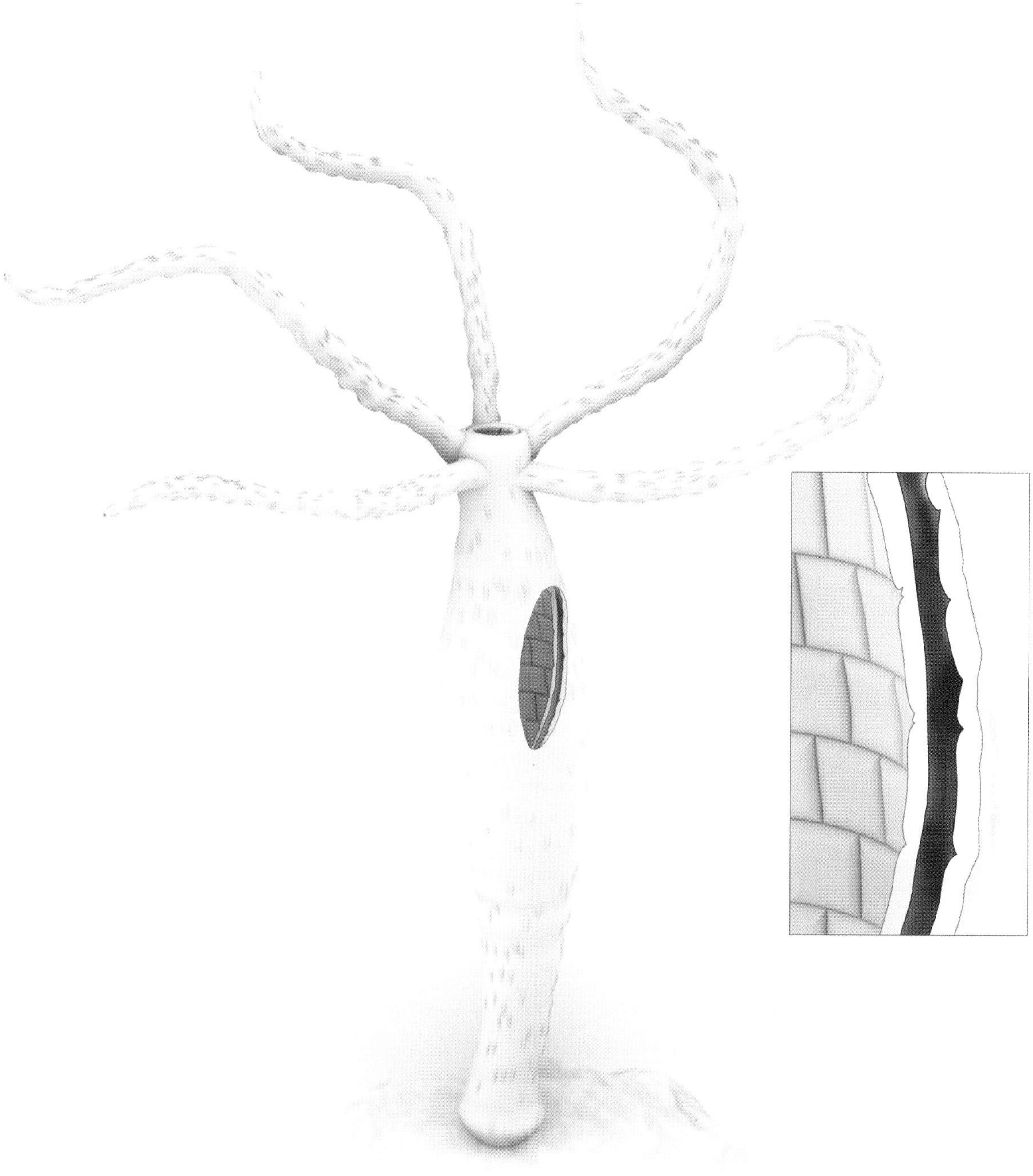

PATRICK MURRAY | YUHAO JI | GUANYU KE

REPRODUCTION

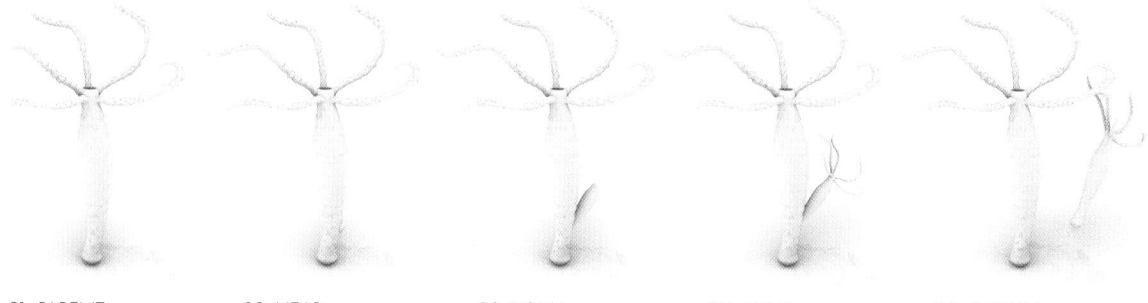

01: PARENT   02: HEAD   03: BODY   04: ARMS   05: DETACH

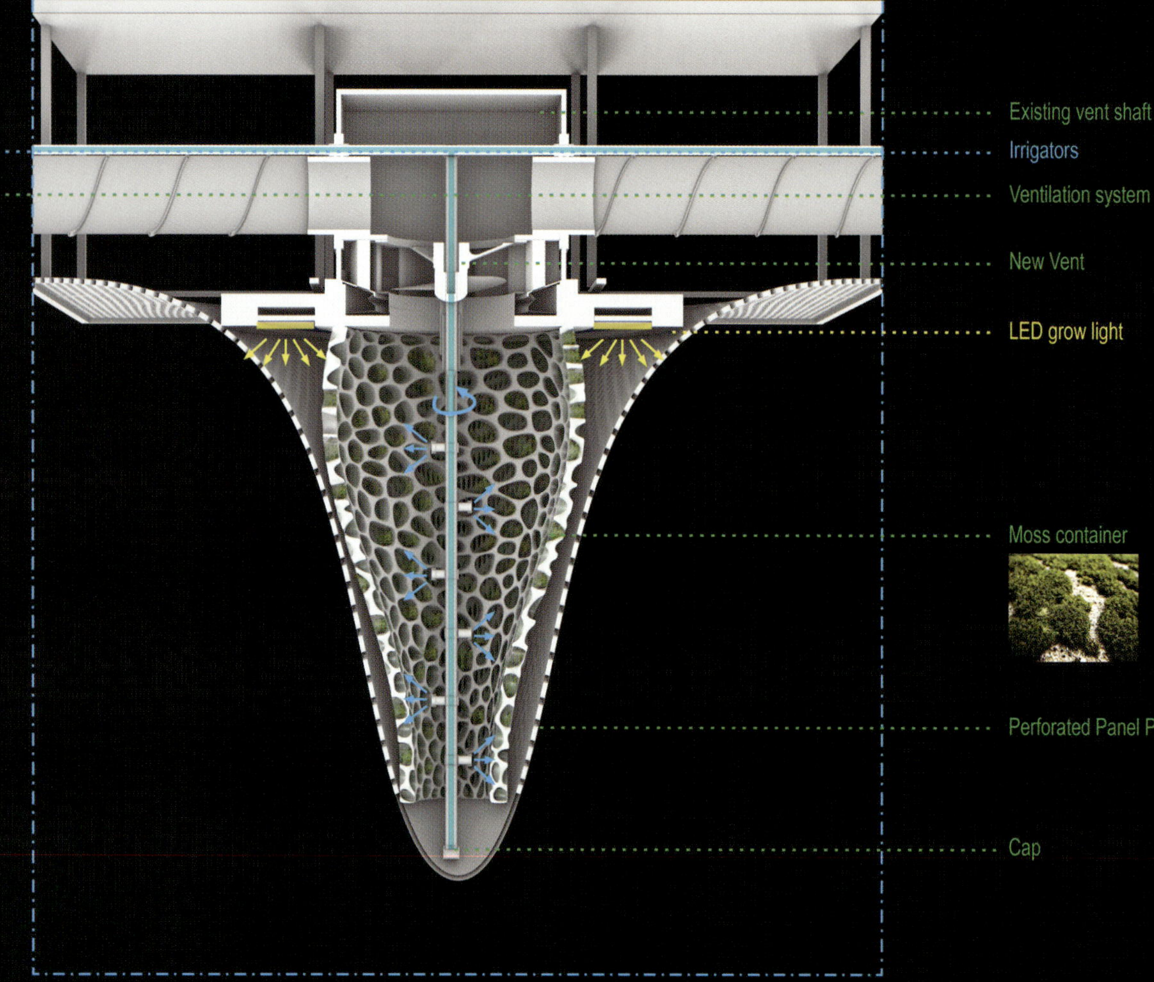

- Existing vent shaft
- Irrigators
- Ventilation system
- New Vent
- LED grow light
- Moss container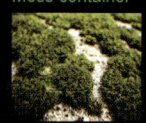
- Perforated Panel P
- Cap

CELLULAR TRANSFORMATIONS

PANDEMIC: 2020
SAFEGUARDS AGAINST COVID-19 RESEARCH

The COVID-19 pandemic has already taken the lives of over 3 million people around the world since early 2020. This virus has altered the social behaviors and interactions of communities all over the world. These projects are attempting to filter air through engineered biological materials with design solutions that enhances the experience of going to restaurants, movie theaters and hospitals. The goal of these projects is to bring back a sense of normalcy in our social and cultural lives and at the same time offer innovative design resolutions that brings technology and biology to the forefront in our daily lives.

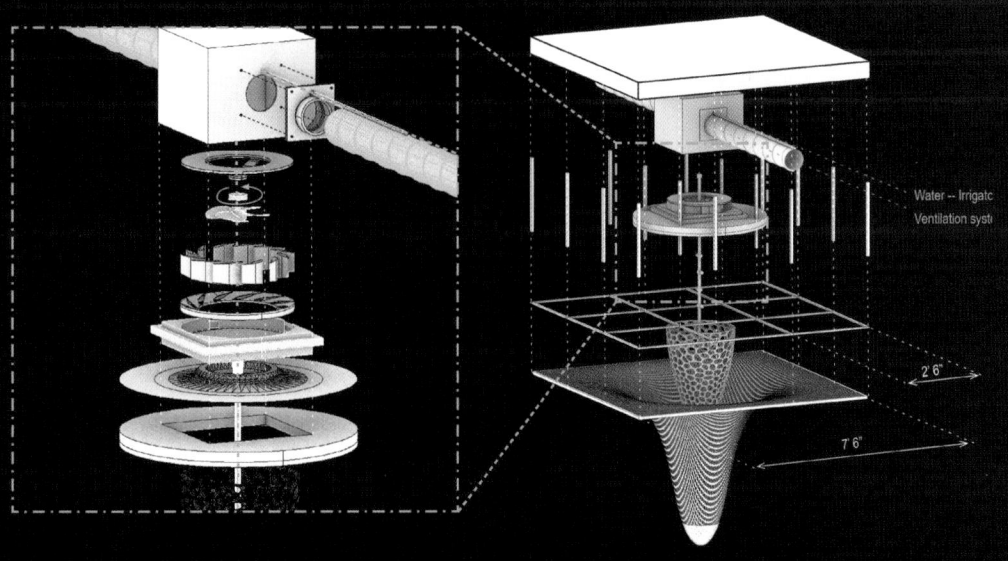

RECLAIMING RESTAURANTS

Throughout the COVID-19 pandemic, the food service industry suffered losses that included the closing of many small restaurants and a significant decline in income for hourly food service workers. While this intervention project does not provide a return to complete normalcy, it would allow restaurants to operate more safely for dine-in business by trapping and containing air-borne pathogens. Introducing a sensor operated panel system between tables creates a separation between parties while still permitting flow throughout the restaurant. With the use of Fuligo septica, a slime mold that feeds on organic material, as well as an improved ventilation system, the intervention also cleans the air as it moves through the space in addition to serving as a safety wall between groups. The properties of Fuligo septica that include rapid growth in response to a food source and an adhesive static charge make it an ideal addition within the intervention to filter and clean the air in the restaurant.

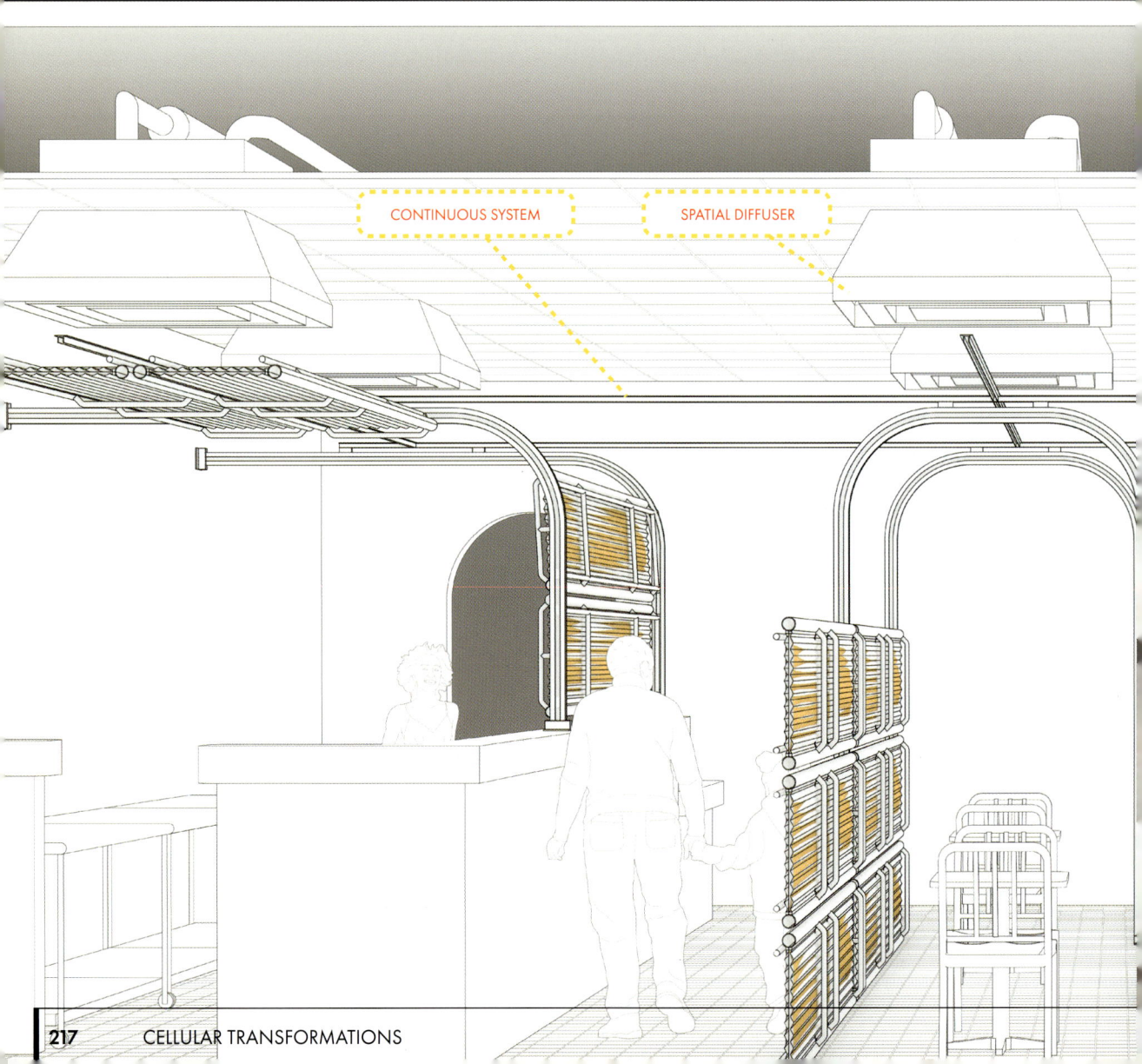

PATRICK MURRAY | YUHAO JI | GUANYU KE

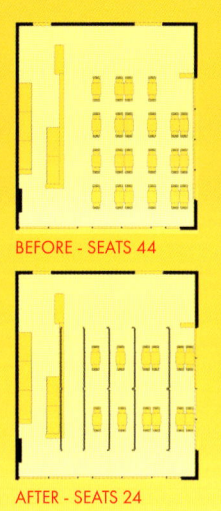

BEFORE - SEATS 44

AFTER - SEATS 24

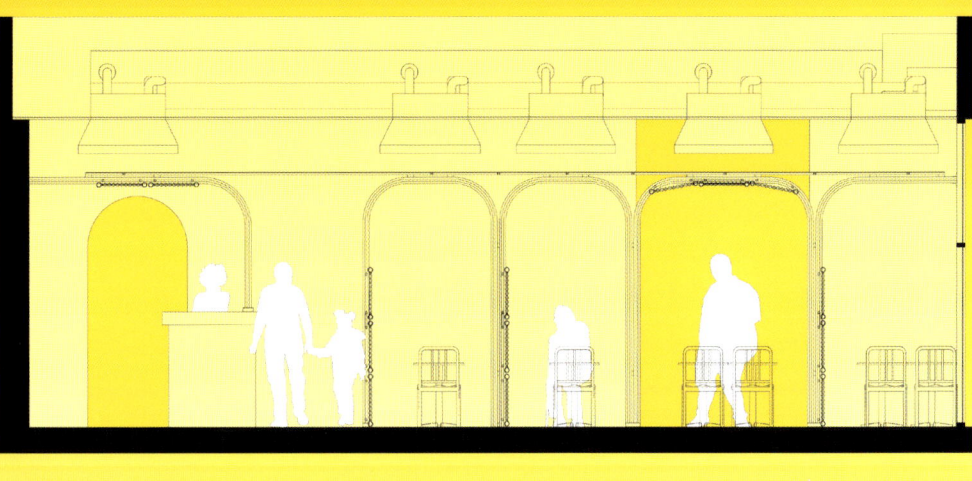

SECTION THROUGH SYSTEM

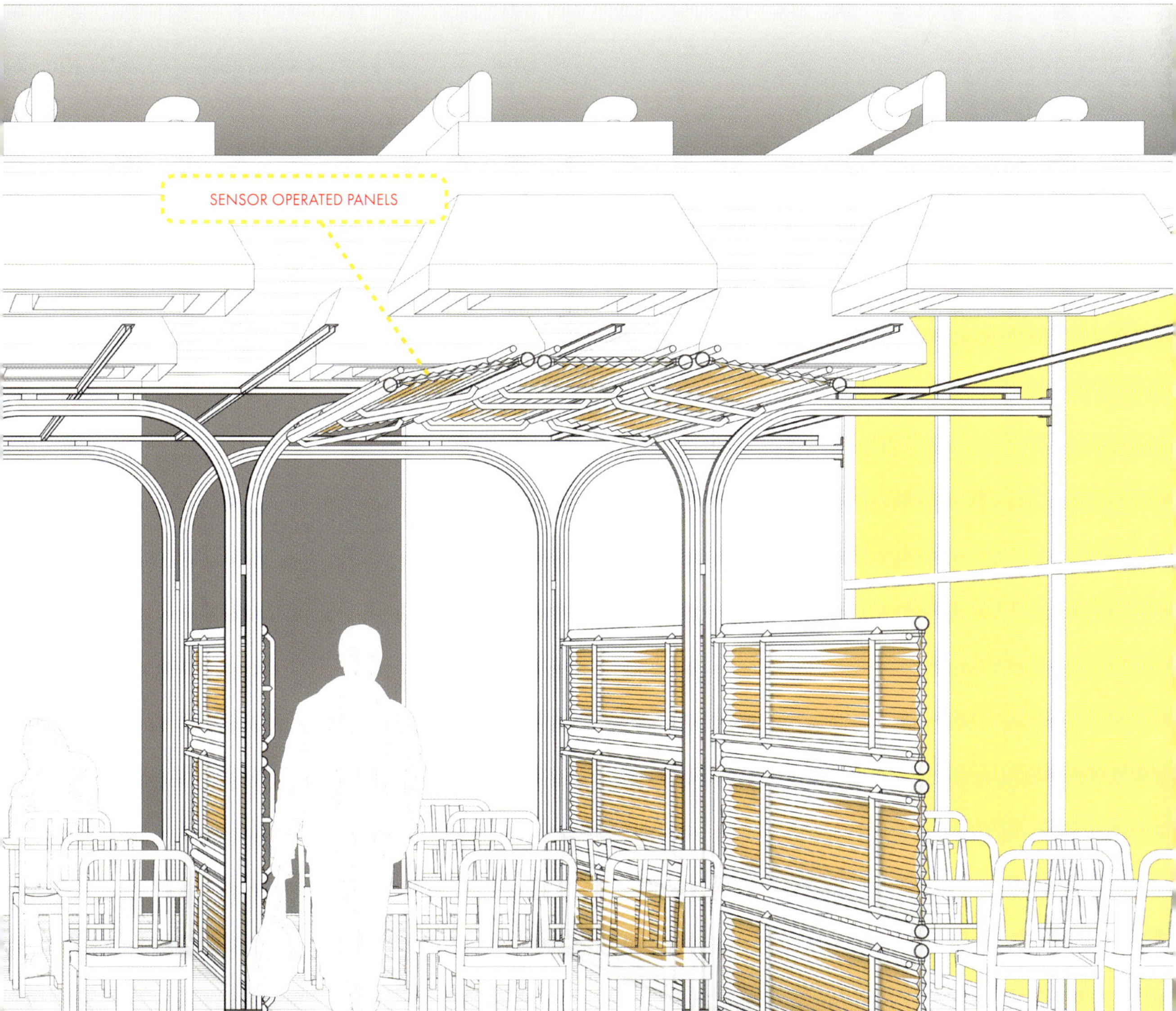

SENSOR OPERATED PANELS

SAFEGUARDS AGAINST COVID-19 RESEARCH

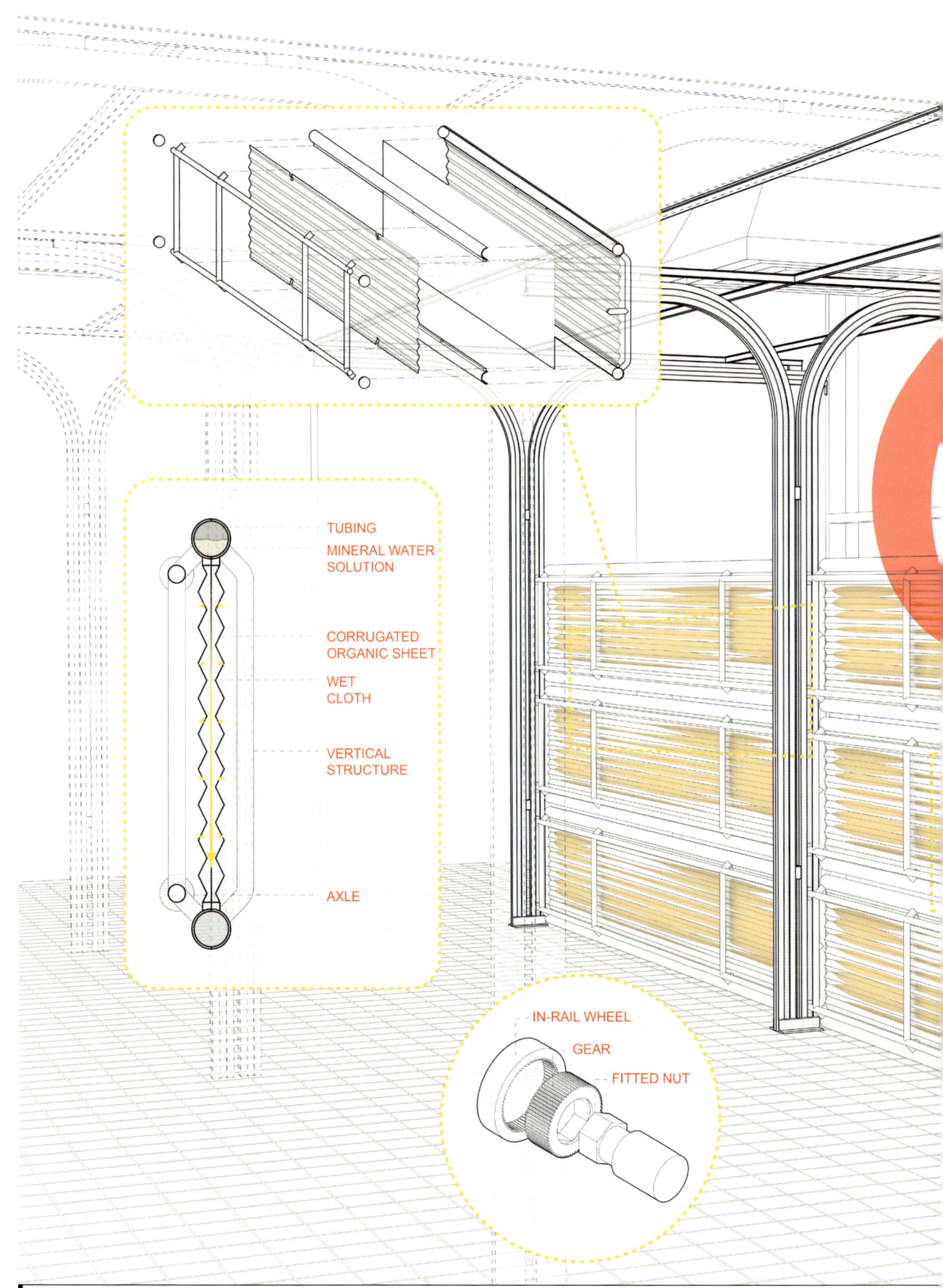

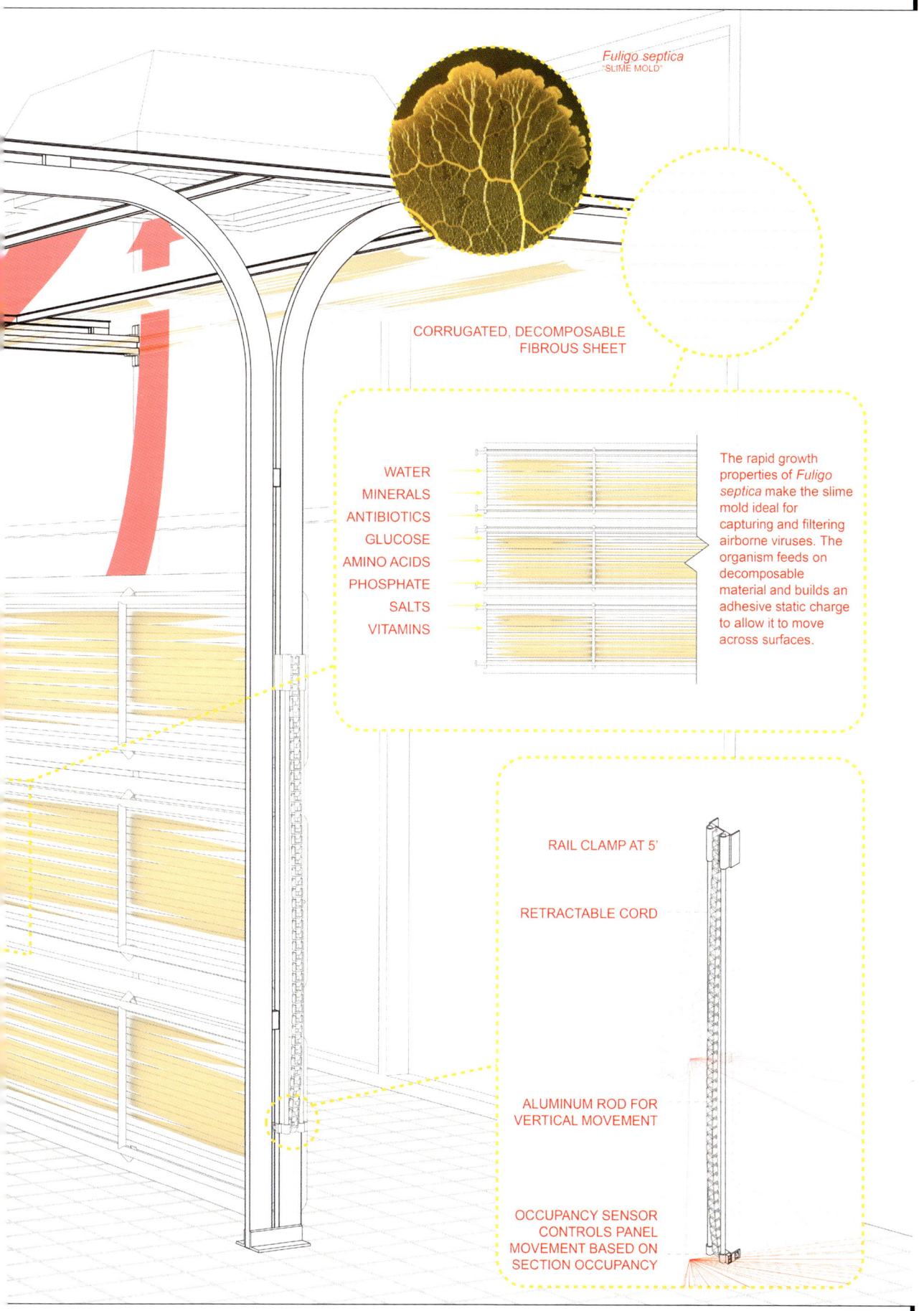

ZHUOXIAN DENG | XINFEI TAO

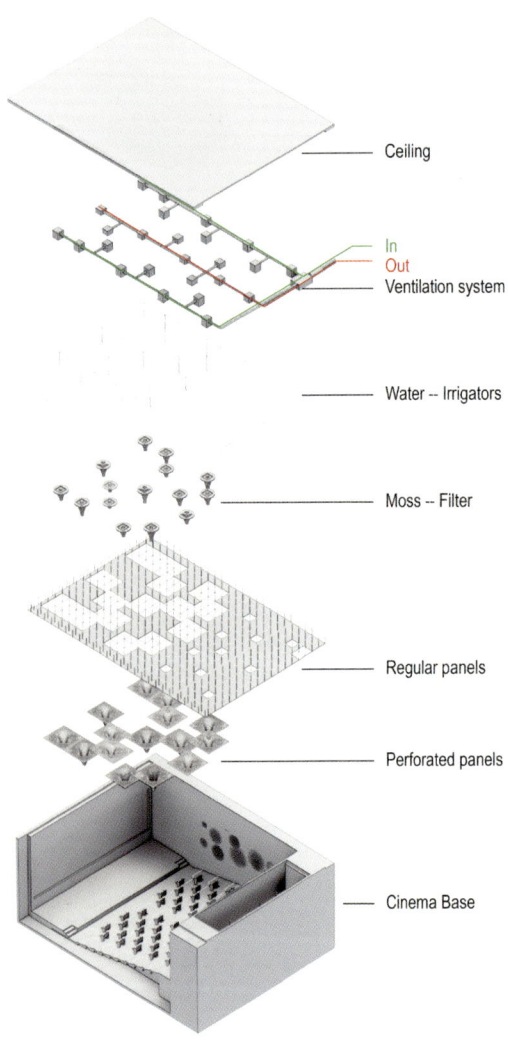

- Ceiling
- In / Out — Ventilation system
- Water -- Irrigators
- Moss -- Filter
- Regular panels
- Perforated panels
- Cinema Base

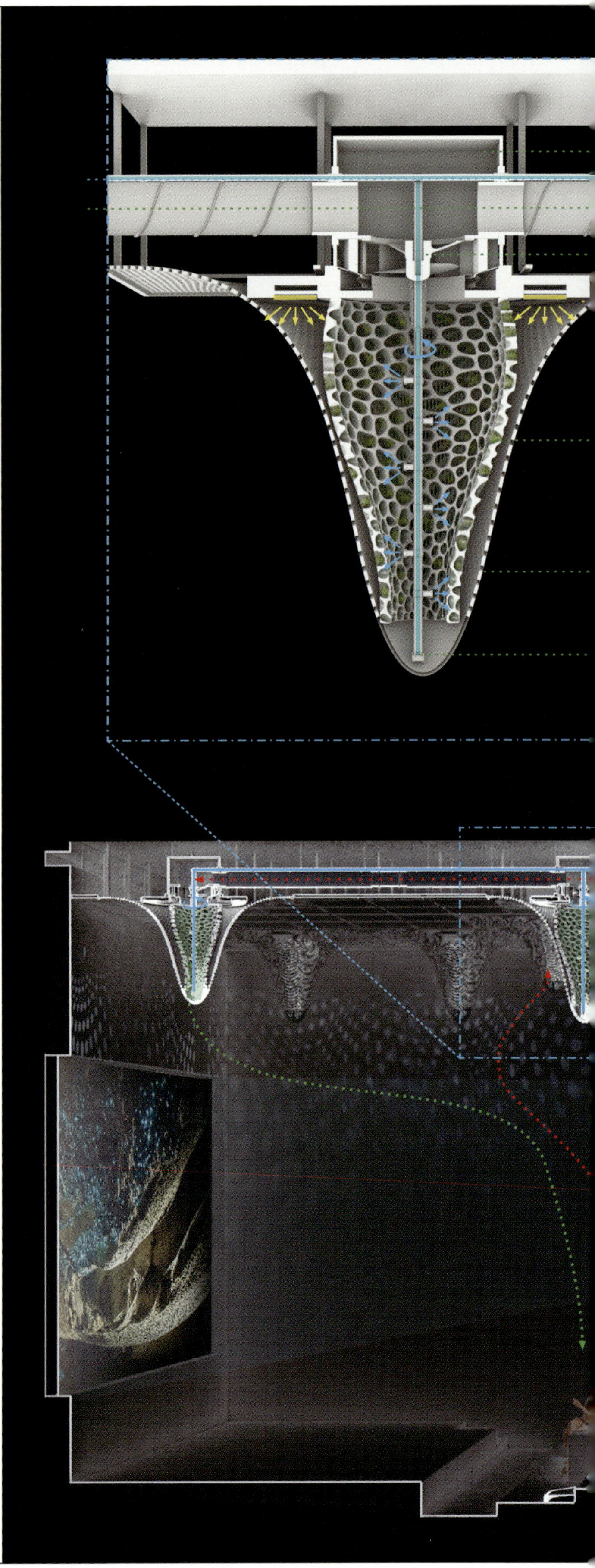

BREATH OF NATURE

The goal of this project is to retrofit a cinema theatre to filter air and provide natural lighting in response to the pandemic. Seats are placed six feet apart to provide safe distance between patrons. A new ventilation system is designed that attaches to the existing vent framework and combines biology with architecture to filter the air using living moss tissue. Lighting is provided by luminous bacteria, Vibrio fischeri, in floor tracks and luminous moss, Schistostega pennata, growing on the wall.

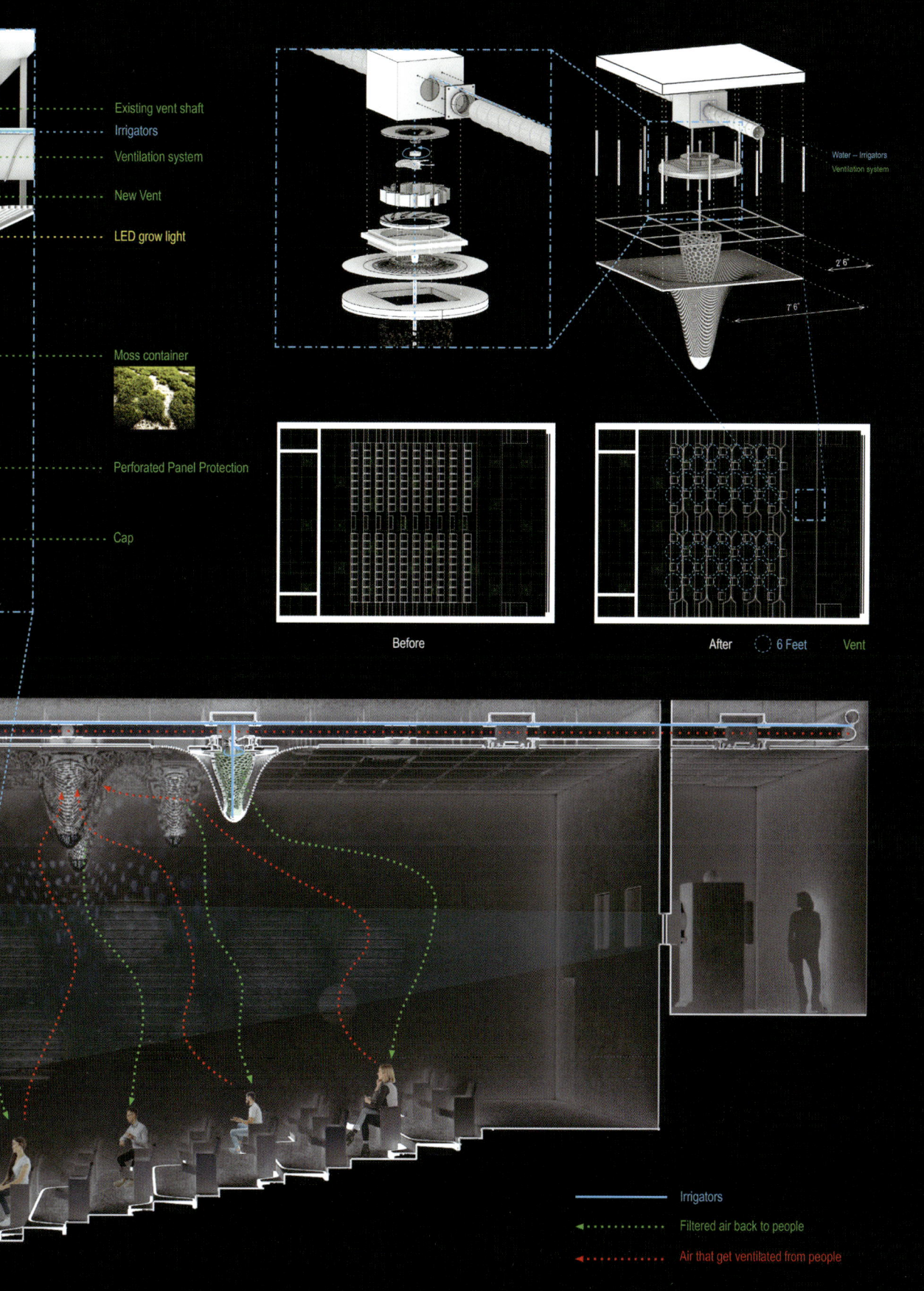

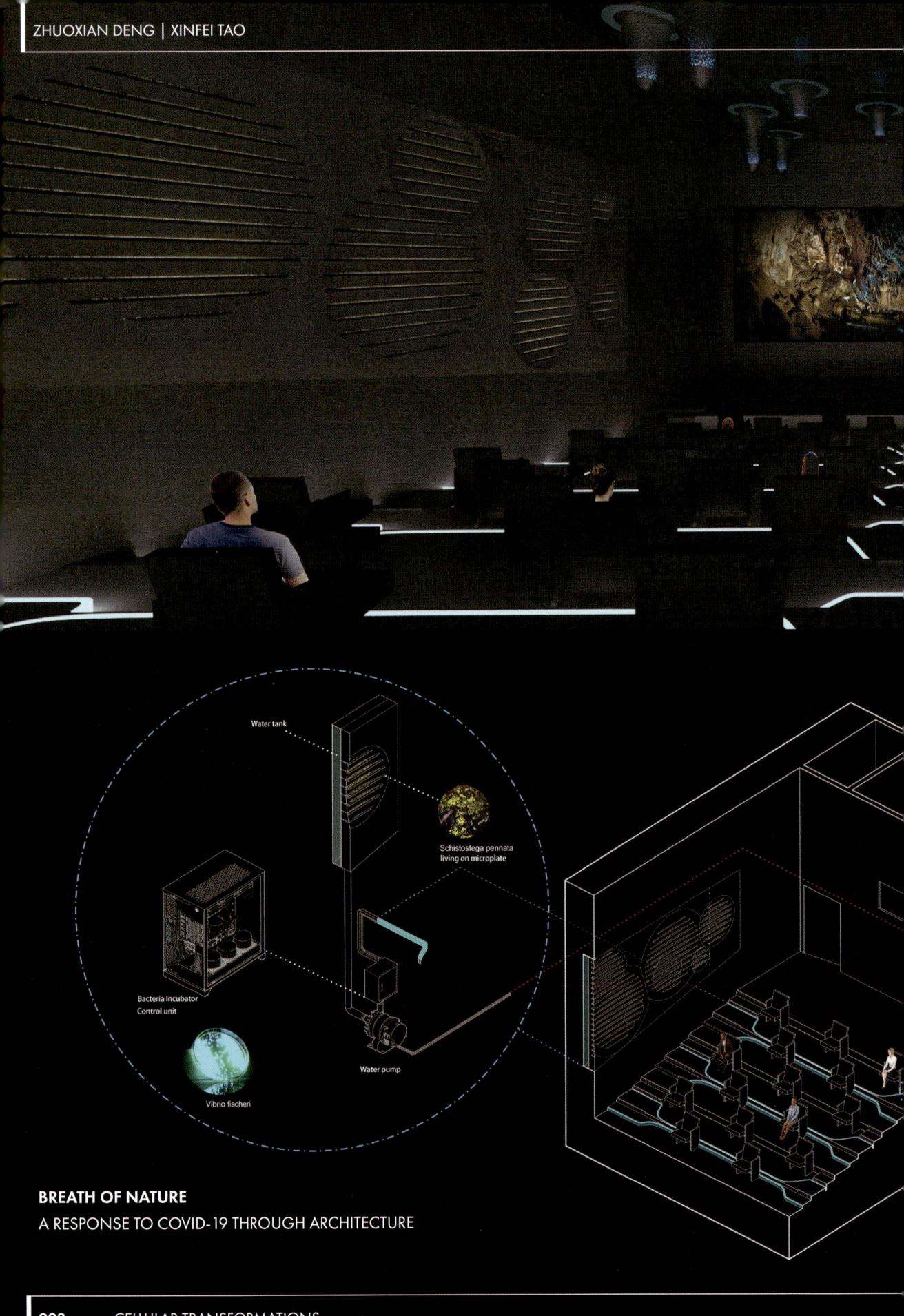

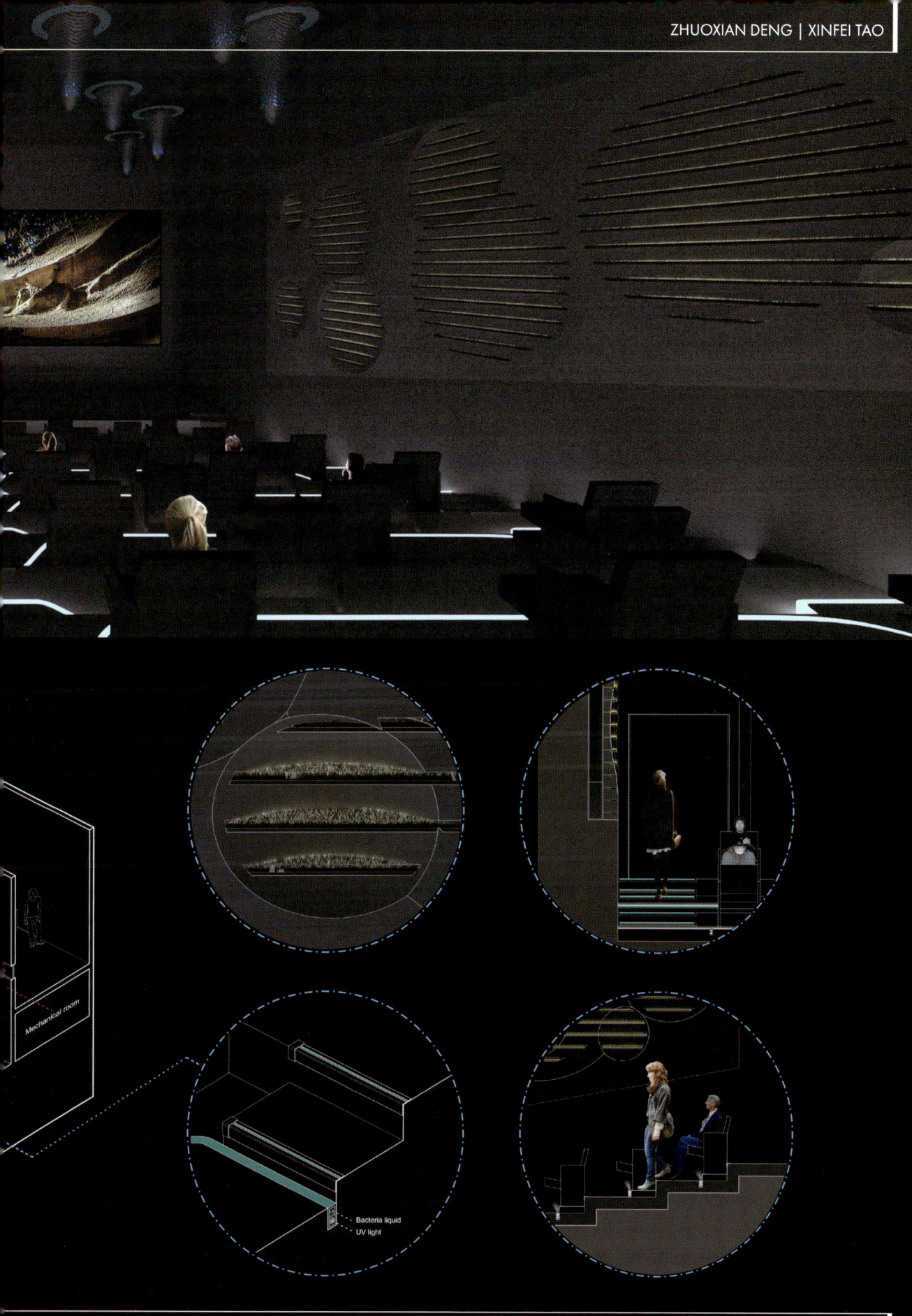

MOBILE HOSPITAL

Mobile Hospital is an emergency field medical facility to treat patients infected with COVID-19 to solve the problem of insufficient number of beds in the hospitals. The prefabricated structure is integrated with plumbing, HVAC, and electrical infrastructures with docking stations for the pod units. Each pod unit holds 2 beds with interior lighting and a ventilation system along with various plants that infuse the air with calming scents for the stressed medical staff. The robotic arm is deployed to transport the pods to the aerial crane helicopter. The bed capsule is cocooned with a protective membrane that separates the medical staff from the infectious patient.

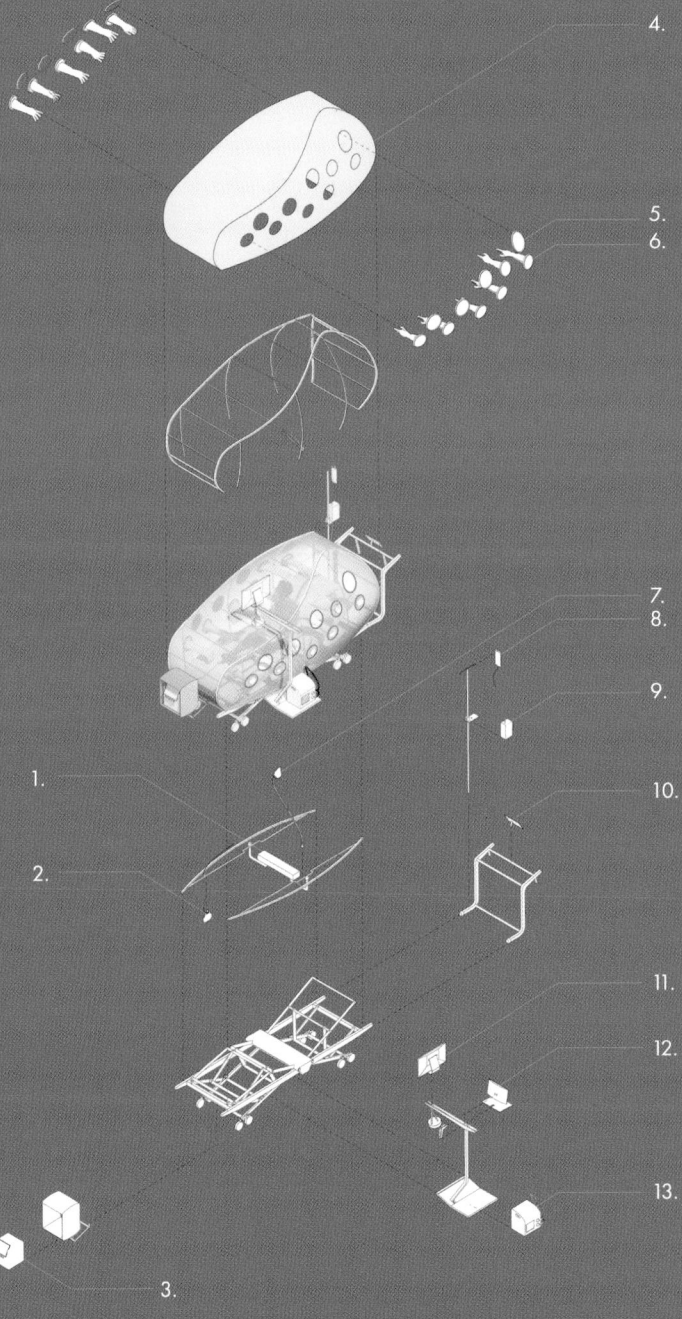

AXONOMETRIC EXPLODED COMPONENT DIAGRAM

ETHAN CHIANG | ZHENGRAN XU

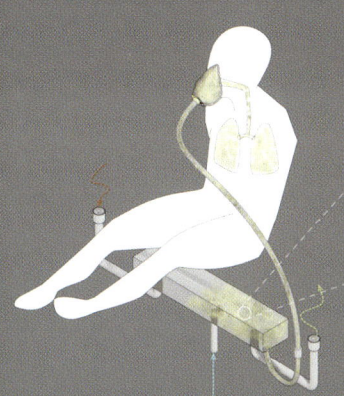

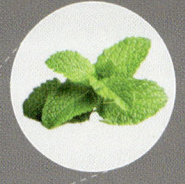

 1. Vaporizer
 2. Catheter
 3. Air Pump
 4. Inflatable Shell

5. Cleatech
6. Oxygen Mask
7. IV Bag
7. IV Pump

9. Control Panel
10. Monitor
11. TV and Table
12. Ventilator

MINT

Use mint leaves for steam therapy. This helps to break down mucus in lungs to improve breathing and provides a pleasant scent that is relaxing.

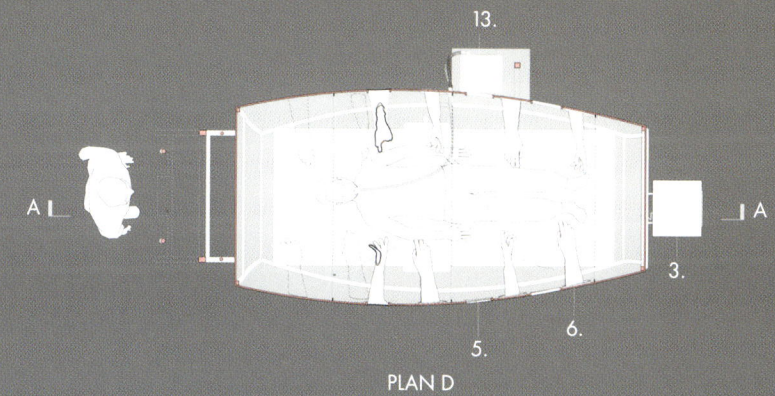

PLAN D

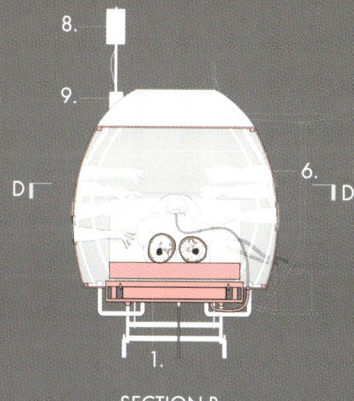

SECTION B

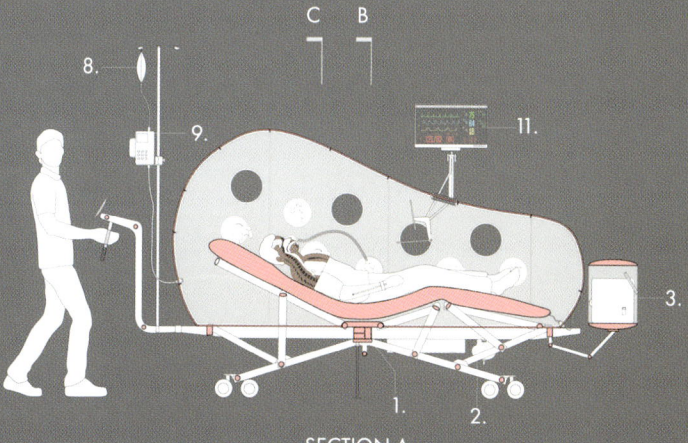

SECTION A

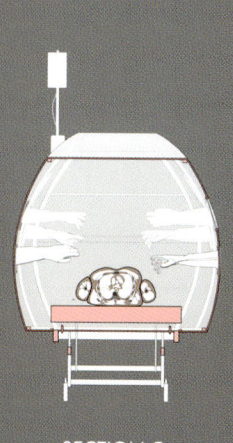

SECTION C

SAFEGUARDS AGAINST COVID-19 RESEARCH

ETHAN CHIANG | ZHENGRAN XU

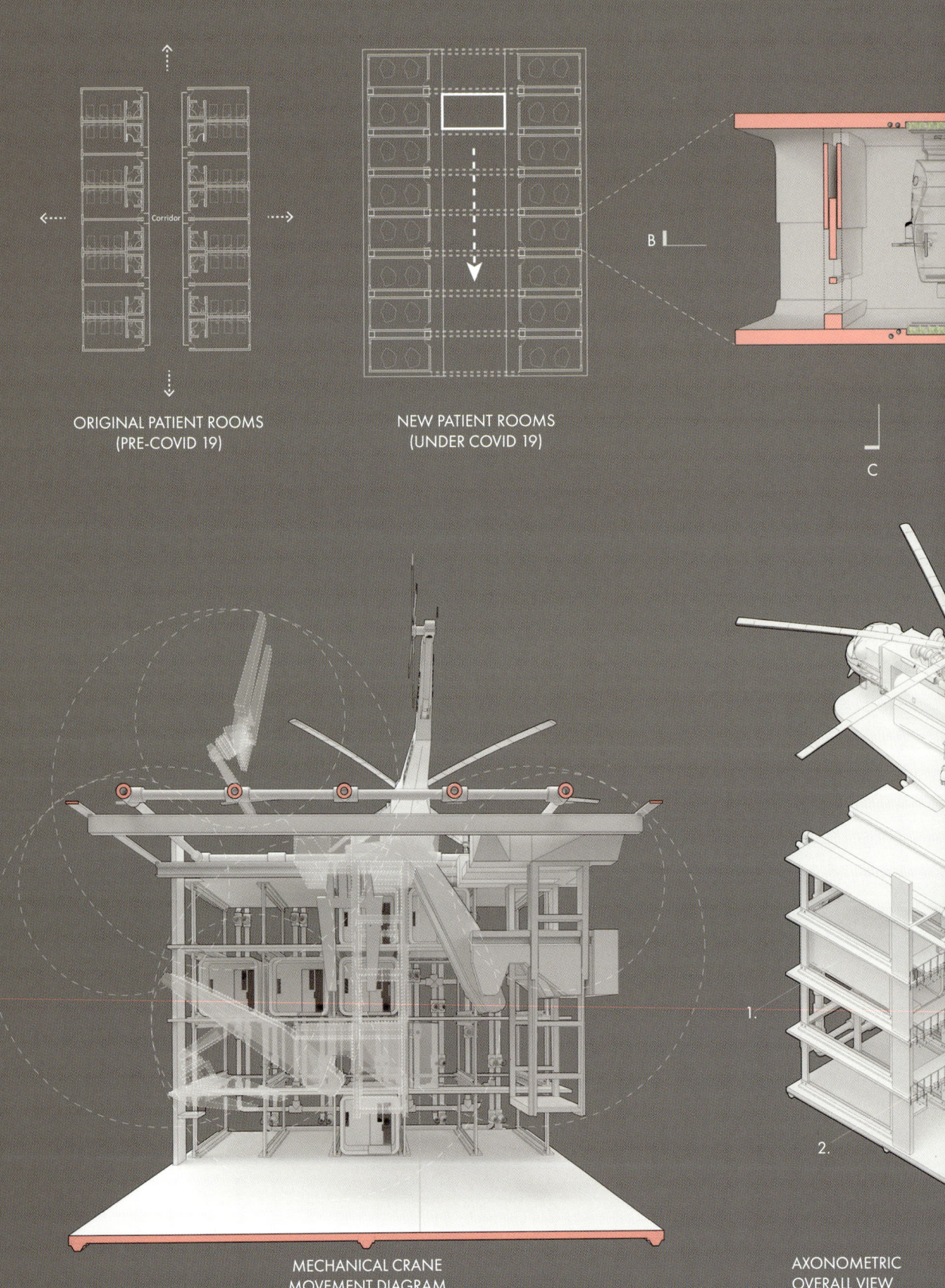

ORIGINAL PATIENT ROOMS
(PRE-COVID 19)

NEW PATIENT ROOMS
(UNDER COVID 19)

MECHANICAL CRANE
MOVEMENT DIAGRAM

AXONOMETRIC
OVERALL VIEW

ETHAN CHIANG | ZHENGRAN XU

UNIT PLAN A

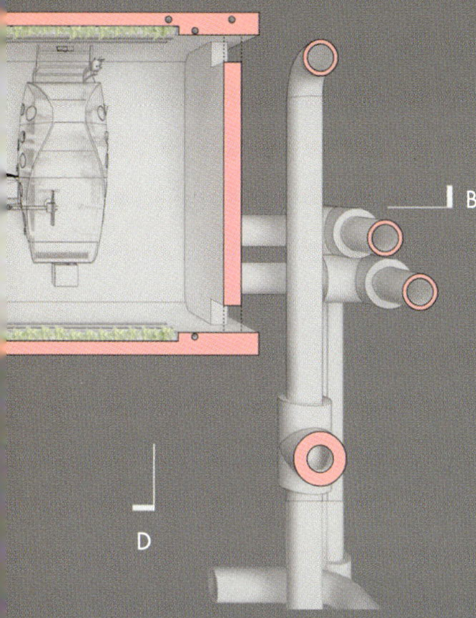

UNIT SECTION A

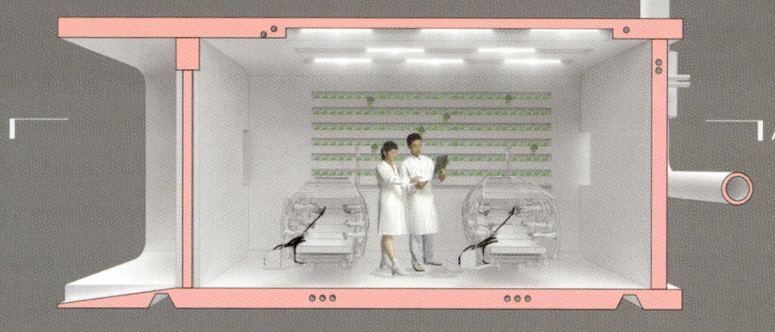

UNIT SECTION C

UNIT SECTION D

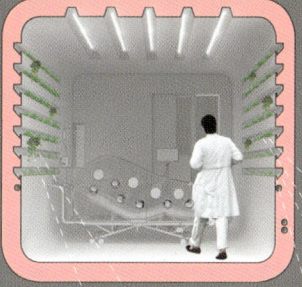
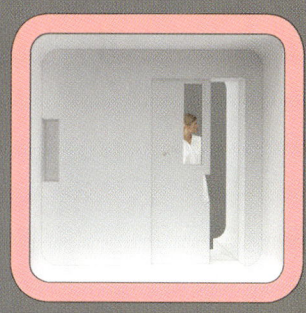

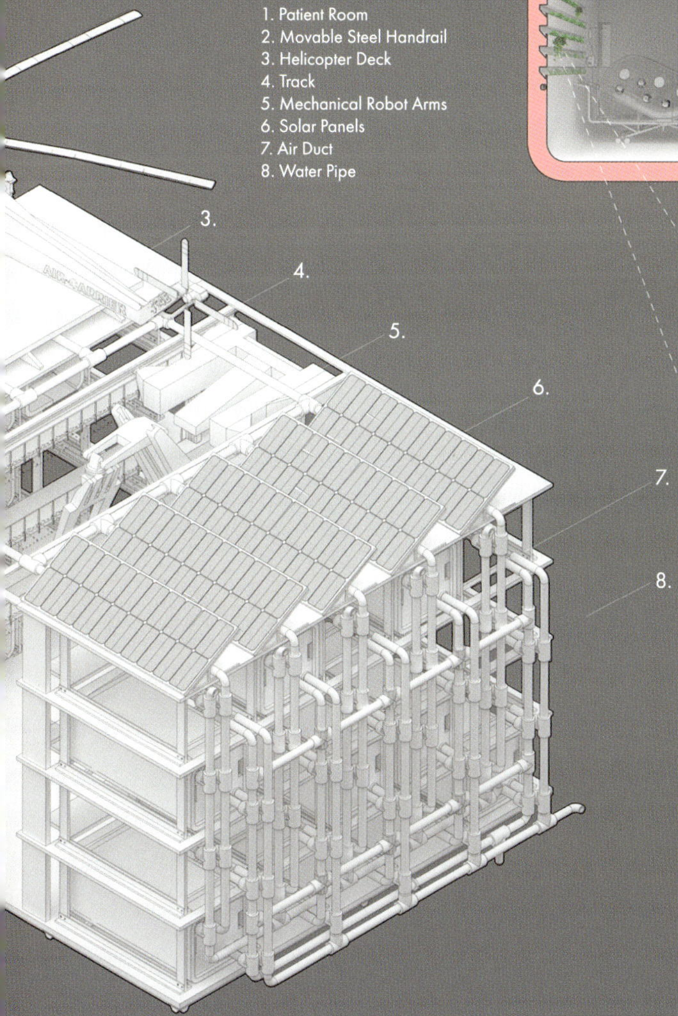

1. Patient Room
2. Movable Steel Handrail
3. Helicopter Deck
4. Track
5. Mechanical Robot Arms
6. Solar Panels
7. Air Duct
8. Water Pipe

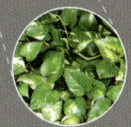
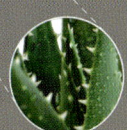

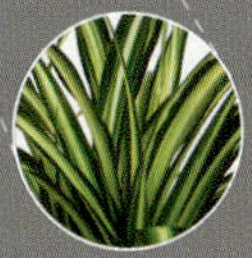

Chlorophytum comosum

Epipremnum aureum

Aloe vera

The NASA Clean Air study found that Chlorophytum comosum (commonly called spider plant) can effectively remove certain household air toxins such as formaldehyde.

This plant (a type of ivy) has been shown to reduce indoor air pollution. The NASA Clean Air study found that it can remove up to 73% of benzene from enclosed environments in a 24-hour period.

Aloe vera is effective at removing harmful volatile organic compounds emitted by a large number of common household products. It can also help reduce microorganisms and dust in the air.

SAFEGUARDS AGAINST COVID-19 RESEARCH

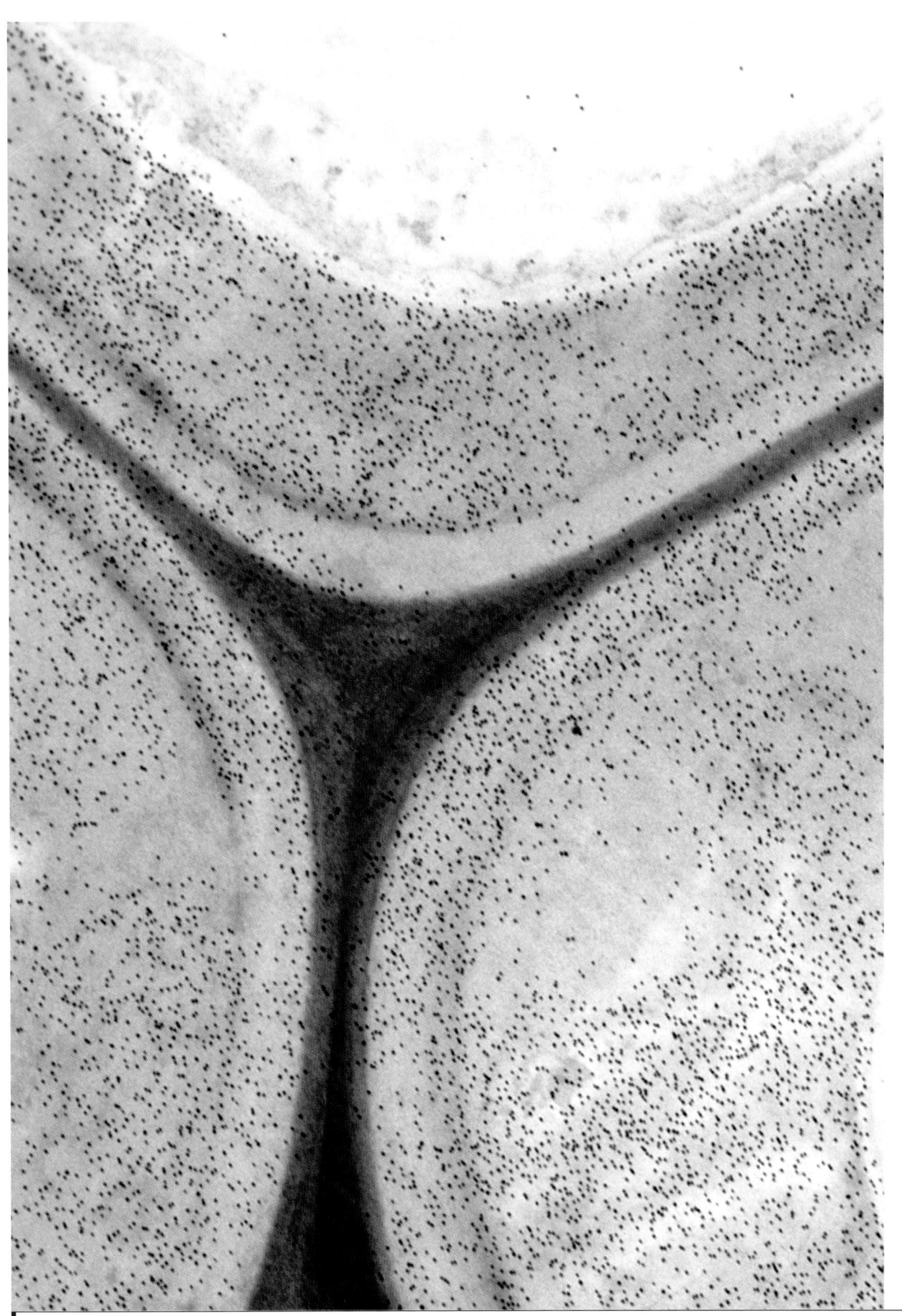

DESIGNING AND STRUCTURING THE INTERDISCIPLINARY
IRIS MEIER

"Perfection is achieved not when there is nothing more to add, but when there is nothing left to take away." This insight by Antoine De Saint-Exupéry cannot necessarily be applied to all great projects of architecture (one must only recall the High Baroque era), but it holds true for much of biological structure. Unlike the human desire to decorate for aesthetic reasons, the selective pressures of evolution have a way of reducing lifeforms to that which is functional. Life does not waste energy, or the respective organism will be poorly adapted and likely not around for long.

With this in mind, I was very curious about the new book by Professors Ram Dixit and Sung Ho Kim, which catalogs and presents in context a multi-year effort to cross-fertilize the fields of architecture and structural biology through college coursework. The class Cellular Transformations has been taught at Washington University for the past 10 years. It brings together architecture and biology majors and challenges them to incorporate principles underlying cellular organization into human-made structures.

Students have to understand and utilize the performance aspects of biological structures for their individual projects that use modern design and making processes including digital media and 3D technologies. The work shows exciting parallels to my own collaboration with Professor of Art Amy Youngs at Ohio State University, where we use coursework to challenge biology and art students to translate an aspect of modern plant biology into artwork accessible to the general public. I can therefore appreciate both the triumphs and the challenges of this type of work.

In the class Cellular Transformations, students actively investigate and apply concepts of biological organization such as self-assembly, dynamics, self-organization, and self-repair. They then develop their own architectural projects through a reflection and transformation process that ultimately leads to new emerging design. The idea is that a multidisciplinary training that integrates science and architecture promotes the conception of new ideas that could be applicable to real-world challenges.

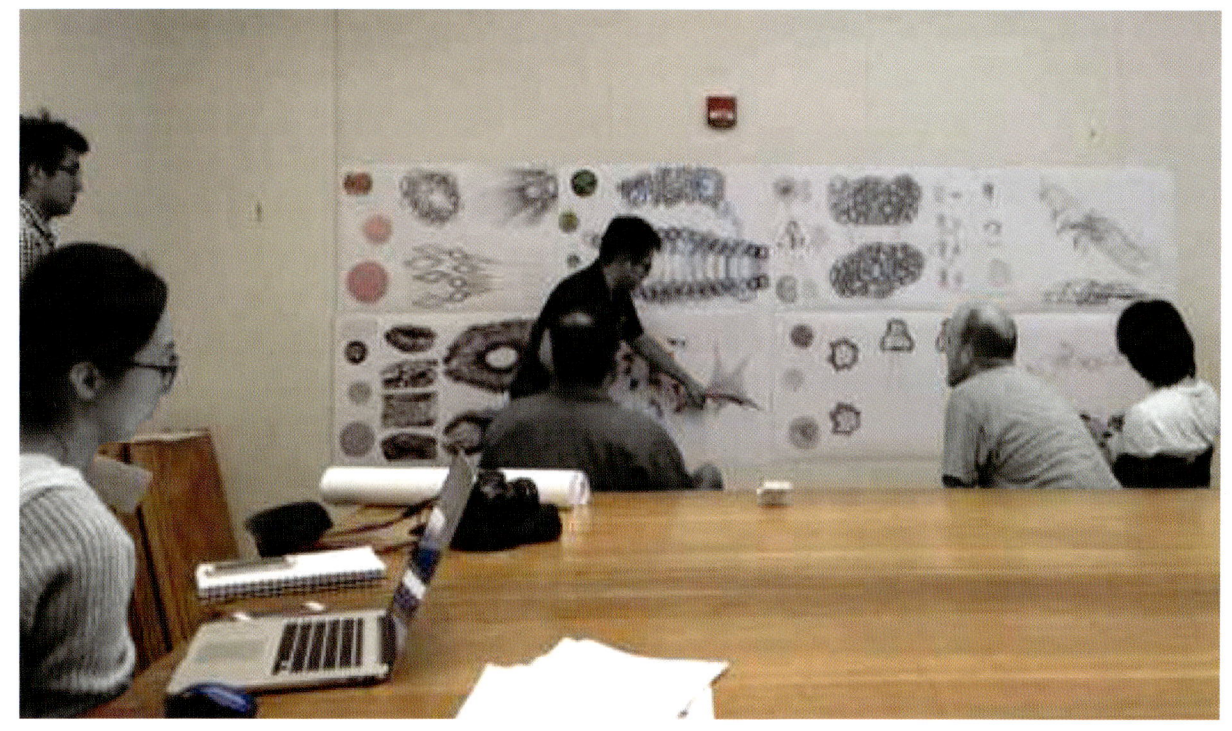

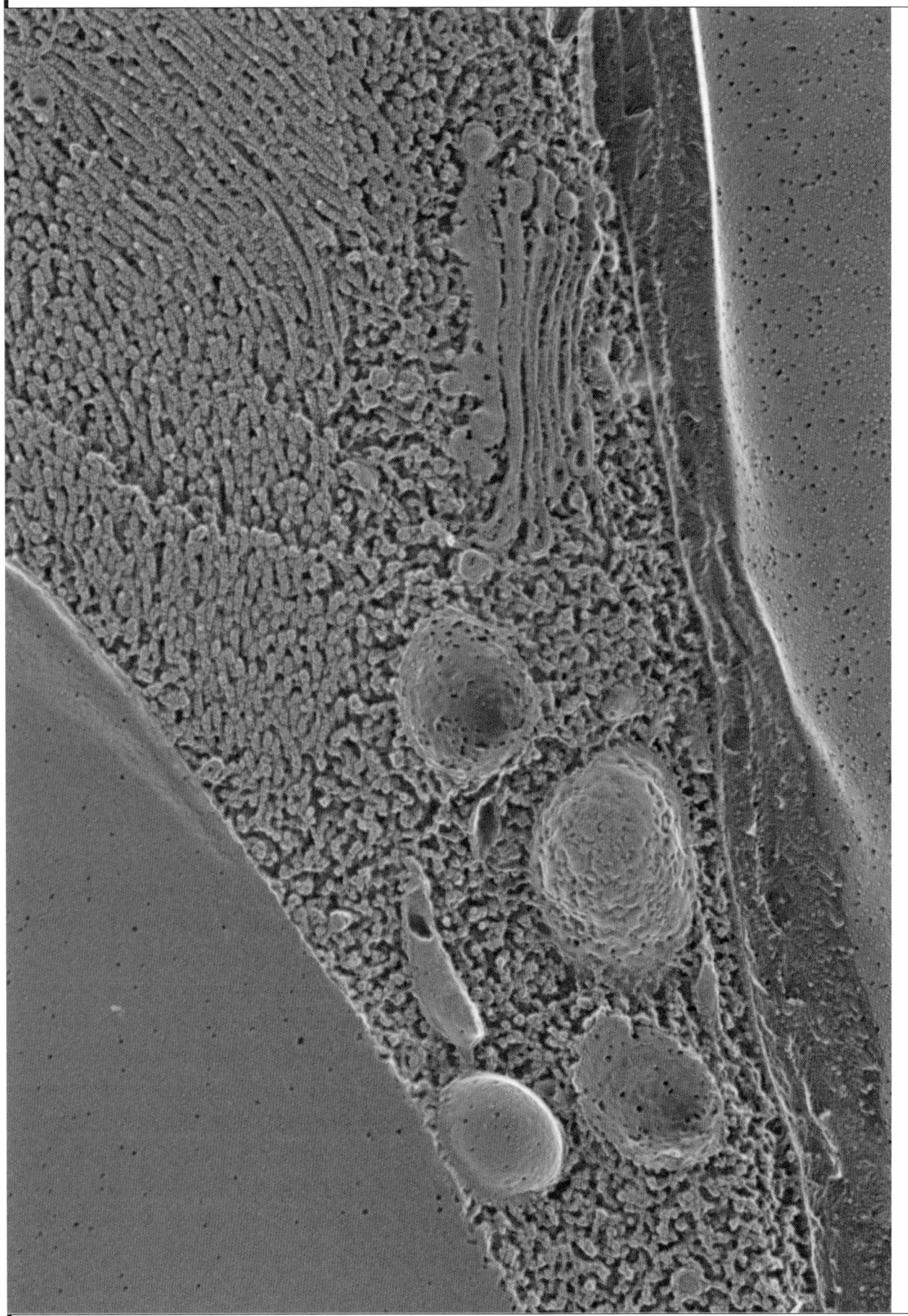

The book first gives an overview of the relevant concepts of structural biology, with several examples drawn from Dr. Dixit's own research work, especially on the microtubule cytoskeleton, one of the cell's "scaffolds". Similarly, skin is then investigated in the context of architectural research. The clear highlight of the book are the student projects. These are organized by year and class taught and thus grouped into the different topics of the respective courses. Throughout, the visuals are stunning and the student work is at a high professional level. There are brief explanatory text sections interspersed, for whole course topics as well as individual student projects. For the latter, I was curious about more, especially as it comes to the motivations and inspirations that drove the individual student projects. Creative work is highly personal, and almost always has an auto-biographic aspect, and to see more of those connections, as expressed by the students, could have added a more personal feeling to the book. However, this too is a question of personal taste and the authors have put together an impressive collection that should inspire and motivate others interested in taking on the challenge of cross-fertilization of science and seemingly unrelated disciplines such as art, architecture, music, poetry, and more.

That there is a need to take on this challenge becomes increasingly apparent. While in the past often driven by the disciplines who wish to engage in a dialogue with science (and sometimes belittled in the science world as quaint pre-retirement projects), science is beginning to learn that this difficult but rewarding communication is by no means a one-way street. In contrast, opening ones viewpoint beyond the familiar – and often beyond the comfortable – lets us, too, discover new questions and thus new scientific ideas. To introduce undergraduate students to it means to operate at exactly the right level, that of the scientist, artist, or architect of tomorrow. A recent feature article in the scientific flagship journal, Nature, about the effect of art-science collaborations on careers highlights its emerging relevance to the scientific community (*Nature* 590, 515-518 (2021)).

In summary, the book is a well-conceived and carefully executed documentation of one of these still-too-rare initiatives and should be a motivational and valuable resource for others with similar activities in mind. De Saint-Exupéry should not have found anything left to take away.

Iris Meier 02.22.2021

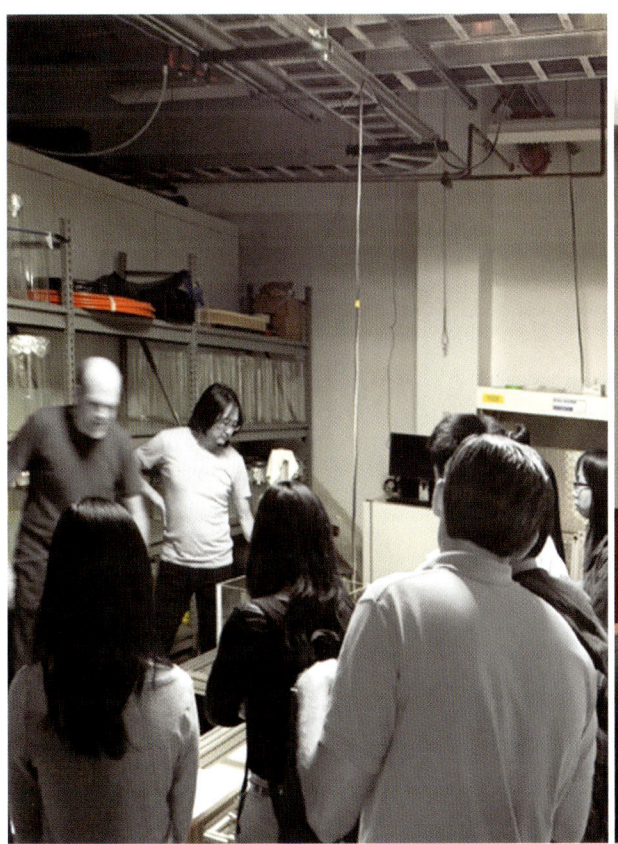
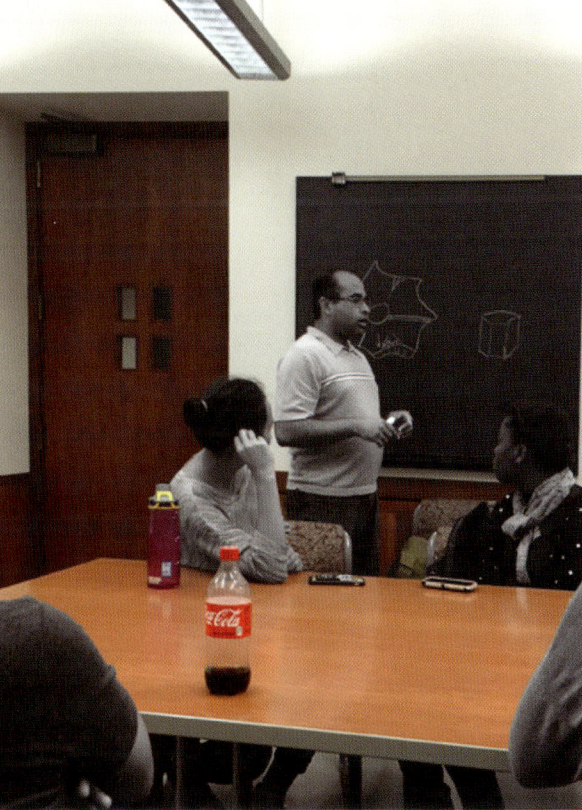

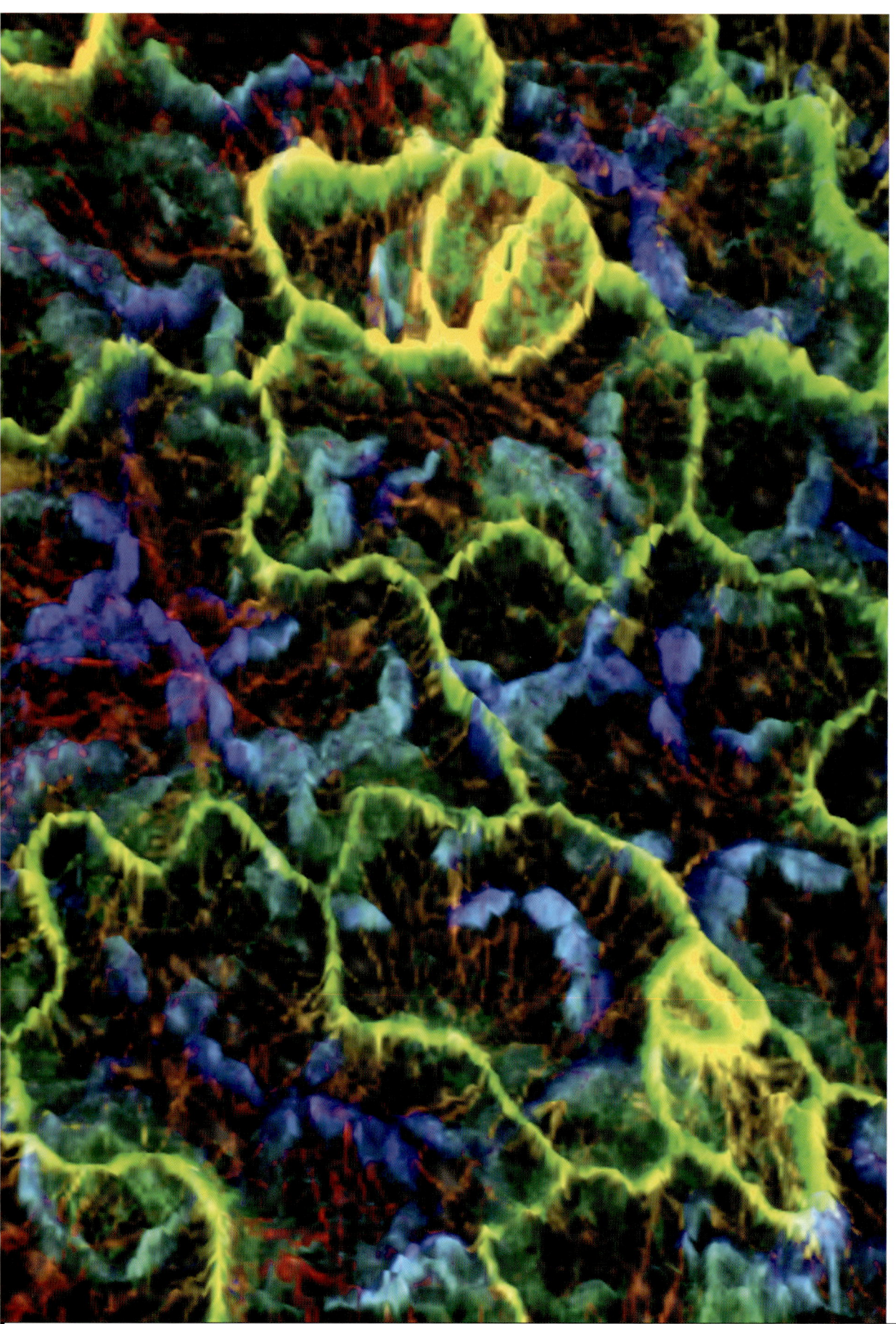

SIMON GILROY
BUILDING NEW PERSPECTIVES

Cellular Transformations looks to fill a key gap for students, researchers and designers alike offering as it does the reader with a new vantage point from the intersection of cell biology, architecture and design. One of my favorite moments in teaching introductory cell biology is starting to describe the cellular process of the biochemistry of energy production by the mitochondrial ATP synthase in terms of a miniature machine with its rods, wheels and gears. The students can begin to visualize cellular processes in these physical terms and suddenly the

Suddenly the events being discussed have moved from the world of the abstract to the relatable, visualized now in the physical terms we all understand and appreciate. Conversely, evolution has already elegantly solved design problems that we struggle with as humans and often in exquisitely beautiful ways. Biology can build the majestic, 100 meter tall tower of a giant redwood tree with self-assembling building blocks that operate at cellular scales at least a million fold smaller than the final titan they create.

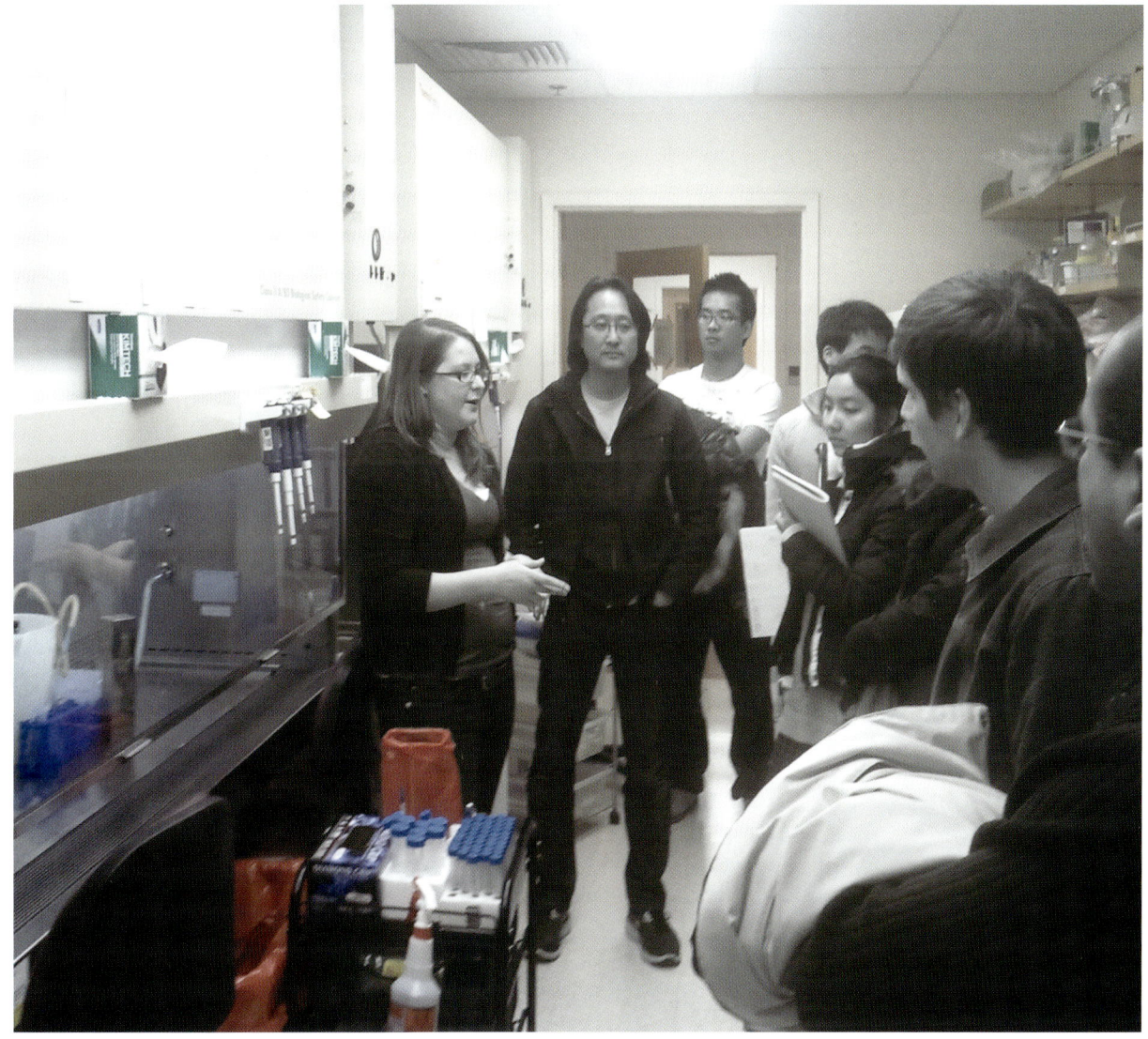

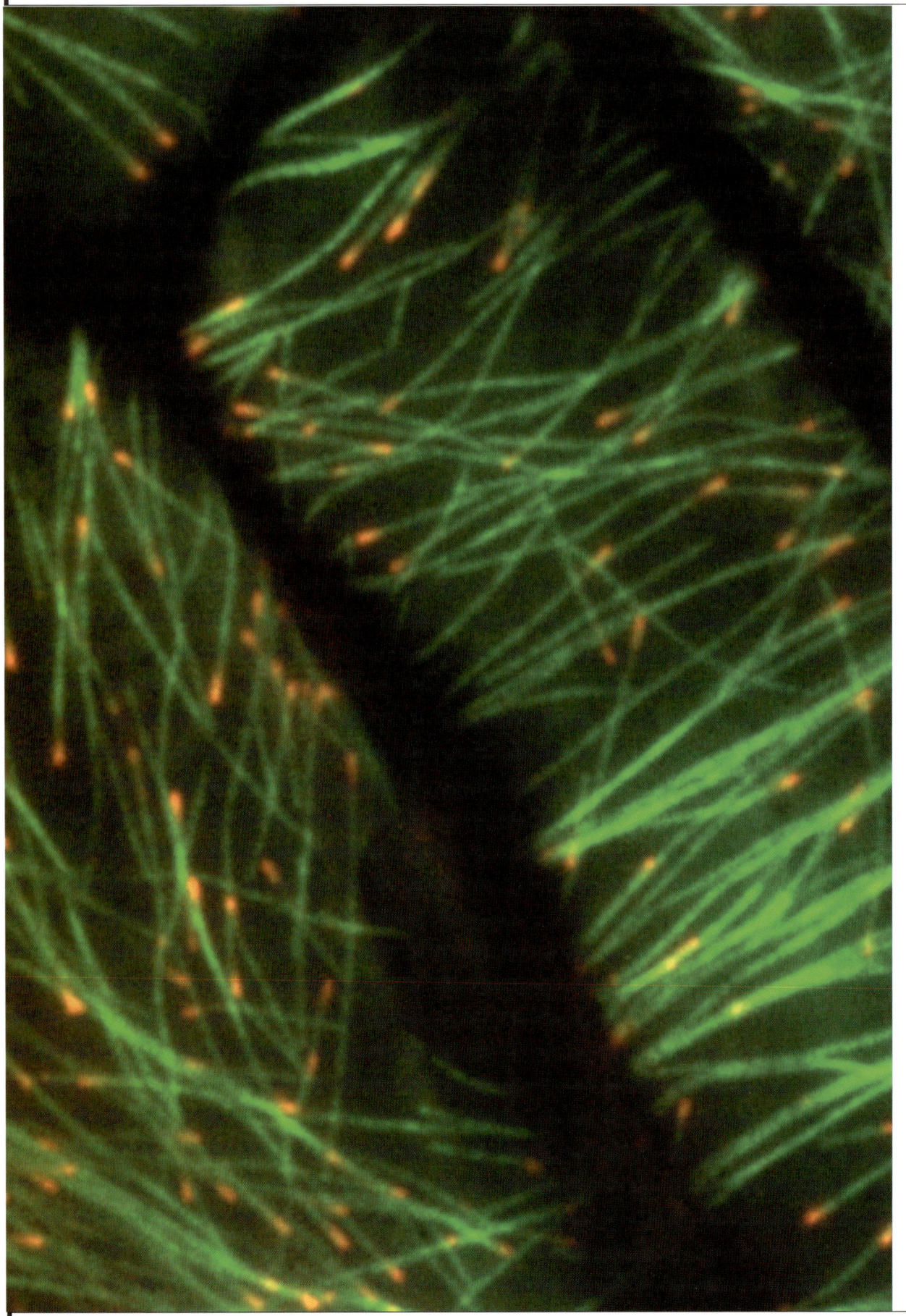

What the *Cellular Transformations* book seeks to do is blend these two worlds, asking the biologist to see through the eyes of an architect and designer and conversely asking the architect to embrace the insights drawn from biological processes. It is through these shifts in perspectives, especially when driven by the fresh approach of students from Dr. Dixit and Kim's class in this area that some truly transformational insights are set to emerge. The examples and ideas throughout the book will offer students a unique opportunity to translate between the languages of biology and architecture. Even established researchers will be offered a new perspective on familiar processes such as seeing how the physical attributes of a substrate or scaffolding designed with architectural principles in mind can then act as a biological control system. Ideas such as drawing on biological functions to design self-assembling, self-healing buildings would have sounded like science fiction only a few decades ago but biological understanding is advancing at a break-neck pace and knowledge of biopolymers, structures and their dynamics is constantly revealing the elegance with which biology solves its challenges. Equipping future pioneers to work at this interface between architecture and biology is a novel and important goal. However, they will need to have gained the broad vision to develop and test new and novel design principles drawn from the biological world and also to then use these insights to further our understanding of the cellular world. There are few books that seek to solidify these ideas into a form that the reader, be they student, researcher or designer can both absorb and use and this is where *Cellular Transformations* makes its key contribution.

Simon Gilroy 03.03.2021

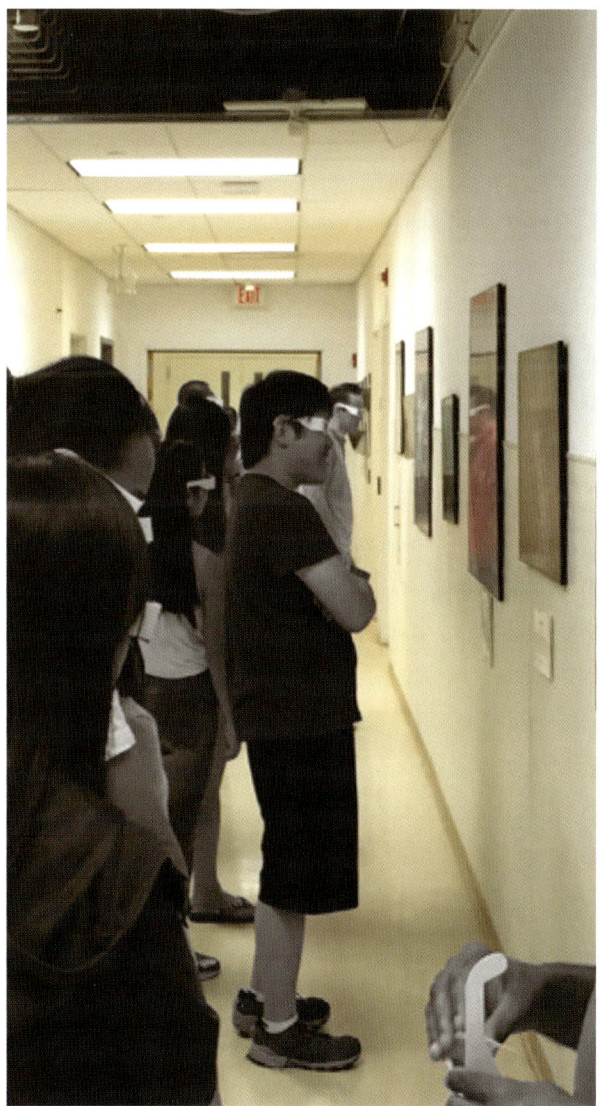
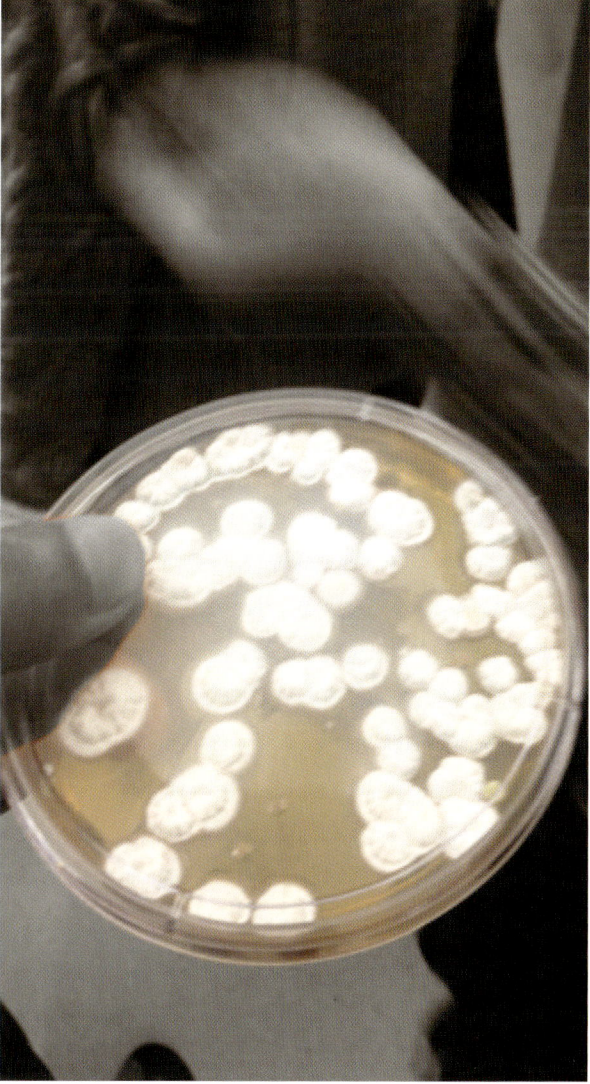

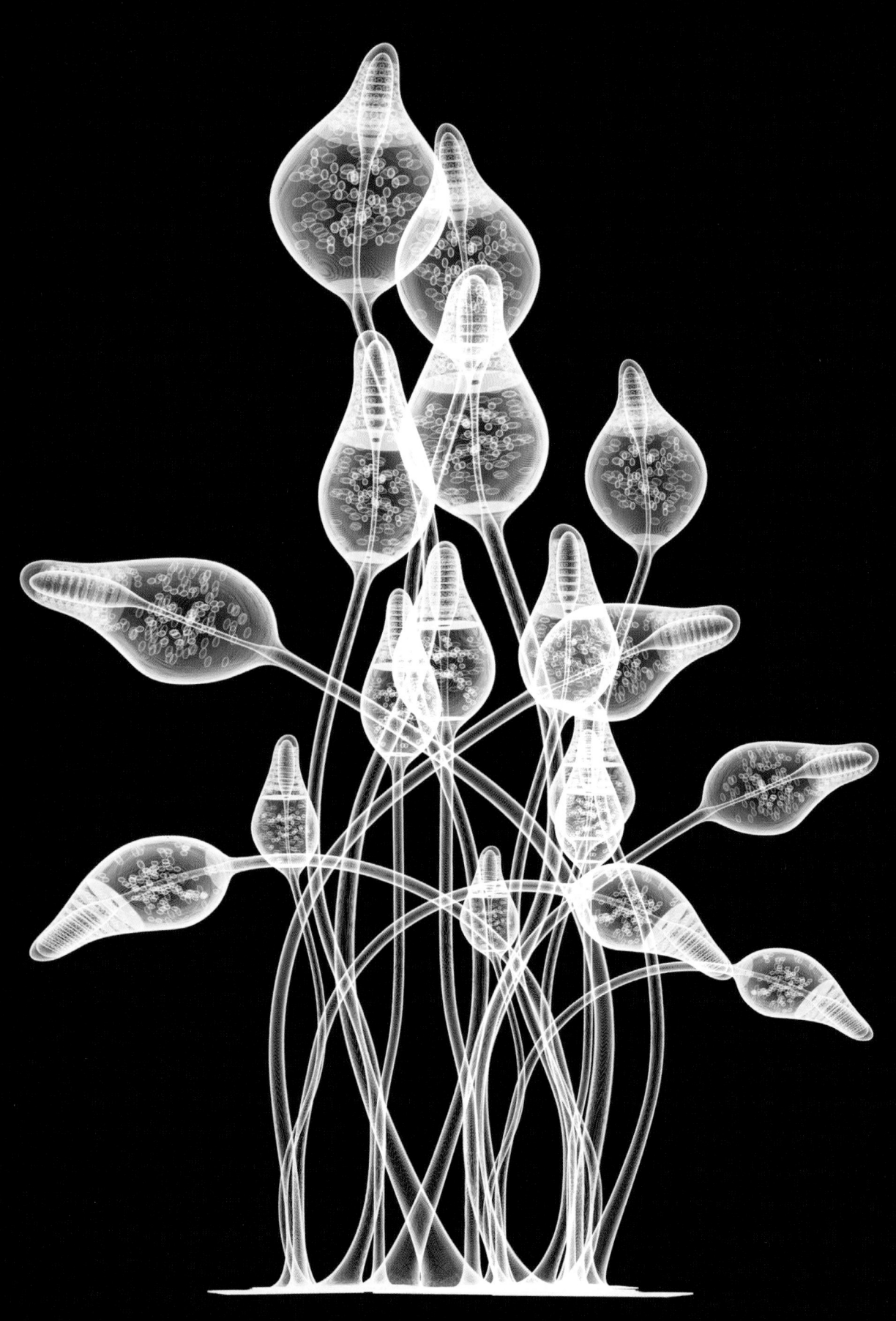

A BIOLOGICAL COMPUTATIONAL MODEL OF DESIGN
BRUCE LINDSEY

"I think the biotech revolution is going to be 10 times more important than the digital revolution, because it allows us to hack the code of life,"... "And we shouldn't be afraid of using this technology to make ourselves healthier."
-Walter Isaacson about Jennifer Doudna and CRISPR

ARCHITECTURE MACHINE

"A design machine must have an artificial intelligence because any design procedure, set of rules, or truism is tenuous, if not subversive, when used out of context..."

In the 1970 book *Architecture Machine*, Nicholas Negroponte, a professor of architecture at MIT and founder of the Media Lab, outlined ideas for "the intimate association of two dissimilar species (man and machine), two dissimilar processes (design and computation), and two intelligent systems (the architect and the architecture machine)." Written before any such machines existed and patterned after ethical robots, a specific class of machines described by cyberneticist Warren McCulloch, Negroponte's *Architecture Machine* was dependent upon an understanding of the environment as an evolving organism as opposed to a designed artifact.

Additionally the interface of the person and machine was predicated on a desire for self-improvement that ascribed intelligence to the artifact or the artificial and was concerned with "problem worrying," not "problem solving" – problem worrying acknowledging the dynamic relationship between problems and solutions in an evolving context. Negroponte goes on to describe that this could happen through a dialogue between the person and the machine and between the machine and the environment. He states that the dialogue between the machine and the environment must be two-fold: First, "an [architecture] machine must receive direct sensory information from the real world," and second be aware of other designers' procedures such that it can provide both "unsolicited knowledge and unsolicited problems." In this way a designer could "tune into controversy," that could challenge the designer's own assumptions preventing the machine from simply being a "yes man."

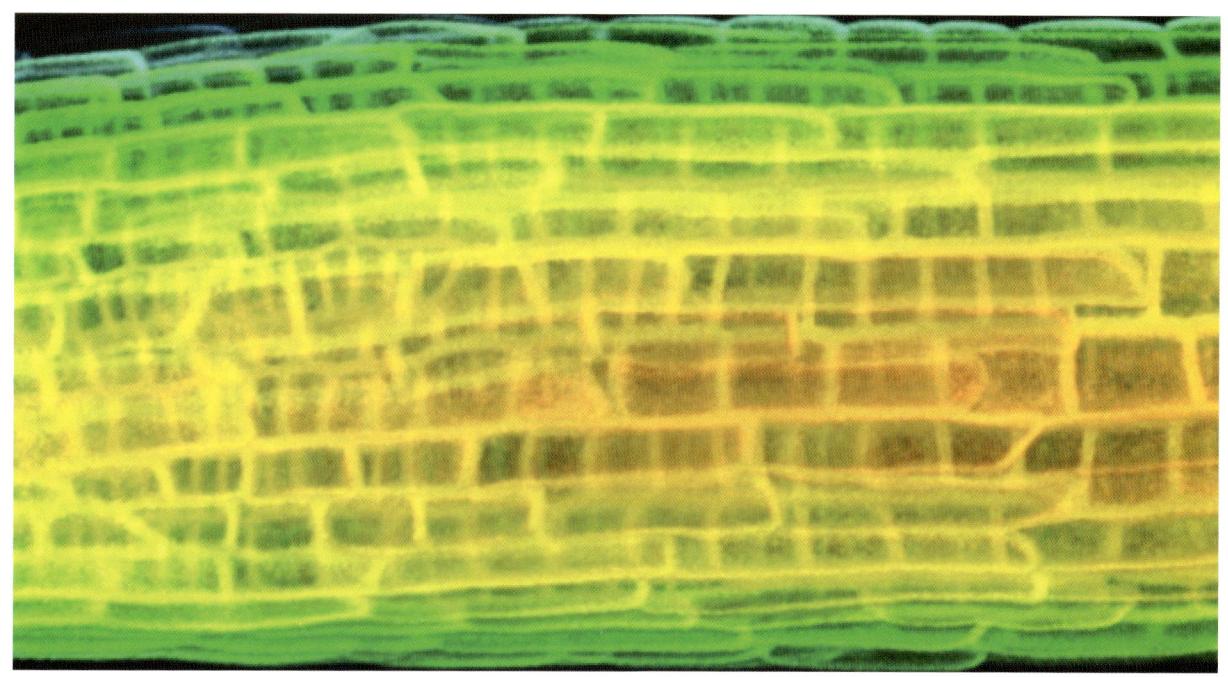

A COMPUTATIONAL THEORY OF MIND

"Design is the process that allows you to find out what you need to know before it's too late."

In his book *The Sciences of the Artificial* (1968), Herbert A. Simon (1916-2001) said that, "everyone designs who devises courses of action aimed at changing existing situations into preferred ones." Simon's background was in political science however he won his Nobel Prize in economics in 1978. He also made significant contributions to the fields of cognitive psychology, management science, and computer science. As an assistant professor of architecture at Carnegie Mellon I attended his 90th birthday in 2006. For nearly ten years I was enamored with Simon often sitting in the back of his classes and each year I would invite him to lecture to my freshman architecture students. He mostly talked about drawing as a means of figuring things out. Drawing figured prominently in his thinking method. Despite this he did not like architects, I found out later reading his autobiography *Models of My Life*, 1996.

I will immodestly try to summarize his Nobel winning work in economics. According to Simon humans and organizations often make decisions based on incomplete information. While individuals and organizations make decisions in different ways they both adopt "working procedures," some of which are unconscious, that try to overcome the problem. He described decision making and by extension design as happening in a space of "bounded rationality." Because an economic model or a design problem cannot be comprehensibly stated the model cannot be optimized but must "satisfice" (good enough). Simon's ideas challenged the prevailing theory that economic modeling could assume, in the aggregate, that humans make rational decisions to maximize individual benefit. Instead humans tentatively specify a goal with available information, assessing the current situation, and then apply a set of operations that reduce the difference. In economics this does not maximize profits. It achieves acceptable economic results while minimizing complications and risk. Simon went on to say

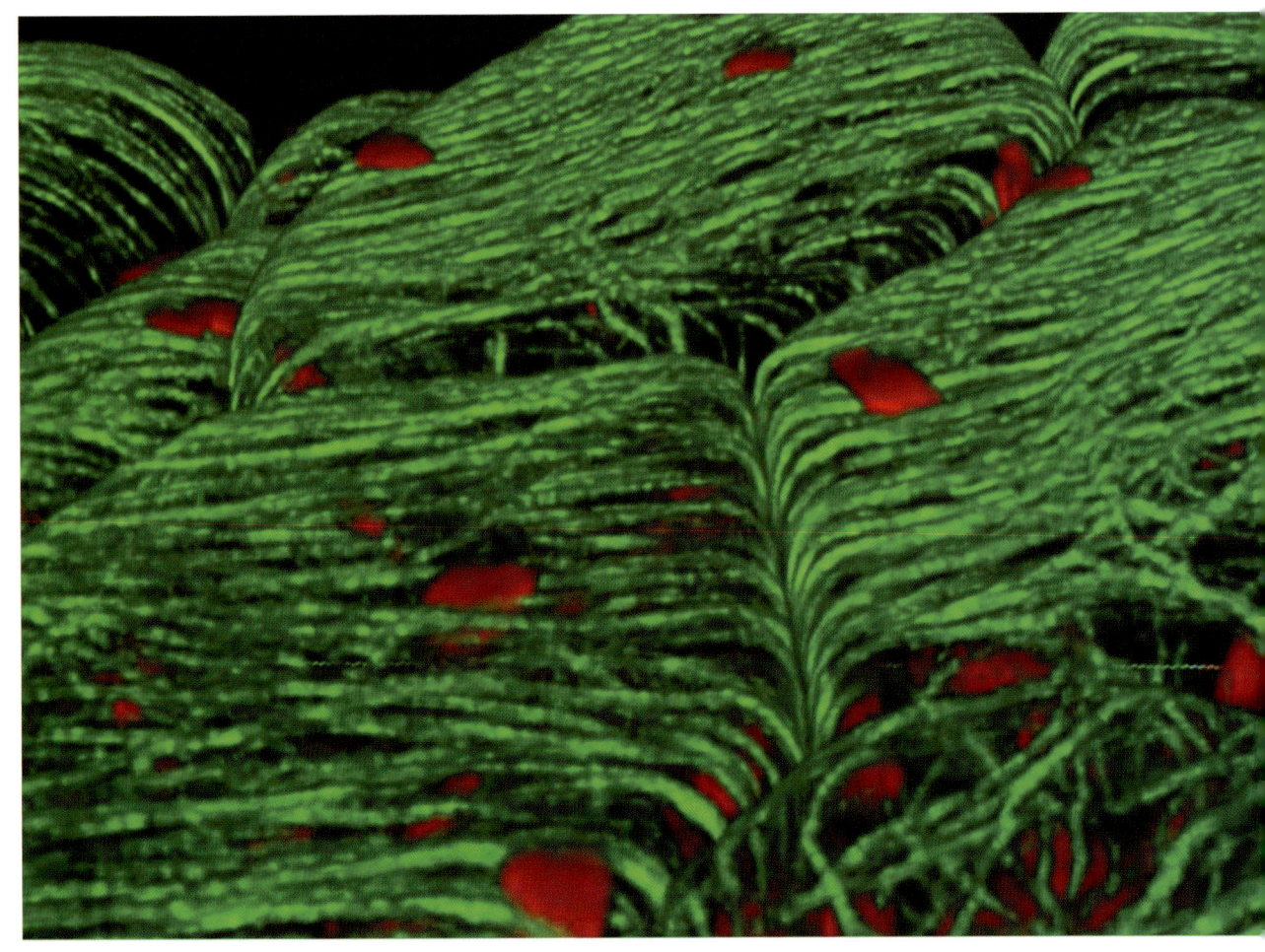

that "everyone designs." Simon, along with his longtime partner Alan Newell (1927-1992), pioneered the use of computers to test theories of how humans think and make decisions even before computers were widely available. In 1954, Simon recalls while consulting with the Rand corporation and seeing a printer print out a map using letters and punctuation that the manipulation of symbols coupled with pattern matching could perhaps simulate the human decision making process. Pattern matching in contrast to pattern recognition allows for a loose fit to be established between two states. Newell describes the moment, "I had such a sense of clarity that this was a new path." In 1956, Simon and Newell with the help of computer programmer Cliff Shaw (1922-1991) wrote a program called Logic Theorist that would come to be known as the first demonstration of artificial intelligence. In January 1956, Simon, his wife, his children, and some graduate students each took 3x5 cards on which Simon had written the program. This effectively made each person a modular component of the program.

Simon recalls, "...here was nature imitating art imitating nature." [Crevier] Newell, Simon, and Shaw using the computer at Rand went on to prove 38 of the 52 theorems from Russell and Whitehead's *Principia Mathematica* using Logic Theorist. Apparently when Simon showed the results to Russell "he responded in delight." [McCorduck] In January 1956 Simon, speaking to a group of graduate students at Carnegie Mellon, stated, "Over Christmas, Al Newell and I invented a thinking machine... [showing] how a system composed of matter can have the properties of mind." With help from MIT computer scientist Marvin Minsky and philosophers Hilary Putnam and Jerry Fordor this work would come to be known as the *computational theory of mind*. Steven Pinker in his book *How the Mind Works* (1997) writes, "The computational theory of mind thus allows us to keep beliefs and desires in our explorations of behavior while planting them squarely in the physical universe. It allows meaning to cause and be caused."

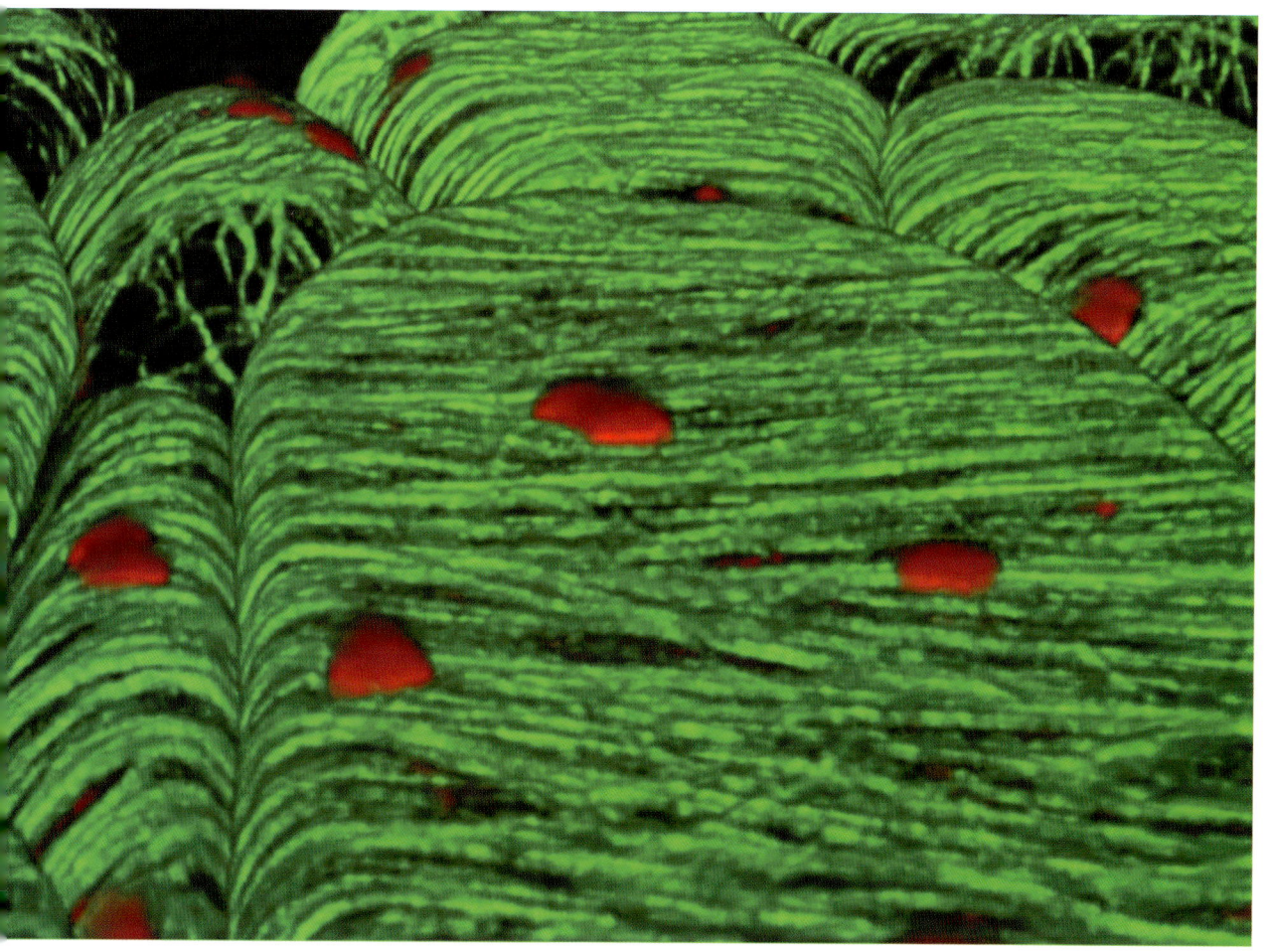

Claude Shannon (1916-2001), known as the father of information theory loved chess. In 1950 he wrote a paper titled "Programming a Computer for Playing Chess." In 1949 he built a chess playing machine himself. Referred to as end-game because the computer could only play the "endgame" with 6 pieces, the endgame, the last of the three parts of a match. The others being the opening book and the middle book. Shannon, a serious mathematician, calculated that if a computer of the day were to calculate for itself all possible moves against an opponent it would take it 10^{90} years to move its first pawn. This fact led to the Shannon Number which is as follows: with 35 possible moves followed by 35 responses over the typical 40 turn match, the possible number of chess games is approximately 10^{120}. It is estimated that there are 10^{70} particles in the visible universe. A computer could figure out all the right moves but it would take a while.

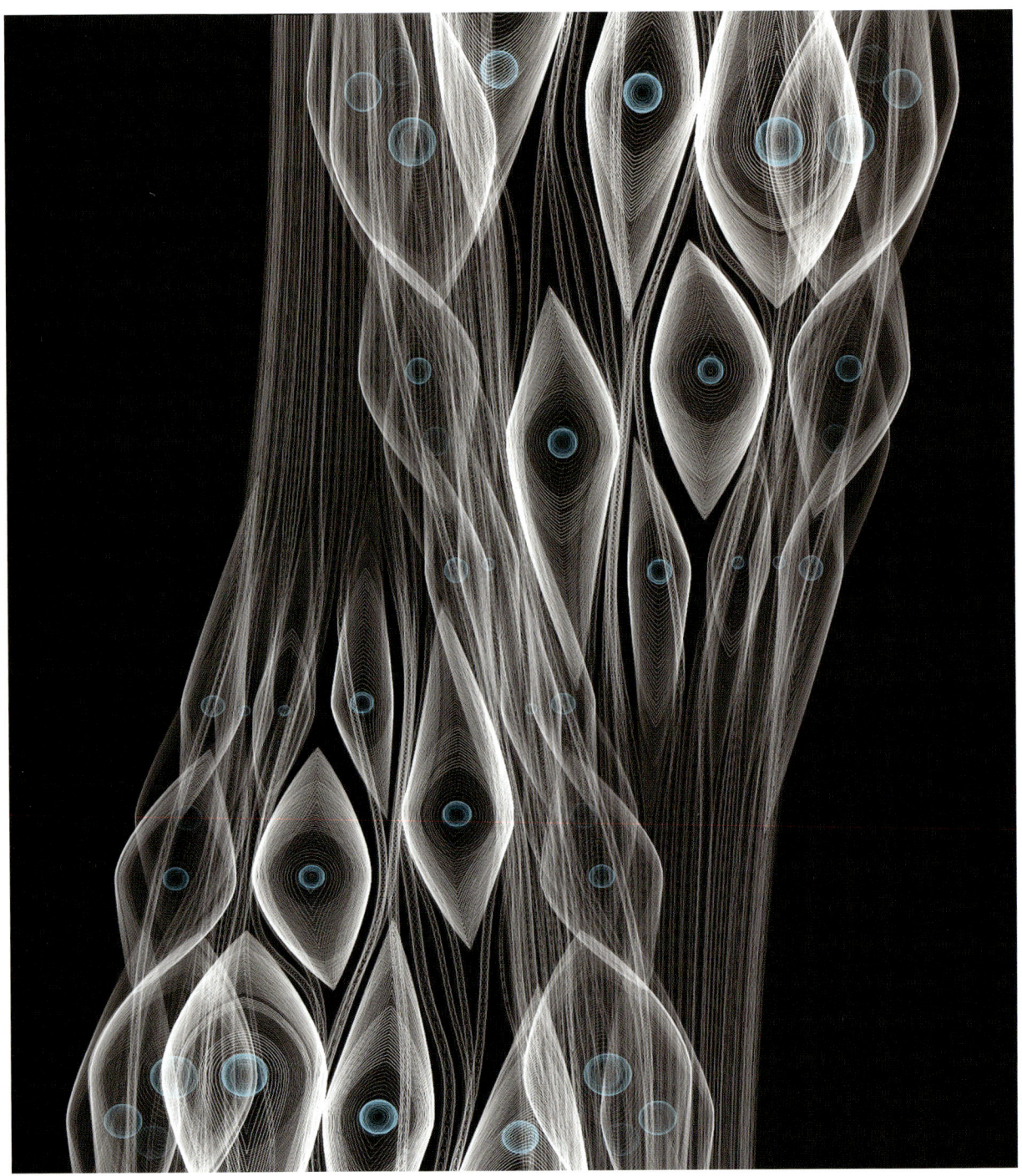

Shannon's paper outlined two strategies for a chess playing machine. The first is based on the machines ability to draw on a large data base of patterns and decide on a possible course of action more quickly than the human opponent. As computers got faster and the data base larger the computer would improve its advantage. The problem is that given any specific opening from the human the computer would play the same game every time. Shannon called this kind of play, "fast and stupid." The second strategy is that the computer would need to learn to adapt over the course of a match. Shannon called this, "slow and smart." Shannon asks, "The Gordian question, more easily raised than answered, is: Does a chess-playing machine of this type think?"

It is tough to say whether Herb Simon loved chess for the game itself or how the game was a perfect example of a bounded decision space. Regardless he was a chess enthusiast and in 1957 predicted that in ten years, a computer would be the world chess champion. In 1958 Simon, Newell, and Shaw's chess program would beat a person. The person had been taught chess one hour before the match. It would take until 1997 for a computer, IBM's Deep Blue, designed by a team led by Feng-hsiung Hsu of Carnegie Mellon, to beat the world chess champion Gary Kasparov in the last game of a 6 game match.

My office in Doherty Hall at Carnegie Mellon was next to the computer science building. In the early 1990's I would routinely see robots and mechanical spiders roaming the halls. At the time there were two competing theories (paraphrased by me) about how to make a computer that could know where it was. The top down theory suggested that you pour as much as you could into a large data base filled with maps and decision trees for determining actions then a digital avatar could go where it chose, go there, and then know where it was. The bottom up theory taped a camera to the robotic spiders head, let it loose to map its own environment like a Roomba vacuum cleaner on the run and when it had a large enough map it could go somewhere it had visited before and then know where it was, relatively speaking of course. The computer Deep Blue was of the top down variety but with a twist. Simon writes in a paper "Implications Of Deep Blue For Artificial Intelligence" shortly after Deep Blue beat Kasparov that, "important progress had been made during the past year in advancing DB's (Deep Blue) chess knowledge and not simply in allowing it to examine more positions. Simon goes on to describe how the "knowledge" of Deep Blue Takes three forms. The first is that DB has a large opening and closing book containing thousands of game trees from actual matches. Second; it is trivial for DB to assign a numerical value to each piece and each position such that different positions can be searched. The third and most important is that DB was able to "characterize' patterns in a way that would allow it to make inferences between one pattern from another altering its evaluation function to the character of the pattern. Given a particular pattern, DB might selectively evaluate more deeply (more examples) rather than trying evaluate as many patterns and positions as possible given the time constraints. Simon speculates that DB was faster and had a larger data base it carried out less searches in the 1997 win then the 1996 loss to Kasparov. Simon in summary states that improved chess knowledge and not faster bigger computers is the answer. Simon states, "... speed is not enough; it must be supplemented by knowledge."

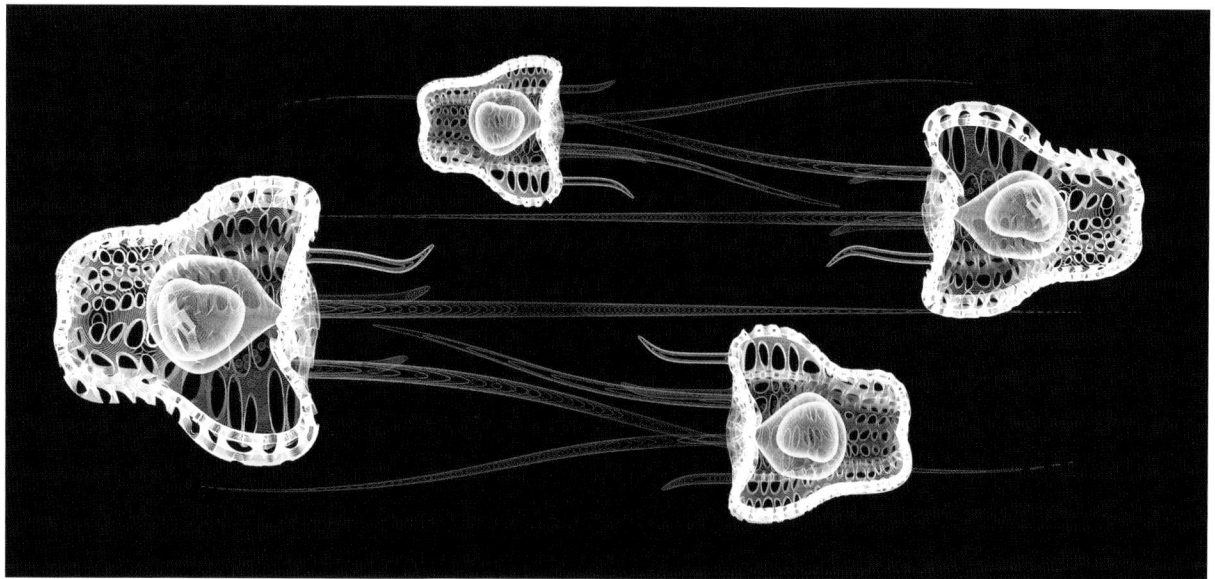

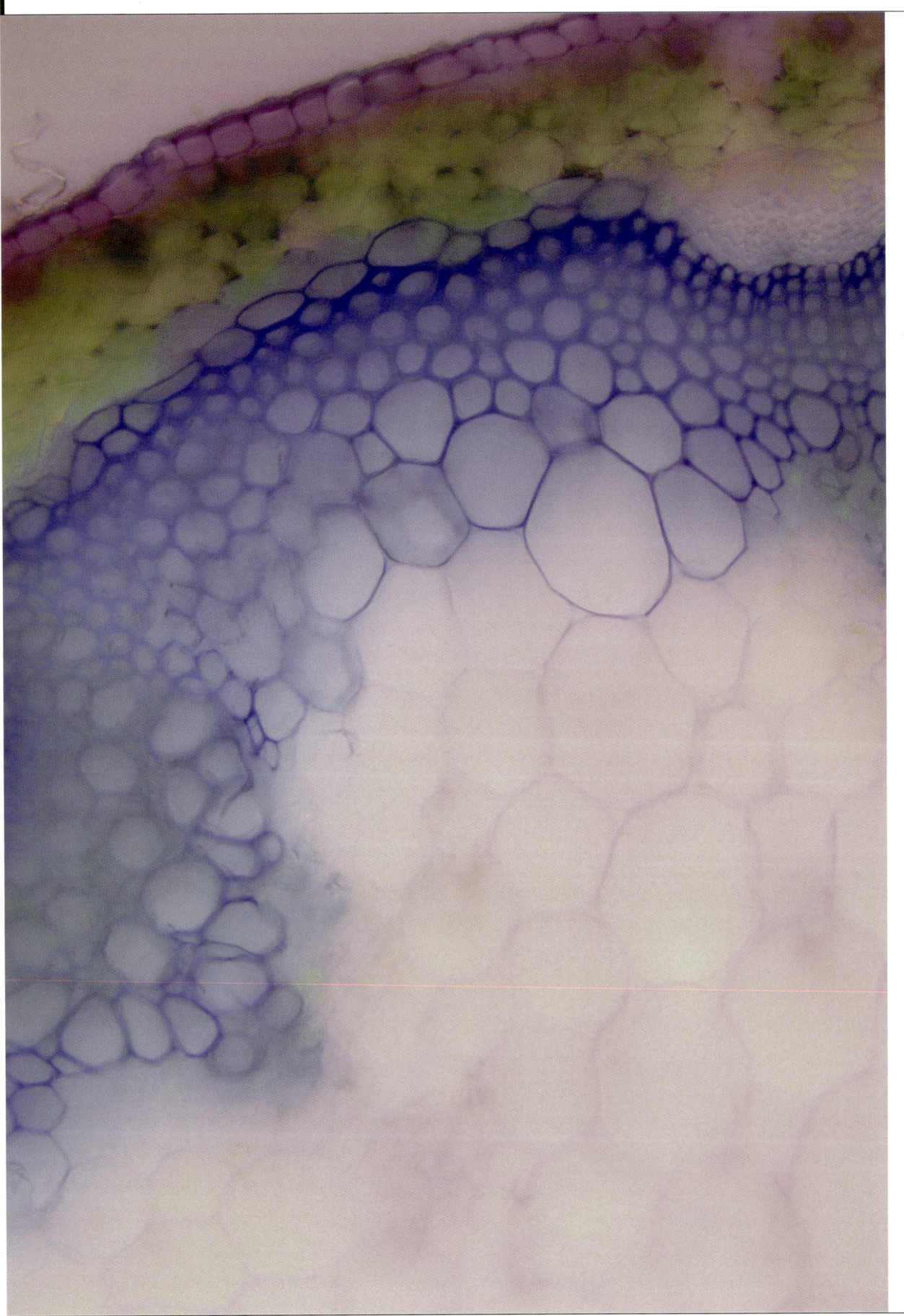

ON GROWTH AND FORM

"Form follows function."-Louis Sullivan
"Form and Function are one."-Frank Lloyd Wright

In 1917 biologist and mathematician D'Arcy Wentworth Thompson (1860-1948) published the 793 page book *On Growth and Form*. British writer and biologist Peter Medawar describes the book as pioneering the use of mathematics in biology and later the field of Biomathematics. Anthropologist Barry Bogin describes Thompson's work as a tour de force that combined natural philosophy, geometry, biology and mathematics to better understand growth and form. Thompson believed that there was an overemphasis of Darwin's theory of evolution and natural selection as the determinate of form and structure in organisms. Using an extensive mathematical and geometric comparative analysis to shed light on the morphogenesis of organisms Thompson hoped to describe a theory aligned with physical laws and the mechanics of how patterns and body structures are formed in plants and animals, morphogenesis being the biological process by which cells become plants and animals. In one of the most influential chapters of the book, chapter XVII, *The Comparison of Related Forms*, Thompson shows through a series of drawings inspired by the artist Albrecht Dürer how the forms of related animals can be described through a series of mathematical and geometric transformations. Inspiring thinkers such as computer pioneer Alan Turing and evolutionary biologist Stephen Jay Gould, Thompson's book has also been very influential with architects such as Le Corbusier, Mies van der Rohe, and Christopher Alexander. Architects Sarah Bonnemaison and Philip Beesley, in the preface to their book *On Growth and Form, Organic Architecture and Beyond* state, "Thompson conceived of form not as a given, but as a product of dynamic forces that are shaped by flows of energy and stages of growth." Organic architecture is a term that has been used often in reference to architecture perhaps most famously by Frank Lloyd Wright. While Wright saw organic architecture as the relationship of a building to its site it was also founded on serving the "whole of life" through common sense and "super-sense" determining "form by way of the nature of materials." [Wright, *The Natural House*]

Simon, in the paper "The Architecture of Complexity" (1962) while not referring to Thompson offers some insight into biological and physical hierarchies and social hierarchies that bridge Thompson's growth and form with context and systems encountered in behavioral sciences. Using the cell as an example, Simon speculates that biological and physical (architecture?) hierarchies are described in spatial terms. "We detect the organelles in a cell in the way we detect the raisins in a cake, they are "visibly" differentiated substructures localized spatially in the larger structure." He goes on to describe that we understand social hierarchies by observing who interacts with whom. In most physical and biological systems intense interaction implies spatial proximity and yet nerve cells and telephone wires permit interaction at a distance meaning spatial proximity is less a determinate of form. Part of Simon's work more generally in artificial intelligence and adaptive systems examining the concepts of feedback and selective information (see Shannon, *The Mathematical Theory of Communication*) Simon, in line with his definition of design points out the distinction between the world as we see it and the world as we act upon it "defines the basic condition for the survival of adaptive organisms.

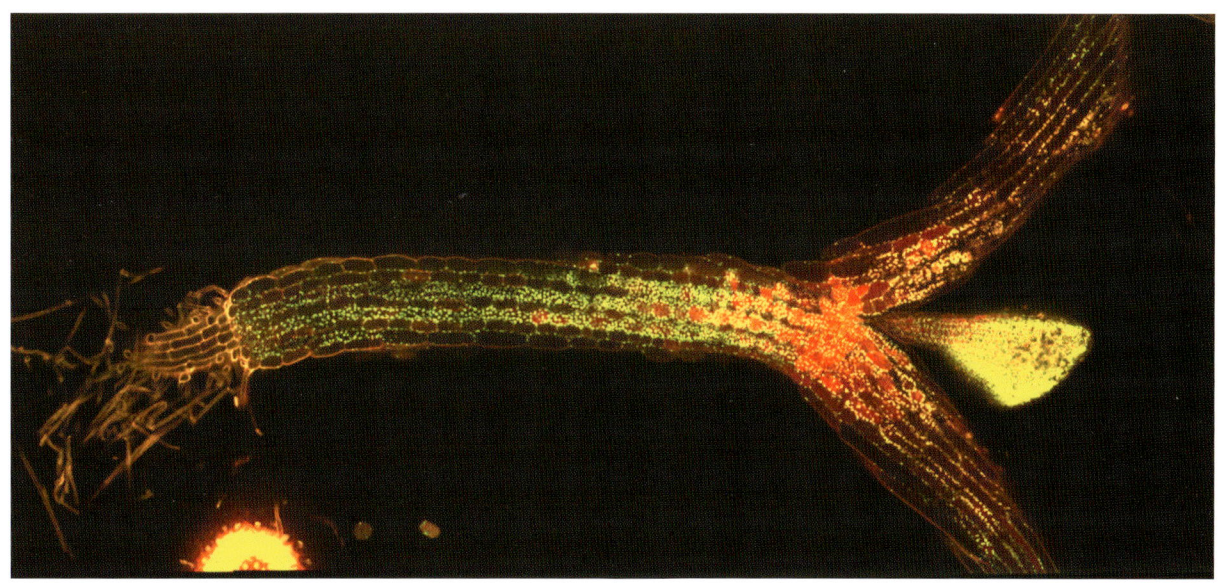

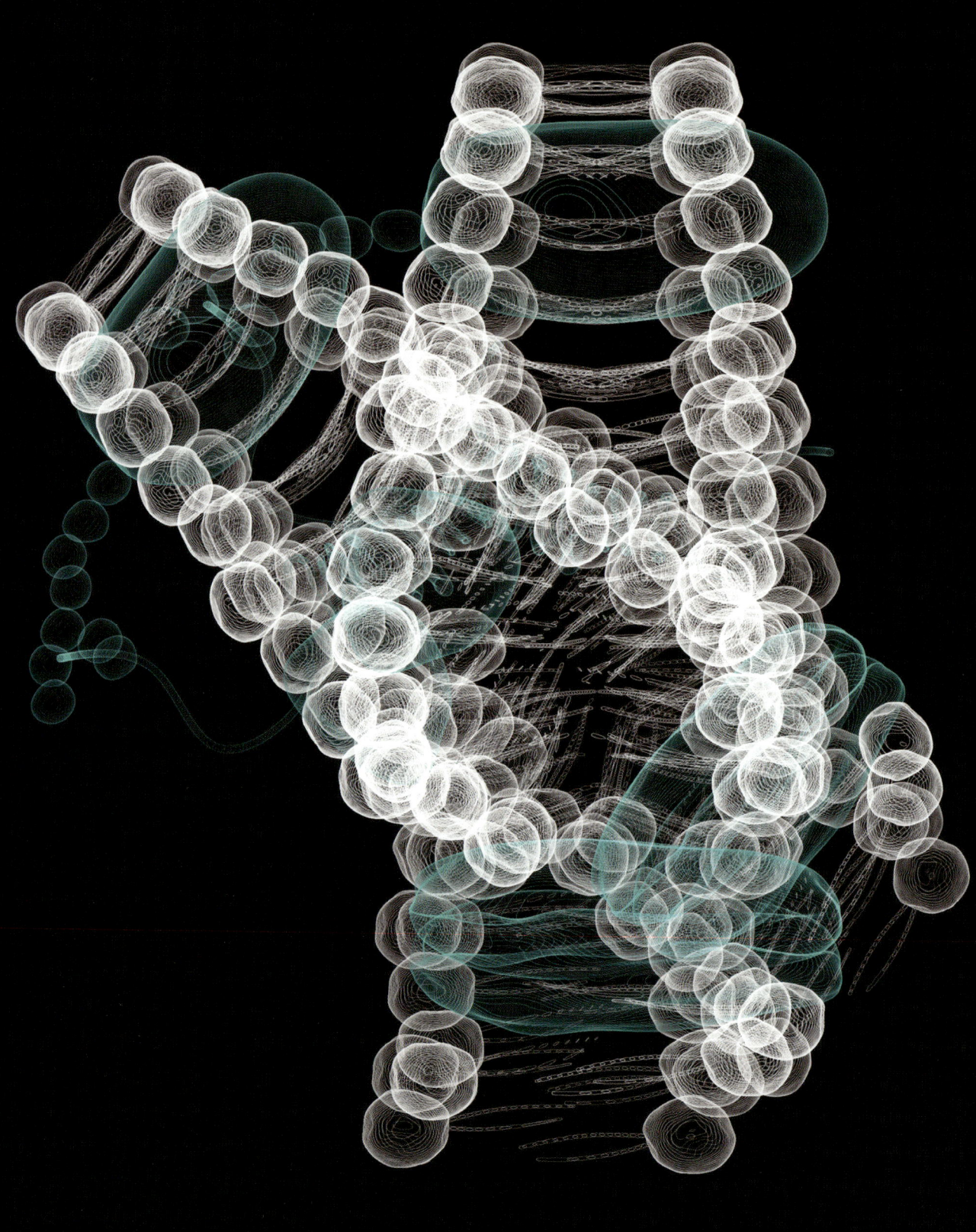

A BIOLOGIST AND AN ARCHITECT WALK INTO A BAR

"I am two with nature." -Woody Allen

There is a beautiful play written by Steve Martin titled *Picasso at the Lapin Agile* (French for nimble rabbit) where Picasso and Einstein have a lengthy argument about the value of genius and talent. A blue-suede-shoed visitor from the future complicates things by demonstrating that genius is not always the product of academic or philosophical understanding. If you have made it this far, thanks for sticking with me as I suggest that the nimble rabbit bar of the book *Cellular Transformations* includes, Herb Simon, Alan Newell, Claude Shannon, D'Arcy Wentworth Thompson, architect Sung Ho Kim, biologist Ram Dixit, a bunch of students, all of age of course. During the course of the evening they build a new architecture machine with the help of Nicholas Negroponte who just showed up. They quickly propose an idea about a biological computational theory of design that would form the software of the architecture machine. The machine hardware would be a biological computer with an enormous opening and end game informed by the database of biology. Both the software and hardware would be fast and smart allowing the architect and biologist to speculate about new combinations of adaptive self-improving systems that would be connected to the environment and by extension to the boogie-woogie of life. The students quickly play out these systems which often show novel relationships of geometry and structure such that they continue to adapt simultaneously from the bottom and the top thwarting even the most unscrupulous global pandemic. Some of the systems (buildings?) have skin. Some breathe. Some sing like Elvis. At some point, well into the night the crew decides that the name machine no longer fits the machine nor themselves. Simon suggests the name Kasparov. Everyone agrees that they will sleep on it.

Bruce Lindsey 03.26.2021

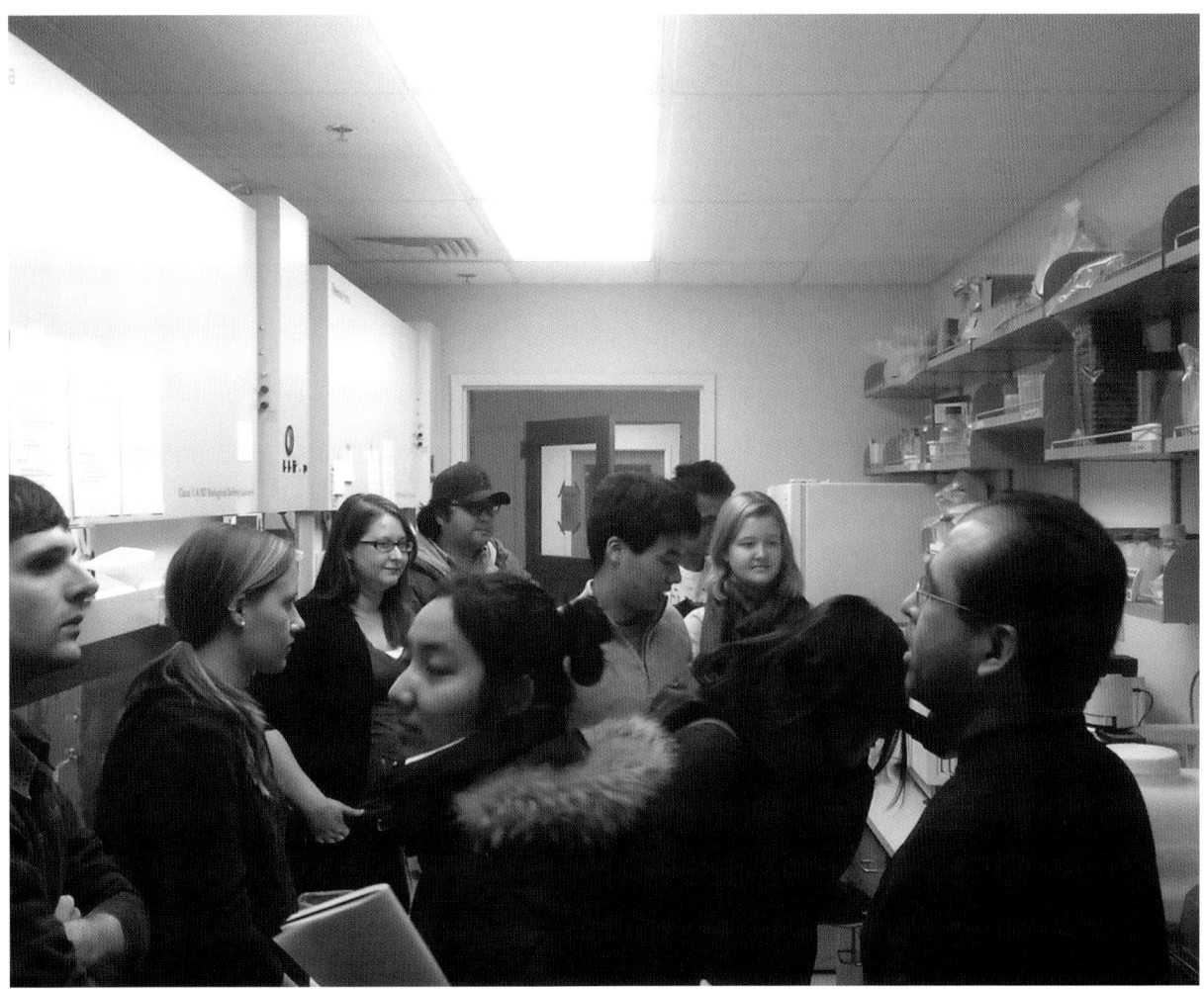

CONTRIBUTORS
BIOGRAPHY

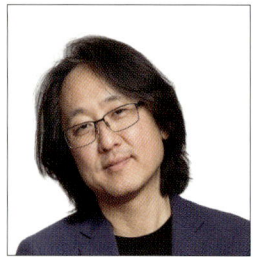

Sung Ho Kim
BFA, BArch, AA Diploma with RIBA I and II, SMArchS

Sung Ho Kim studied drawing and sculpture as a teenager at the Art Students League of New York and Harvard Graduate School of Design Career Discovery Program. He received a Bachelor of Fine Arts and Bachelor of Architecture from Rhode Island School of Design and an AA Diploma from Architectural Association of London, UK with Royal Institute of British Architects Part I and II. He also received his Master in Science in Architecture Studies from Massachusetts Institute of Technology. He was a project designer for Nasrine Seraji in Paris, France and Wellington Reiter in Cambridge, Massachusetts. He served as a principal researcher for the Interrogative Design Group at Center for Advanced Visual Studies at MIT. Sung Ho taught at Rhode Island School of Design and was an Assistant Professor at Northeastern University. He was a Visiting Professor at Aristotle University of Thessaloniki in Greece and Konkuk University in Seoul, Korea. Currently, he is a tenured Full Professor of Architecture and engaged in research with Biology and Computer Science at Washington University in St. Louis. He was a founding Director of Axi:Ome llc of Providence, RI from 2001 and has been Co-Director of Axi:Ome llc of St. Louis with Heather Woofter since 2003.

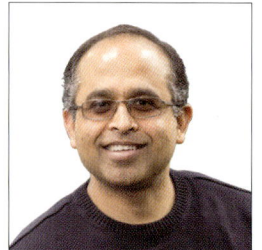

Ram Dixit
BS, PhD

Ram Dixit, PhD, received his Bachelor of Science in Biochemistry from the State University of New York at Stony Brook where he conducted research with Dr. Abraham Krikorian on somatic embryogenesis from carrot cell suspension cultures. He then moved upstate to Cornell University where he worked with Dr. June Nasrallah to study cell-cell communication during plant reproduction and received a Ph.D. in plant molecular biology in 2000. During his Ph.D. work, Ram got interested in the inner workings of cells that produce shape and execute various cellular functions. He did postdoctoral work with Dr. Richard Cyr at Penn State University where he used fluorescence microscopy and computational modeling to characterize the dynamics and organization of plant cortical microtubules. He then joined Dr. Erika Holzbaur's lab at the University of Pennsylvania to study molecular motor proteins and microtubule tip-binding proteins using single-molecule imaging and functional reconstitution experiments. Ram joined the Biology Department at Washington University in St. Louis as an Assistant Professor in 2008 and is currently a Full Professor of Biology. He serves as faculty director of the BioSURF program at Washington University, as co-director of the Plant and Microbial Biosciences graduate program, and as associate director of education for the NSF-funded Science and Technology Center for Engineering Biology.

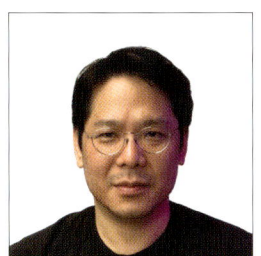

Andrew Yoo
BS, MS, PhD

Andrew Yoo, PhD, received his Bachelor of Science degree in Physiology from McGill University and his Masters of Science degree in Experimental Medicine (Neurology) from the University of British Columbia. During his time at Columbia University, he received his Ph.D. in Cellular, Molecular, and Biophysical Studies. In addition, he was a Postdoctoral fellow at Stanford University where he studied Chromatin biology and cell fate programming. Andrew joined the Department of Developmental Biology at Washington University School of Medicine in 2011 and is currently an Associate Professor. His lab works on developing cell reprogramming methods to generate human nerve cells by directly converting skin cells, and modeling neurodegenerative disorders using patient-derived neurons. Andrew Yoo's work has been recognized by many awards including WUSM Distinguished Investigator Award, Ellison Medical Foundation New Investigator in Aging Award, NIH Director's New Innovator Award and Presidential Early Career Award for Scientists and Engineers from the White House.

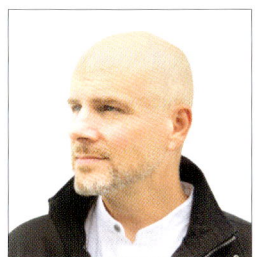

Mitchell Joachim
BA, MArch, MAUD, PhD, AIA

Mitchell Joachim, Co-Founder of Terreform ONE and an Associate Professor of Practice at NYU. Formerly, he was an architect at the offices of Frank Gehry and I.M. Pei. He has been awarded a Fulbright Scholarship and fellowships with TED, Moshe Safdie, and Martin Society for Sustainability, MIT. He was chosen by Wired magazine for "The Smart List" and selected by Rolling Stone for "The 100 People Who Are Changing America". Mitchell won many honors including; Lafarge Holcim Acknowledgement Award, Ove Arup Foundation Grant, ARCHITECT R+D Award, AIA New York Urban Design Merit Award, 1st Place International Architecture Award, Victor Papanek Social Design Award, Zumtobel Group Award for Sustainability, Architizer A+ Award, History Channel Infiniti Award for City of the Future, and Time magazine's Best Invention with MIT Smart Cities. He's featured as "The NOW 99" in Dwell magazine and "50 Under 50 Innovators of the 21st Century" by Images Publishers. He co-authored four books, "Design with Life: Biotech Architecture and Resilient Cities," "XXL-XS: New Directions in Ecological Design," "Super Cells: Building with Biology," and "Global Design: Elsewhere Envisioned". His design work has been exhibited at MoMA and the Venice Biennale. He earned: PhD at Massachusetts Institute of Technology, MAUD Harvard University, M.Arch Columbia University with honors.

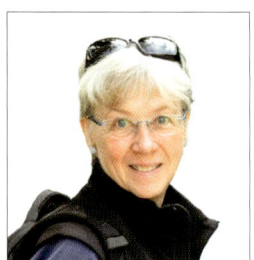

Iris Meier
MS, PhD

Iris Meier did her Ph.D. work in the Department of Biophysics at Heinrich Heine University Duesseldorf, Germany, working on bacterial repressor-operator complexes. After postdoctoral training at The Max Planck Institute in Cologne, Germany and UC Berkeley, USA in plant molecular biology, she has led her research group at the University of Hamburg, Germany, the DuPont Experimental Station, USA, and - since 1999 - The Ohio State University, where she is a Full Professor in the Department of Molecular Genetics. Her lab has - with collaborators - discovered protein complexes that link the plant nucleoplasm with the cytoplasm and that affect nuclear morphology, nuclear movement, and a variety of plant traits, including male fertility, stomatal function, and nodulation. Her research now focuses on understanding their biochemical, cellular, and organismal roles and on comparing their structure-function relationships with analogous complexes in animals and fungi. In addition, she has initiated and is continuously developing an art-science project that involves a cross-disciplinary course for undergraduate students who develop art to visualize current topics of plant biology and present them to the broader public.

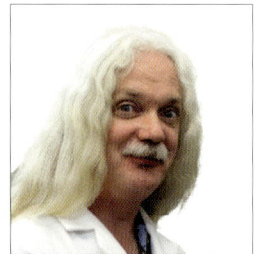

Simon Gilroy
BA, PhD

Simon Gilroy Ph.D., received a Bachelor of Arts in Botany from Cambridge University in the U.K in 1984. He then moved to Edinburgh University to pursue his Ph.D. with Tony Trewavas, working on trying to understand the internal control networks that allow plants to sense and respond to environmental stresses. Here he discovered his lifelong fascination with developing approaches to visualize the real time dynamics of plant signaling processes. He received his doctorate in plant biochemistry in 1987 and stayed in Edinburgh for his first postdoc and then moved to the University of California at Berkeley to work with Dr. Russel Jones, using a combination of biochemistry and fluorescence microscopy to probe the intricacies of hormone signaling during seed germination. In 1993 Simon joined the Biology Department at PennState University as an Assistant Professor and in 2007 moved to the University of Wisconsin at Madison where he is a Full Professor in the Botany Department. His research continues to probe the signaling networks that plants use to sense and respond to their environment, with projects studying a range of stresses from herbivory and mechanical stimulation to flooding. He has also taken these approaches and applied them to a new frontier working with NASA on projects designed to reveal how plants respond to unique stresses of growing in space.

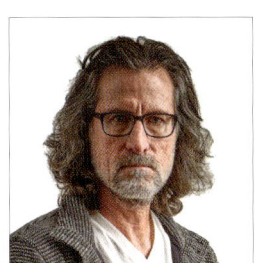

Bruce Lindsey
BFA, MFA, MArch, RA

Bruce Lindsey is the E. Desmond Lee Professor for Community Collaboration in the College of Architecture in the Sam Fox School of Design & Visual Arts at Washington University in St. Louis. Lindsey served as Dean of the school from 2006-2017. Lindsey's research has focused on beginning design education, and digital tools and their application to design and construction. His book *Digital Gehry: Material Resistance Digital Construction* published by Birkhauser in 2001 explores the use of technology in the design and delivery process of Frank Gehry's architectural office. Lindsey's has received numerous awards for his architecture and design work and Lindsey's work as a crafts person and photographer has been exhibited in venues such as the American Crafts Museum in New York City, Carnegie Museum of Fine Arts, Pittsburgh, and the Kimball Arts Center in Park City Utah. A native of Idaho, Lindsey holds a bachelor's and master's degree from the University of Utah and a master's degree in architecture from Yale University.

CELLULAR TRANSFORMATIONS
BETWEEN ARCHITECTURE AND BIOLOGY

The Arts and Sciences are fundamentally intertwined human endeavors that are artificially and unhelpfully treated as separate entities by society and our educational institutions. Cellular Transformations grew out of our desire to bridge these two disciplines at Washington University in St. Louis. This convergence is especially important to solve the many urgent problems facing humanity. We have witnessed how a global pandemic can wreak havoc on our social, healthcare, political, racial, and economic systems. Successfully overcoming these challenges demands bold new ideas that we believe emerge when students collaborate across disciplines. In short, our vision is innovation through integration. The future of higher education lies in the unification of fields to harness our collective knowledge into the next breakthrough discoveries and technologies.

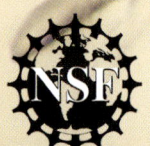 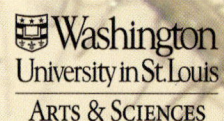 Department of Biology